TRANSFUSION MEDICINE:
LOOKING TO THE FUTURE

Éditions John Libbey Eurotext
127, avenue de la République, 92120 Montrouge, France
Tél : 33(0)1.46.73.06.60
http : //www.jle.com
e-mail : contact@jle.com

John Libbey and Company Ltd
42-46 Hight Street
Esher
Surrey
KT 10 9 QY
United Kingdom

© 2006, John Libbey Eurotext, Paris

ISBN 2-7420-0614-1

Unauthorized duplication contravenes applicable laws.

TRANSFUSION MEDICINE: LOOKING TO THE FUTURE

Editors :

Patrick Hervé
Jean-Yves Muller
Pierre Tiberghien

Translated by :

Agnes Jacob

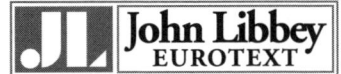

This book is dedicated
– to blood and cell donors without whom the future would not be possible:
their generosity and availability are greatly appreciated;
– to all personnel working in transfusion centers, health institutions
and affiliated organizations.
We acknowledge and gratefully recognize their commitment to this collective effort.
We trust that these advances will benefit the patients placed in our care.

Table of Contents

List of Authors	XI
Glossary	XIII
Preface S. Veil	1
Introduction J. Cinqualbre	3
Transfusion, a Matter of Cells: Review of the Past Three Decades P. Hervé, P. Tiberghien	5

Transfusion Safety:
Certainties, Uncertainties and New Directions

The Concept of Safety in Blood Transfusion J.-H. Trouvin	16
Residual Risks in Transfusion: a Strategic Perspective J. Coste	24
Toward Universal Pathogen Inactivation in Blood Cells J.-P. Cazenave	34
Nanotechnologies Revolutionize the Biological Qualification of Blood Donations M. Hoummady, P. Morel	45

Biotechnologies and Transfusion: what Prospects?

Ex vivo Production of Blood Cells: the Role of Erythrocytes
L. Douay, M.-C. Giarratana. 59

Cytokines and Erythrocyte and/or Platelet Saving Strategy
N. El Kassar, A. Schmidt-Tanguy, M.-L. Bidet, N. Ifrah 72

Reducing Immunogenicity of Labile Blood Products
and Creating Universal Erythrocytes
J.-Y. Muller, J. Chiaroni. 86

Contribution of New Technologies to Blood Cell Collection and Preparation
G. Andreu, A. Chabanel, B. Pelletier 101

Blood Substitutes: Challenge or Marginality?
P. Menu, M. Toussaint-Hacquard, J.-F. Stoltz 112

Cellular Engineering in Transfusion Medicine

The Cell: a Legally Distinct Entity
J.-R. Binet 126

Cellular Engineering and Transfusion: a Continuum?
P. Tiberghien. 142

Stem Cells and their Therapeutic Promise for Tomorrow's Regenerative Medicine
A. Turhan, A.-L. Bennaceur Griscelli 150

Gene Transfer: from the Laboratory to Clinical Practice
F. Rolling, M. Weber, G. Folléa, Ph. Moullier. 163

Evolution of Transfusion Medicine in its Sociological, Ethical and Cultural Environment

The Ethics of Donation: an Established or Evolving Practice?
D. Sicard. 176

New Fields of Expertise: what Priorities for Tomorrow?
B. Cuneo, Ph. de Micco. 182

Quality Assurance and Transfusion Medicine: what Are the Tools,
what Is at Stake?
G. Folléa, C. Lefort 190

Transfusion Medicine in the Europe of Tomorrow
G. Folléa 201

Transfusion Medicine and Hospitals: the Need for Cooperation
J.-Y. Muller, Ph. Richebe, V. Betbèze, P. Fialon, G. Janvier 221

By Different Roads: Blood Banks *versus* Transfusion Medicine
Interview F. Décary and P. Hervé 238

Transfusion Medicine in Ten Years: Fiction or Reality?
P. Hervé, J.-Y. Muller 249

List of Authors

Andreu G., MD, PhD, Medical and Scientific Director, French National Blood Service ; EFS, 20, avenue du Stade de France, 93218 La Plaine-Saint-Denis, France.

Bennaceur-Griscelli A.-L., MD, PhD, Professor of Hematology, Laboratory of Biological Hematology / Embryonic Stem Cell Program, University of Paris XI - Paul-Brousse Hospital, and INSERM U 362 ; Institut Gustave-Roussy, 12, avenue Paul-Vaillant-Couturier, 94804 Villejuif, France.

Betbèze V., Blood Safety Unit, University Hospital of Nantes, 9, quai Moncousu, 44093 Nantes Cedex 01, France.

Bidet M.L., MD, Assistant Manager, Pays de la Loire-French National Blood Service ; EFS - Pays de la Loire, 16, boulevard Mirault, 49103 Angers Cedex 02, France.

Binet J.-R., Doctor in Law, Lecturer, Faculty of Law, University of Besançon, 5, rue Léonel de Moustier, 25000 Besançon, France.

Cazenave J.-P., MD, PhD, Professor of Hematology-Transfusion, University Louis-Pasteur, Director, Alsace-French National Blood Service ; EFS - Alsace, 10, rue Spielman, 67065 Strasbourg Cedex, France.

Chabanel A., Sc. D, Responsible for Blood Component Processing and QC Division, Medical and Scientific Direction, French National Blood Service ; EFS, 20, avenue du stade de France, 93218 La Plaine-Saint-Denis, France.

Chiaroni J., MD, PhD, Assistant Manager, Alpes-Méditerranée-French National Blood Service ; EFS - Alpes-Méditerranée, 149, boulevard Baille, 13392 Marseille Cedex 5, France.

Coste J., PhD, Scientific Director, Pyrénées-Méditerranée-French National Blood Service ; EFS - Pyrénées-Méditerranée, 240, avenue Emile-Jeanbrau, 34094 Montpellier Cedex 5, France.

Cuneo B., Consulting sociologist, 11, place Denfert-Rochereau, 75014 Paris, France.

Décary F., MD, PhD, MBA, President and Chief Executive Officer HEMA-QUEBEC, 4045, boulevard Côte-Vertu, Saint-Laurent (Québec) H4R 2W7.

Douay L., Prof., MD, PhD, Head of Hematology Laboratory, Pierre et Marie Curie University and Hôpital Trousseau, 26, avenue du Dr Arnold-Netter, 75571 Paris Cedex 12, France.

El Kassar N., MD, PhD, Pays de la Loire-French National Blood Service ; EFS - Pays de la Loire, 16, boulevard Mirault, 49103 Angers Cedex 02, France.

Fialon P., MD, Victor Segalen University Bordeaux 2, University Hospital of Bordeaux, avenue de Magellan, 33604 Pessac Cedex, France.

Folléa G., MD, PhD, Director, Pays de la Loire-French National Blood Service ; EFS - Pays de la Loire, 34, boulevard Jean-Monnet, 44011 Nantes Cedex 01, France.

Giarratana M.-C., Research Engineer, Pierre et Marie Curie University, CHU Saint-Antoine, 27, rue de Chaligny, 75571 Paris Cedex 12, France.

Hervé P., Prof., MD, President of French National Blood Service ; EFS, 20, avenue du Stade de France, 93218 La Plaine-Saint-Denis Cedex, France.

Hoummady M., PhD, Chairman and CEO, Nanobiogene, Belfort Technopole, 6, avenue des Usines, 90000 Belfort, France.

Ifrah N., MD, PhD, Professor of Hematology, UPRES EA 3863, Faculty of Medicine, rue Haute de Reculée, 49045 Angers Cedex, France.

Janvier G., MD, PhD, Chairman and Professor of Anesthesiology and Critical Care Medicine, Victor Segalen University Bordeaux 2, University Hospital of Bordeaux, avenue de Magellan, 33604 Pessac Cedex, France.

Lefort C., Pharmacist, Haemovigilance Manager and Quality Assurance Vice-Manager, Pays de la Loire-French National Blood Service ; EFS - Pays de la Loire, 34, boulevard Jean-Monnet, 44011 Nantes Cedex 01, France.

Menu P., MD, Associated Professor, Henri Poincaré University, LEMTA UMR CNRS 7563, and Faculty of Medicine, 9, avenue de la Forêt de Haye, 54505 Vandoeuvre-lès-Nancy, France.

Micco Ph. de, MD, PhD, General Manager, Alpes-Méditerranée-French National Blood Service ; EFS - Alpes-Méditerranée, 149, boulevard Baille, 13392 Marseille Cedex 5, France.

Morel P., MD, PhD, Bourgogne-Franche-Comté-French National Blood Service ; EFS - Bourgogne-Franche-Comté, 1, boulevard A. Fleming, 25020 Besançon Cedex, France.

Moullier Ph., MD, PhD, Scientific Director, Pays de la Loire-French National Blood Service and INSERM U 649 ; EFS-Pays de la Loire, 34, boulevard Jean-Monnet, 44011 Nantes Cedex 01, France.

Muller J.-Y., MD, PhD, Professor of Immunology, University Hospital of Nantes, 9, quai Moncousu, 44093 Nantes Cedex 01, France.

Pelletier B., MD, Head of Blood Collection Organization, Medical and Scientific Direction, French National Blood Service ; EFS, 20, avenue du Stade de France, 93218 La Plaine-Saint-Denis Cedex, France.

Richebé Ph., MD, Assistant Professor, Victor Segalen University Bordeaux 2, University Hospital of Bordeaux, avenue de Magellan, 34604 Pessac Cedex, France.

Rolling F., PhD, Research Associate, INSERM U 649, University Hospital of Nantes, 9, quai Moncousu, 44093 Nantes Cedex 01, France.

Schmidt-Tanguy A., MD,UPRES EA 3863, Faculty of Medicine, rue Haute de Reculée, 49045 Angers Cedex, France.

Sicard D., MD, Professor of Internal Medicine, President of National Ethic Consultative Council of France, Department of Internal Medicine, University Hospital Cochin, 27, rue du Faubourg Saint-Jacques, 75679 Paris Cedex 14, France.

Stoltz J.-F., PhD, Professor of Hematology, Director of Cell and Tissue Therapy Unit, University Hospital, 9, avenue de la Forêt de Haye, 54505 Vandoeuvre-lès-Nancy, France.

Tiberghien P., MD, PhD, Professor of Medicine, Director, Bourgogne-Franche-Comté-French National Blood Service, University of Franche-Comté EA 2284 / IFR 133 and INSERM U 645 ; EFS - Bourgogne-Franche-Comté, 1, boulevard A. Fleming, 25020 Besançon Cedex, France.

Turhan A., MD, PhD, Professor of Hematology, Head, Division of Laboratory Hematology/Oncology, Research Director, UPRES EA 3805, University of Poitiers - Hôpital Jean-Bernard, and Cell Therapy Program, Institut Gustave-Roussy, 1-39, rue Camille-Desmoulins, 94805 Villejuif, France.

Toussaint-Hacquard M., Assistant Professor, Henri Poincaré University, and Hematology Laboratory, University Hospital, 9, avenue de la Forêt de Haye, 54505 Vandoeuvre-lès-Nancy, France.

Trouvin J.-H., Professor of Pharmacology, Head, Directorate for Evaluation of Medicinal Products and Biologicals, French Health Regulatory Agency, AFSSAPS, 143, boulevard A. France, 93283 Saint-Denis Cedex, France.

Weber M., MD, PhD, Professor of Ophtalmology, University Hospital of Nantes, place Alexis Ricordeau, 44093 Nantes Cedex 01, France.

Glossary

AAV	Adeno Associated Virus
AFS	Agence Française du Sang
AFSSAPS	French Health Regulatory Agency
AIDS	Acquired Immune Deficiency Syndrome
BFU-E	Burst-Forming Unit Erythrocyte
BSE	Bovine Spongiform Encephalopathy
CFU-E	Colony Forming Unit Erythrocyte
CMV	Cytomegalovirus
CSF	Colony Stimulating Factor
EBA	European Blood Alliance
EFS	French National Blood Service
FAH	Fumaryl Acetoacetate Hydrolase
FDA	Food and Drug Administration
G-CSF	Granulocyte Colony Stimulating Factor
GFP	Green Fluorescent Protein
GM-CSF	Granulocyte Monocyte – Colony Stimulating Factor
GMP	Good Manufacturing Practices
HBV	Hepatitis B Virus
HCV	Hepatitis C Virus
HGV	Hepatitis G Virus
HHV	Human Herpes Virus
HIV	Human Immunodeficiency Virus
HLA	Human Lymphocyte Antigen
HTLV	Human T-Cell Leukemia Virus
IL	Interleukin
InVS	Institut de Veille Sanitaire
LBP	Labile blood product
LFB	Fractionation and Biotechnologies Laboratory
MAPC	Multipotent Adult Stem Cell
MGDF	Megacaryocyte-Growth Development Factor
MLV	Murine Leukemia Virus
RBC	Red blood cells
SARS	Severe Acute Respiratory Syndrome
SCF	Stem Cell Factor
SP	Side Population
TPO	Thrombopoietin
TRALI	Transfusion Related Acute Lung Injury
TSE	Transmissible Spongiform Encephalopathy
UVA	Ultra Violet A
vCJD	Variant Creutzfeldt-Jakob Disease
VEGF	Vascular Endothelial Growth Factor
WB	Whole blood
WNV	West Nile Virus

Preface

Giving blood or cells is one of the most generous gestures a person can make to benefit a stranger, without regard for race or religion. This truly humane act was severely tarnished twenty years ago by a tragedy which affected many patients contaminated by the HIV virus.

It became obvious that the French transfusion system had to be restructured. The process was started in 1992; it led to the creation of the "Agence française du sang"(French Blood Agency) and to the introduction of a "blood" law in January 1993.The entire transfusion system was reorganized; technical facilities were connected together so as to allow them access to the most efficient technologies. Plasma fractionation was entrusted to a new institution, the " Laboratoire français du fractionnement et des biotechnologies"(French Fractionation and Biotechnologies Laboratory). At the same time, we maintained a tightly knit network of transfusion sites near donors and patients.

The French Blood Agency focused its work on testing, safeguards and good transfusion practices. The government considered it essential that the same high standard of transfusion safety be maintained throughout the national territory.

No other medical field has undergone such profound changes in so short a time. A series of health crises(AIDS, hepatitis C, prions, the Nile virus in the south of France)contributed to creating the conditions for constant improvement of transfusion safety. Blood donors deserve high praise. They sailed through all these upheavals serenely. Their loyalty and reliability remained unshaken. They continue to give their blood, their platelets, their plasma and sometimes their bone marrow for transplantation. This practice of giving a little of oneself serves to renew our faith in human nature in a world where we often hear of violence, selfishness and indifference.

The introduction of the "blood" law and the creation of the "Etablissement français du sang"(EFS) raised the question of the extent of activities entrusted to blood establishments. Should they concentrate exclusively on transfusion and leave all other activities(biology labs, health care centers, cell and tissue engineering, research and development...)to hospitals? Or, on the contrary, should some of these establishments be entrusted with carrying out such activities? The Director General of Health at the time and successive presidents of the Agency decided to keep all these activities within the mission of the EFS.

Today, the field of transfusion has regained its credibility and can rely on its full potential to face the future and define its strategy.

Transfusion medicine is well equipped to maintain high quality transfusion safety and to engage in the development of biotechnologies. This clearly defined policy aims at creating new types of know-how and at encouraging all forms of donation regularly in the media.

Employment management by objectives will lead to the acquisition of new skills. The continued search for greater efficiency will provide transfusion medicine with the means of reaching its objectives. These are the commitments transfusion medicine of the future must make to donors, patients and the field of health care.

Simone Veil
Former Minister of Health

Introduction

Will we ever succeed in freeing blood from the narrow confines in which many authors, from Melville to Goethe - through the character of Faust - imprisoned it long ago? After chaotic beginnings, modern transfusion is founded on principles established over a century ago, and which have never been questioned: the ABO blood group discovered by Landsteiner in 1900, and the principle of preserving on citrate, which was a great step forward compared to the previous practice of simultaneous "arm to arm" donation! Starting in the 1930s, DeBakey, Jouvelet and Jeanneney competed to develop imaginative methods of administering fresh or stored blood. Since the publication of *L'Oeuvre de la transfusion d'urgence*, by Tzanck and Gosset, no one can doubt the benefits of this natural therapy originating in the human body, and whose efficiency has not been approached by modern science since. For example, we have not yet found an alternative for even the basic oxygen-carrying function. Without transition, transfusion entered a new era by replacing plasma fractionation with cellular engineering. In the process, expectations have been raised in regard to making transfusion a universal tool able to correct various visceral deficiencies.

Foreseeing that transfusion was certain to play a major role in medical practice, a great medical statesman, Eugène Aujaleu, Director of national health services, provided it with a legal framework (Law of 1952) which, a half a century later, remains a model of concision, pragmatism and lucidity. Rooted in the efficiency of transfusion services, the French sector of haematology, pioneered by Andral and then Hayem, flourished around people like Bernard, Bessis, Caen, Dausset, Goudemand, Michon, Peters, Waitz and many others…, and their worthy successors. What other medical field can claim such prestigious bases?

And yet, just when Faustian fears were about to be dispersed, an event occurred which put an abrupt end to this cycle of progress, bringing into question even the most basic foundations of the field. Once again, blood was to become frightening. We all know the reason: for the sake of greater variety of therapeutic agents - and in order to achieve enhanced safety for recipients -, one opted for reduced final preparations issued from huge quantities. As the minimalist architect Mies van der Rohe liked to say: "Less is more". Amazingly enough, this aesthetic principle took on a very peculiar meaning in this context : less final product, greater risk! We envisioned wider possibilities of use, and therefore reduction of risk, and instead we found ourselves confronted with greater exposure and therefore increased danger. In addition, we were faced with the challenge of new organisms having novel modes of reproduction and invasion, and we were insufficiently prepared, without enough mastery of methods and production processes. This situation was to end in tragedy.

As Didier Sicard wrote, "we (went from) transfusion as the paradigm of medical ethics, to transfusion as the paradigm of medical risk". Once again, we lost confidence. It became fashionable to be indignant about "comfort transfusions" which nevertheless were very helpful to post-gastrectomy patients and patients recovering from malnutrition. Clinicians started to sing the praises of "autotransfusion", to the exclusion of everything else. Allogeneic human blood products lost their mythical value; the era of synthetic products was inaugurated. What had become of those dissenting voices on modernity with numerous medication recalls and subsequent marketing bans on "blockbuster drugs" used by millions of people on the planet?

It is in the light of these facts that we express our thanks for the timely project proposed by Patrick Hervé, Jean-Yves Muller and their colleague Pierre Tiberghien, who is the voice of the new generation. We welcome their edited work "**Transfusion Medicine : Looking to the Future**", and appreciate their perspective, as well as that of the other contributors, all of whom were selected for their expertise.

The themes were also carefully chosen to present a balanced overview. In fact, the table of contents reads like a logical summary of the field : the state of the art, the possibilities, the desirable prospects... that often tend toward an ideal. Thus, contributions to the book can be classified in three categories : i) the future of transfusion, through stricter controls; ii) the future of transfusion, through risk reduction; iii) the future of transfusion... by imagining alternative solutions.

There is no doubt that safety is the main concern. Not a theoretical or a hysterical concern: a concrete concern. The first part of the book is entirely devoted to it; it is described in detail, with discussion of cross-over detection, global inactivation of pathogenic agents and production of erythrocytes with attenuated immunogenicity or with universal potential. A review of the entire field is presented, along with analysis of mandatory producer-user connections.

Reflexion on building the future is pervasive, and the project is undertaken with obvious enthusiasm. By launching cell engineering, the authors open an even wider perspective than that created by Cohn when he introduced the plasmatic fractionation revolution. Starting out modestly with the use of technologic means of selective sampling of blood donations, this innovative engineering can be applied to the handling of peripheral lineages, to the optimisation of stem cell samples and, soon, to their transformation.

The book goes on to discuss the role of transfusion in this new paradigm, its relation to European geopolitics, its accomplishments and the conditions required for developing its full potential... before concluding with a courageous attempt at foreseeing the next decade. I would not presume to comment on this "Picture of transfusion in ten years", except to say that it reads like the mastery of daring. We cannot guess what the future of blood transfusion will be, but we can say that, today, it illustrates the words of Miguel de Unamuno : "Others would do better. I just do." And therein lies its substancial merit.

Jacques Cinqualbre, MD
Professor of Surgery (Louis Pasteur University, Strasbourg)
Former President and founder, French Blood Agency

Transfusion, a Matter of Cells: Review of the Past Three Decades

Patrick Hervé, Pierre Tiberghien

Sequence of the First Discoveries

In transfusion medicine, the diversity of discoveries and their applications made successive stages overlap, and the uneven advancement of knowledge placed different types of events in the same timeframe. The 20th century was a period when genius and innovation existed side by side with scandal and tragedy [1].

Transfusion entered the modern age with the discovery of blood groups, made by Karl Landsteiner in 1900. However, awareness of the importance of this discovery came later.

It was in 1930 that Landsteiner won the Nobel Prize for his work [2]. In 1918, Beth and Vincent developed a technique of rapid blood typing. In 1940, Landsteiner and Wiener discovered the Rhesus group [3].

In 1950, Dausset (Nobel Prize 1980), Payne and Van Rood described the HLA system [4]. The genetic system involved in foreign tissue rejection is the major histocompatibility complex which codes highly polymorphic cellular surface molecules [5].

In 1914, when Hustin discovered citrated blood, a great step forward was made in the field.

The success of the first transfusion using citrated blood was due to the fortunate accident of compatible blood types. Had there been incompatibility, the complications would have been blamed on sodium citrate.

Arnault Tzanck, the first person to have the idea of creating transfusion centres [6], was the founder of the "Œuvre de la transfusion sanguine d'urgence" in Paris, in 1928. The purpose of this first transfusion center was to gather and select donors in response to needs, while maintaining the generous image of blood donation. The first transfusion centre using preserved blood was created in 1934.

In 1943, an important advance was made in the "long" term preservation of blood: the introduction of the ACD solution (acid citrose dextrose) by Loutit and Mollison [7]. Preservative mixtures evolved in four major stages: 1957, discovery of CPD (citrate phosphate dextrose), making it possible to preserve blood for twenty-one days; 1962, when adenine was added, the conservation period was extended to thirty-five days; 1978, the introduction of the saline/ adenine/ glucose solution (SAG) increased the rate of post-transfusion survival; finally, the SAG-mannitol mixture allowed blood preservation for forty-two days, the legal period still in effect today [8-10]. Current research is working on the preparation of new preservative mixtures that will make it possible to prolong this period by fifteen days.

The introduction of plastic containers for whole blood collection in 1952 was a great step forward [11, 12]. They were the original version of the equipment used today. This discovery led to the development of biotechnologies applied to blood transfusion. All these advances gave transfusion medicine the tools it needed to develop, innovate and expand the field of its activities.

In the last four decades, we have seen a gradual transition from the therapeutic use of whole blood to the use of blood components, so as to transfuse patients only with the cells required for the treatment of a specific pathology [13-16]. This was the first chapter in the story of "cell therapy", which places the cell, whatever its origin and function, at the center of the new technologies (apheresis, cell sorting, cryopreservation, cell expansion...).

The story we want to tell is that of the successive stages of these discoveries, that led up to today's transfusion medicine, and justify its future ambition: the development of cell engineering technologies making it possible to diversify the applications of cell therapy.

Cells Like the Cold

Thanks to the discovery of the cryptoprotective properties of glycerol, erythrocytes can be frozen in plasma containing 15% of glycerol, and can be stored for three months at -80 °C [17]. In 1951, Mollison performed the first transfusion of frozen-and-thawed erythrocytes. During the 1980s, platelet freezing techniques were developed, and two methods of cryopreservation were tested: one using dimethyl sulfoxide (DMSO), and the other using glycerol [18, 19]. Frozen platelet survival studies *in vivo* showed dimethyl sulfoxide to be superior.

The publication of Pegg's work in 1964 gave great impetus to the cryobiology of hematopoietic stem cells intended for clinical use [20]. Long term preservation of hematopoietic stem cells in liquid nitrogen (- 196 °C) was demonstrated [21]. In 1978, Appelbaum reported successful hematopoietic reconstitution after transfusion of cryopreserved bone marrow in lymphoma patients treated with myeloablative therapy [22].

In 1977, Fliedner's group described a preclinical bank model of hematopoietic stem blood cells and of cryopreserved mononuclear cells [23]. Cryobiology made it possible to create protocols for autologous hematopoietic stem cell transplantation [24-26]. But we do not yet have a technique for the cryopreservation of granulocytes.

Advent of Cell Apheresis Techniques

The use of blood components in clinical treatment developed with the use of plastic equipment. At first, developing more or less automated techniques for cell collection was motivated by the need to obtain compatible HLA platelets in sufficient quantities, from the same donor, to treat an immunized patient. In 1971, a group of Boston scientists created the first methods of semi-automatic apheresis adapted to platelets [27-29]. Today, apheresis is performed using semi-automatic cell separators. The donor's blood is anticoagulated and flows through the separator to achieve separation of the different blood components (plasma, erythrocytes, platelets). The desired component is stored in a side pocket and the reconstituted blood is reinfused in the donor. At the start of 2006, there are eight types of cell separators marketed by five different companies; they are differentiated according to the component they are designed to separate: platelets, granulocytes, lymphocytes, plasma, stem blood cells. All functions of the separator, such as the addition of the anticoagulant, the conditions of centrifugation, the separation of the cellular component, are controlled by a microprocessor. New devices are being developed to improve automated control, safety and quality of the separated cellular components.

Blood Stem Cell Transplantation: an Ideal Field for Biotechnologies Applications

In 1968, Good successfully performed the first autologous transplantations to treat severe combined immune deficit. Autologous transplantations benefited greatly from the work of the Seatle group [30, 31]. Thomas received the Nobel Prize for his work in 1990. In France, autologous transplantations have developed since 1978, led by the pioneering work of the Paris-St. Antoine group [32]. Given the complications specific to the two types of transplantations: risk of relapse for autologous transplantations and risk of graft-*versus*-host reaction for allografts, technologic innovations made it a priority to reduce, even eliminate, these risks.

Much research was devoted to the deletion and elimination of residual disease in grafts of autologous hematopoietic stem cells. The first approach consisted of treating grafts with *ex vivo* chemotherapy. 4-hydroperoxycyclophosphamide (Asta-Z) was discovered in 1968 [33]. It is the substance used most by the Baltimore and Paris-St Antoine teams, despite delayed hematologic reconstitution [34, 35]. Availability of monoclonal specific malignancy antigen antibodies allowed cell sorting by means of immuno-absorption columns, of immunotoxins that combine a toxin like ricin with a monoclonal antibody [36], or of the immunomagnetic selection technique used specifically for neuroblastoma [37]. These methods of *ex vivo* treatment of blood stem cell grafts encouraged the development of various quality control tests, cultures of hematopoietic progenitors, phenotype identification by flux cytometry, long term culture, molecular biology and microbiologic safety. The effectiveness of *ex vivo* chemotherapy in terms of event-free survival has not been demonstrated due to the lack of randomized trials.

Reduction of T-lymphocytes found in a blood stem cell graft, in view of preventing graft reaction against the host, was the first application of biotechnology in an allogeneic setting. Complement-dependent cytolysis with monoclonal anti-T antibodies was the first stage of this application [38]. A few years later, the use of immunotoxins was tested [39, 40]. Unfortunately, T-cell depletion causes two major complications: greater incidence of hematologic reconstitution failure, and higher rate of relapse, especially in chronic myeloid leukemia [41].

Identification of the CD34 antigen on cells responsible for hematopoietic reconstitution was an important breakthrough, whose 20th anniversary was celebrated recently [42, 43]. Biomedical equipment was designed in order to allow immunologic purification of CD34+ cells. This immuno-selection makes it possible to deplete accessory cells such as T-lymphocytes, monocytes or contaminating tumor cells [44]. CD34+ cell count makes it possible to estimate the functional quality of autologous and allogenic grafts.

The number of CD34 + cells collected and reinjected can predict the time frame for hematologic reconstitution.

Immuno-selection by magnetic sorting of CD34 + cells is the accepted technique for T-cell depletion in allogeneic settings, and for reduction of residual disease in CD34 – tumor pathologies in autologous settings [45]. However, the consequences of immunodepletion well beyond simple T-cell depletion of the graft (for example, depletion of natural killer cells or of immunoregulatory cells) are still to be assessed.

Potential of Hematopoietic Cytokines

In 1906, the first identified cytokine, hematopoietin, became a substance of clinical interest. It was at the centre of the most important technological advance in the fifteen-year history of cell engineering and development of new cell therapy products. This advance involved the development of hematopoietic growth factors obtained through genetic engineering. Used at first, starting in 1987, to accelerate hematopoiesis after increasing doses of chemotherapy, hematopoietic cytokines were to acquire many other uses. At the end of the 1980s, blood stem cell graft practices entered a new phase. Mobilisation of hematopoietic stem cells in peripheral blood after treatment with hematopoietic cytokines, in an autologous setting, led to the use of stem blood cells obtained by apheresis for transplantation purposes [46-48]. A few years later, these cells were going to be introduced gradually into allogeneic settings.

The availability of growth factors encouraged new approaches in the handling of blood stem cells. For example, hematopoietic progenitors can be expanded *ex vivo* to produce more mature progenitors, able to reduce the post-transplantation neutropenia and thrombocytopenia period. More rapid graft take will reduce the need for adjuvant transfusion, bringing us closer to autologous transplants performed in ambulatory care [49, 50]. Applications of *ex vivo* cell expansion in the presence of growth factors are numerous: expansion / maturation of lymphocytes for adoptive immunotherapy, production of clones of specific viral infection lymphocytes [51], expansion of megakaryocytes to produce platelets as an adjunct to transfusion, expansion of normal cells at the expense of abnormal cells as a purging process. The possibility of obtaining functional erythrocytes in great quantities from placental stem cells was demonstrated in 2002.

Diversity of Hematopoietic Stem Cell Sources

The two principles regarding a single medullary source of hematopoietic stem cells and a required HLA genetic identity have been invalidated in the 1980s [52, 53]. Apheresis and availability of hematopoietic cytokines have allowed rapid development of hematopoietic stem blood cell transplantations [54]. In 1989, Broxmeyer identified placental blood as a source of hematopoietic stem cells [55]. The same year, the first placental blood transplantation was performed in Paris, followed five years later by the organization of an international network of banks for unrelated cryopreserved placental blood grafts [56]. This international network is composed of 36 banks which store 170,000 grafts. In the past ten years, 6,000 placental blood graft transplantations were performed, out of a total of 350,000 myeloid and hematic blood stem cell grafts. Pluripotent hematopoietic stem cells abound in placental blood. Hematologic reconstitution is closely related to the number of injected cells [57].

Today, there are several categories of donors of allogeneic hematopoietic stem cells: genotypically matched sibling, partly identical family member, unrelated partly or totally phenotypically matched donor.

Toward the Medicine of the Future : Stem Cell Engineering

In the past few years, many studies have demonstrated the presence of stem cells within various "adult" tissues or organs, suggesting that the stem cells of a given tissue are able to differentiate into cells of another tissue. This unique characteristic was given the name "stem cell plasticity" [57]. Adult and embryonic stem cells have differentiation and proliferation capacities that could serve to treat different pathologies. Several types of cells have great potential in cell therapy settings. In addition to hematopoietic stem cells, we can cite mesenchymal cells, described by Friedenstein in 1980 [58] and by Owen in 1985 [59]. These cells can differentiate into different tissues (osteogenetic, chondrogenetic, angiogenetic…).

Although their functional properties are not completely known, mesenchymal stem cells are pluripotent and are likely to be able to be cryptopreserved. They are not immunogenic and in allogeneic settings they are capable of immunomodulation. In 2002, the Verfaillie group developed a culture system capable of producing multipotent adult progenitor cells (MAPC) [60]. In their system, multipotent adult progenitors can differentiate into cells with meso, ecto and endodermic characteristics. It has, however, been difficult, but possible, to produce such cells in other laboratories.

Embryonic stem cells are derived from the internal cellular mass of embryos. These totipotent cells, commonly called ES cells, have been extensively studied in animals; they have immense potential for regenerating organs, due to the diversity and number of cell types that can be produced [61, 62]. They can be preserved and expanded *in vitro*, to provide an inexhaustible source of cells that can be used in reconstructive medicine. The new French bioethics law bans all research on therapeutic cloning. This type of research is subject to controversy in many countries. Europeans started introducing legislation regarding biomedical research ethics at the end of the 1980s. In the future, the only research legal in France will be the study of embryonic cell lineages already established, and this research will be conducted only in certain selected laboratories [63].

Cellular Engineering of Erythrocytes and Immunologic Transfusion Safety

Efforts to convert ABO blood groups started over 30 years ago. The method consists of converting A or B erythrocytes to O erythrocytes, by enzyme treatments, in conditions that make it possible for them to be used in transfusion [64, 65]. In order to achieve this, two things are required:

– removing sufficient antigens so that the treated erythrocytes can be tolerated by the recipient as native O erythrocytes;
– preserving the capacity of treated erythrocytes to function normally.

Screening of numerous alpha-galactosidases led the pioneering teams to select a B-enzyme without sialidasic activity. Erythrocytes treated with these enzymes can be frozen without producing functional changes.

Another approach of interest for transfusion safety is surface modification of erythrocytes using pegylation. Polyethylene-glycol can conceal erythrocytic antigens, making possible incompatible transfusions in recipients immunized to these antigens. This approach gave rise to many studies during the 1990s [66]. Polyethylene-glycol cannot conceal all red cell antigens, to make red cells "universal". It has been shown recently that polyethylene-glycol can produce specific immunization [67]. Polyethylene-glycol immunogenicity could bring into question the antigenic camouflage of erythrocytes.

Cellular Immunotherapy: Passion and Disappointment

Better understanding of the role of cellular immunity in the control of diseases such as viral infections and cancers, as well as the development of methods of production of immunocompetent cells, have led to the introduction of cellular immunotherapy. It was in the allogeneic hematopoietic transplantation setting that adoptive immunotherapy (immunocompetent cell transfer) was most developed. By showing that, in mice, leukemia could be cured by the administration of allogeneic lymphocytes, in 1952 Barnes et al. lay the foundations for an important therapeutic effect: the graft-*versus*-leukemia effect, a reaction widely used today in the field of hematopoietic transplantation [68], but which is, unfortunately, linked with a potentially lethal complication: graft-*versus*-host disease [69].

In effect, the donor's T lymphocytes, in a hematopoietic graft or administered separately at a distance from the graft, trigger an allogeneic response directed against host tissues, with the possible occurrence of a graft-*versus*-host reaction; against host residual hematopoietic cells, with a preventive effect on graft rejection; or against malignant hematopoietic cells (and perhaps solid tumors as well), with a powerful antitumoral effect: the graft-*versus*-leukemia reaction.

A relapse rate two or three times higher after T lymphocyte depleted hematopoietic transplantation and, above all, the effectiveness, in certain malignant hemopathies, of donor T lymphocyte administration after relapse at a distance from the hematopoietic graft (> than 70% of complete lasting remissions after relapse in chronic myeloid leukemia), made it possible to demonstrate the effective antitumoral action of T lymphocytes [70]. Minor histocompatibility antigens, resulting from genetic disparity between donor and recipient, are the main target of these alloreactive T lymphocytes. Recently, it was demonstrated that donor natural killer lymphocytes can sometimes also exert a powerful alloreactive antitumoral effect and facilitate graft take, while possibly preventing the occurrence of a graft-*versus*-host effect [71].

In an autologous setting, the results of adoptive antitumoral immunotherapy have been much more disappointing so far, with the exception of tumors associated with the Epstein-Barr virus. In the case of the latter, using T cytotoxic lymphocytes directed against the Epstein-Barr virus can give excellent results [72]; however, the methods needed to produce these effects are complex and do not lend themselves to routine use. Limited knowledge concerning potential antigenic targets, very active immunosuppression mechanisms at tumoral sites, and limited *in vivo* survival associated with the absence of tumoral localization of immunocompetent cells, are factors that have contributed to the relative inefficiency of approaches using so-called LAK (blood lymphocytes cultivated in the presence of IL-2) TIL(cultivated tumor infiltrating T-lymphocytes) cultivated *ex vivo* [73]. More recently, the association of an "immunosuppressor" treatment to deplete lymphocytes regulating endogens before the administration of T lymphocytes directed against tumoral antigens has given promising results [74]. Better mastery of the methods of production of cytotoxic lymphocytic populations (or, on the contrary, "regulatory" populations) specifically targeting the relevant antigens (viral, tumoral or minor histocompatibility antigens or, on the contrary, "autoimmune" antigens) should lead to the advent of these innovative approaches in the near future. The use of specialized cells for presentation of antigens to the immune system, such as dendritic cells to induce an *in vivo* immune antitumoral response, is another process which has been studied for over ten years.

Better phenotypical and functional characterization of specialized cells in the presentation of the antigens used, as well as their level of maturation, and optimization of the methods of administration (use of adjuvants, mode and schedule of administration), are stages to be developed further before we can fully assess the therapeutic potential of such "cellular vaccines" [75].

The Promise of Gene Therapy

Gene transfer for therapeutic purposes (gene therapy) has also known considerable progress, both in the fields of cellular therapy (gene therapy *ex vivo*) and *in vivo* gene therapy (*in vivo* administration of the transgene +/- its vector). Depending on the target cell and on the desired effect, the gene transfer method (virus, liposomes...) allows genomic integration (stability of expression) or epigenetic integration. The goal of *ex vivo* gene therapy is to endow target cells (hematopoietic stem cells, immunocompetent cells, fibroblasts) with new abilities: to compensate a deficit, to reinforce an immunocompetence, to confer susceptibility to a prodrug ... A first success was achieved by the Alain Fisher team (Necker), when it demonstrated that *ex vivo* gene therapy (retroviral gene transfer into hematopoietic stem cells) could "cure" children with severe immunodeficiency [76]. Unfortunately, the manifestation in several of these children of leukemias triggered in part by oncogene activation during insertion mutagenesis [76] was a reminder of the potential toxicity of such approaches, and of the obvious need to make further advances in this promising new field.

Quality Control Programs:
European Pressure to Achieve "the Medicinal Cell"?

In the past ten years, quality control programs have developed intensively in all transfusion organizations, particularly in France, in response to the tragedy of blood contaminated by the AIDS virus. The epidemic involving this new virus led health authorities to introduce quality control systems applying specifically to blood transfusion. This process culminated, in France, in the acquisition of an Iso/9001 certification by most transfusion establishments by the end of 2005.

Good practices of blood collection and of preservation and storage of mononuclear blood cells, of hematopoietic stem blood cells and of hematopoietic stem cells of placental origin, have been the focus of several public inquiries in the second half of 1995, and were approved by the Board of Directors of the "Etablissement français des greffes" in June 1996.

Current French regulations are based on three laws: the law of May 28, 1996 (DMOSSS) which applies to cell and gene therapies as treatment practices; the law of January 4, 1993 (called the Blood Law) and the law of July 24, 1994, with their respective application directives.

Quality control must cover all stages of production, from the product obtained from blood collection to the end product, including storage and transport conditions. Quality control validates documentation, and insures implementation of control procedures and of authorized control methods. In order for a quality control system to be effective, it must exert control over natural biologic variations, over preparation techniques and over the regulation of blood products or cell therapies. Traceability of blood products and cell therapy "lots" products is mandatory.

In Conclusion

The history of blood transfusion is a fabulous human adventure in the course of which medical and scientific expertise came together by chance or by design to give birth to a new medical discipline. The originality of these successive stages where applied research dominated consists in the extraordinary therapeutic potential of blood and myeloid cells. This potential concerns numerous pathologies, many of which are outside the field of hematology. The next decade faces the challenge of pursuing the development of this therapeutic potential. No matter how complex the technology brought into play, the donor remains the essential player in the story, just as he has been from the beginning. This medical and scientific adventure must go hand in hand with the application of rigorous ethical principles.

References

1. Bay C. *Histoire de la transfusion : le XXe siècle, le génie et l'innovation côtoient le scandale et la tragédie.* Thèse doctorat en médecine 1995, Université de Franche-Comté 95-013, 195 p.
2. Landsteiner K, Wiener AS. An agglutinable factor in human group recognizable by immune sera for rhesus blood. *Proc Soc Exp Biol Med* 1940 ; 43 : 223.
3. McKusick. From Karl Landsteiner to Peter Agre : 100 years in the history of blood group genetics. *Transfusion* 2004 ; 44 : 1370-6.
4. Terasaki PI, Dausset J, Payne R, et al. *History of HLA : ten recollections.* Los Angeles : UCLA Tissue Typing Laboratory, 1990.
5. Powis SH, Trowsdale J. Human major histocompatibility complex genes. *Behring Inst Mitt* 1994 ; 94.
6. Tzanck A. *Problèmes théoriques et pratiques de la transfusion sanguine.* Paris : Masson, 1933, 212 p.
7. Loutit JF, Mollison PL. Advantages of a disodium-citrate-glucose mixture as a blood preservative. *Br Med J* 1943 ; ii : 744-5.
8. Högman CF, Hedlund K, Zetterstrom H. Clinical usefulness of red cells preserved in protein-poor media. *N Engl J Med* 1978 ; 299 : 1377-81.
9. Nakao M, Nakao T, Arimatsu Y, Yoshikawa H. A new preservative medium maintaining the level of adenosine triphosphate and the osmotic resistance of erythrocytes. *Proc JPn Acad* 1960 ; 36 : 43.
10. Hervé P, Lamy B, Peters A, et al. Preservation of human erythrocytes in the liquid state biological results with a new medium. *Vox Sang* 1980 ; 39 : 195-204.
11. Sack T, Gibson J, Buckley E. The preservation of whole ACD blood collected, stored and transfused in plastic equipment. *Surg Gynecol Obstet* 1952 ; 95 : 113-9.
12. Amouch PJ. Conservation du sang en sacs plastiques. Application à la préparation des concentrés globulaires. *Transfusion* 1964 ; 7 : 23-5.
13. Genetet B, Mannoni P. *La transfusion.* Paris : Flammarion, 1978.
14. Slichter SJ, Harker LA. Preparation and storage of platelet concentrates. *Br J Haematol* 1976 ; 34 : 395-419.
15. Mollison PL. *Blood transfusion in clinical medicine.* 6th Oxford Blackwell Scientific Publications, 1979.
16. Lane TA, Anderson KC, Goodnough LT, et al. Leukocyte reduction in blood component therapy. *Ann Intern Med* 1992 ; 117 : 151-62.

17. Smith AU. Prevention of hemolysis during freezing and thawing of red blood cells. Lancet 1950 ; 2 : 910-3.
18. Hervé P, Potron G, Droulé C, et al. Human platelets frozen with glycerol in liquid nitrogen : biological and clinical aspects. Transfusion 1981 ; 21 : 384-9.
19. Kim BK, Tanque L, Baldini MG. Storage of human platelets by freezing. Vox Sang 1976 ; 30 : 401-9.
20. Pegg DE. Freezing of bone marrow for clinical use. Cryobiology 1964 ; 1 : 64-71.
21. Malini TI, Pegg DE, Perry VR, et al. Long term storage of bone marrow cells at liquid nitrogen and dry ice temperature. Cryobiology 1970 ; 7 : 65-9.
22. Appelbaum FR, Herzig GP, Ziegler JC. Successful engraftment of cryopreserved autologous bone marrow in patients with malignant lymphoma. Blood 1978 ; 52 : 85-95.
23. Fliedner TM, Korbling M, Calvo W, Herbst E. Cryopreservation of blood mononuclear leukocytes and stem cells suspend in a large fluid volume : a preclinical model for a blood stem cells bank. Blut 1977 ; 35 : 1.
24. Dicke KA, Spitzer G, Peters L, McCredie KB. Autologous bone marrow transplantation in relapsed adult acute leukaemia. Lancet 1979 ; 3 : 514-7.
25. Gorin NC, Hervé P, Aegertu P, et al. Autologous bone marrow transplantation for acute leukaemia in remision. Br J Haematol 1986 ; 64 : 385-9.
26. Reiffers J, Gaspard MH, Maraninchi D, et al. Comparison of allogeneic or autologous bone marrow transplantation in patients with acute myeloid leukaemia in first remission : a prospective controlled trial. Br J Haematol 1989 ; 72 : 57-61.
27. Tullis JL, Tinch RJ, Baudanza P, et al. Plateletpheresis in a disposable system. Transfusion 1971 ; 11 : 368-77.
28. Graw RG, Herzig GP, Eisel RJ, Perry S. Leukocyte and platelet collection from normal donors with the continuous flow blood cell separator. Transfusion 1971 ; 11 : 94-101.
29. Szymanski IO, Patti K, Kliman A. Efficacy of the latham blood processor to perform plateletpheresis. Transfusion 1973; 13 : 405-11.
30. Thomas ED, Storb R, Clift RA, et al. Bone marrow transplantation. N Engl J Med 1975; 292 : 832-43.
31. Weiden PL, Flournoy N, Thomas ED, et al. Antileukemic effect of GVH disease in human recipients of allogeneic marrow grafts. N Engl J Med 1979 ; 300 : 1068-73.
32. Gorin NC. Autologous bone-marrow transplantation in acute myelocytic leukaemia. Lancet 1977 ; 1 : 1050.
33. Yeager AM, Kaiser H, Santos GW, et al. Autologous bone marrow transplantation in patients with acute myelogenous leukemia using ex-vivo treatment with 4-hydroperoxycyclophosphamide. N Engl J Med 1968 ; 315 : 141-7.
34. Sharkis SJ, Santos GW, Colvin M. Elimination of acute myelogeneous leukemic cells from marrow and tumor suspensions in the rat with 4-hydroperoxy-cyclophosphamide (4-HC). Blood 1980 ; 55 : 521-3.
35. Gorin NC, Douay L, Laporte JP, et al. Autologous bone marrow transplantation using marrow incubated with ASTA Z 7557 in adult acute leukemia. Blood 1986 ; 67 : 1367-76.
36. Casellas P, Canat X, Fauser AA, et al. Optimal elimination of leukemic T cells from human bone marrow with T 101-ricin-A chain immunotoxin. Blood 1985 ; 65 : 289-95.
37. Kemshead JT, Ugelstad J. Magnetic separation techniques : their applications to medicine. Mol Cell Biochem 1985 ; 67 : 11-8.
38. Hervé P, Cahn JY, Flesch M, et al. Successful GVHD prevention without graft failure in 32 HLA identical allogeneic bone marrow transplantation with marrow depleted of T-cells by monoclonal antibodies and complement. Blood 1987 ; 69 : 388-93.

39. Martin PJ, Hansen JA Torok-Storb B, et al. Effects of treating marrow with a CD3 –specific immunotoxin for prevention of acute graft-versus-host disease. *Bone Marrow Transplant* 1988 ; 3 : 437-44.
40. Cavazzana-Calvo M, Fromont C, Le Deist F, et al. Specific elimination of alloreactive T-cells by an anti-IL-2 receptor B chain specific immunotoxin. *Transplantation* 1990 ; 50 : 1-7.
41. Kernan NA. Graft failure following transplantation of T cell depleted marrow. In : Burakoff SJ, Deeg HJ, Ferrara J, Atkinson K, eds. *Graft-vs-host disease : immunology, pathophysiology and treatment*. New York : Marcel Dekker, 1990 : 557-68.
42. Civin CL, Strauss LC, Brovall C, et al. Antigenic analysis of hematopoiesis III. A hematopoietic progenitor cell surface antigen defined by a monoclonal antibody raised against KG-1a cells. *J Immunol* 1984 ; 133 : 157-65.
43. Chabannon C. Happy anniversary, CD34. *ISCT Telegraft* 2004 ; 11 : 9-10.
44. Shpall EJ, Jones RB, Franklin WA, et al. Transplantation of enriched CD34+ autologous marrow into breast cancer patients following high dose chemotherapy : influence of CD34+ peripheral blood progenitors and growth factors on engraftment. *J Clin Oncol* 1994 ; 12 : 28-36.
45. Carlo Stella C, Cazzola M, De Fabritis P, et al. CD34-positive cells : biology and clinical relevance. *Haematologica* 1995 ; 80 : 367-87.
46. Goodman JW, Hodgson GS. Evidence for stem cells in the peripheral blood of mice. *Blood* 1962 ; 19 : 702-14.
47. Richman CM, Wiener RS, Yankee RA. Increase in circulating stem cells following chemotherapy in man. *Blood* 1976 ; 47 : 1031-9.
48. Bronchud MH, Potter MR, Morgenstern G, et al. In vitro and in vivo analysis of the effects of recombinant human G-CSF in patients. *Br J Cancer* 1988 ; 58 : 64-9.
49. Frei R, Heimfeld S, Yu Z, et al. Ex-vivo expansion of human CD 34+ hematopoietic progenitor cells. *Exp Hematol* 1994 ; 22 : 726-7.
50. Reiffers J, Caillot C, Dazey B, et al. Abrogation of post-myeloablative chemotherapy neutropenic by ex-vivo expanded autologous CD34-positive cells. *Lancet* 1999 ; 354 : 1092-3.
51. Riddell S, Watanabe K, Goodrich J, et al. Restoration of viral immunity in immuno-deficient humans by the adoptive transfert of T-cell clones. *Science* 1992 ; 257 : 238-41.
52. Hansen JA, Clift RA, Thomas ED. Transplantation of marrow from an unrelated donor to a patient with acute leukaemia. *N Engl J Med* 1980 ; 303 : 565-7.
53. Ash RC, Casper JT, Chitambon CR, et al. Successful allogeneic transplantation of T-cell depleted bone marrow from closely HLA matched unrelated donors. *N Engl J Med* 1990 ; 322 : 485-94.
54. Gianni AM, Siena S, Bregni M, et al. Autologous bone marrow transplantation for acute leukaemia in remission. *Br J Haematol* 1986 ; 64 : 385-9.
55. Broxmeyer HE, Douglas GW, Hangoc G, Cooper S, Bard J, English D, Arny M, Thomas L, Boyse EA. Human umbilical cord blood as a potential source of transplantable hematopoietic stem/progenitor cells. *Proc Natl Acad Sci USA* 1989 ; 86 : 3828-32.
56. Rubinstein P, Rosenfield R, Adamson JW, et al. Stored placental blood for unrelated bone marrow reconstitution. *Blood* 1993 ; 81 : 1679-90.
57. Orkin SH, Zon LI. Hematopoiesis and stem cells : plasticity versus developmental heterogeneity. *Nat Med* 2002 ; 3 : 323-8.
58. Friedenstein AJ. Stromal mechanisms of bone marrow : cloning in vitro and retransplantation in vivo. In : Thienfelder S, Rodt H, Kolb HJ, eds. *Immunology of bone marrow transplantation*. Berlin : Springer-Verlag, 1980 : 19-20.
59. Owen M. Lineage of osteogenic cells and their relationship to the stromal system. In : Peck WA, ed. *Bone and mineral research*, vol.3. New York : Elsevier, 1985 : 1-25.

60. Jiang Y, Jahagirdar BN, Lee Reinhardt R, *et al.* Pluripotency of mesenchymal stem cells derived from adult marrow. *Nature* 2002 ; 418 : 41-9.
61. Weissman IL. Stem cells : units of development, units of regeneration and units in evolution. *Cell* 2000 ; 100 : 157-68.
62. Magli MC, Levantini E, Giorgetti A. The developmental potential of somatic stem cells in mammalian adults. *J Hemathother Stem Cell Res* 2000 ; 9 : 961-9.
63. Barrat CLR, StJohn JC, Afnan M. Clinical challenges in providing embryos for stem-cell initiatives. *Lancet* 2004 ; 364 : 115-8.
64. Schenkel-Brunner H, Tuppy H. Enzymatic conversion of human O into A erythrocytes and B into AB erythrocytes. *Nature* 1969 ; 223 : 1271-3.
65. Goldstein J, Siviglia G, Hurst R, *et al.* Group B erythrocytes enzymatically converted to group O survive normally in A, B and O individuals. *Science* 1982 ; 215 : 168-70.
66. Scott MD, Murad KL, Kampouran F, *et al.* Chemical camouflage of antigenic determinant : stealth erythrocytes. *Proc Natl Acad Sci USA* 1997 ; 94 : 7566-71.
67. Armstrong JK, Wenby RB, Meiselman JH, *et al. In vivo* survival of poly(ethylene-glycol)-coated red blood cells in the rabbit. *Blood* 2003 ; 102 : 94 (abstr).
68. Horowitz MM, Gale RP, Sondel PM, *et al.* Graft-versus-leukemia reactions after bone marrow transplantation. *Blood* 1990 ; 75 : 555-62.
69. Ferrara JL. Pathogenesis of acute graft-versus-host disease: cytokines and cellular effectors. *J Hematother Stem Cell Res* 2000 ; 9 : 299-306.
70. Kolb HJ, Schattenberg A, Goldman JM, *et al.* Graft-versus-leukemia effect of donor lymphocyte transfusions in marrow grafted patients. *Blood* 1995 ; 86 : 2041-50.
71. Ruggeri L, Capanni M, Urbani E, Perruccio K, Shlomchik WD, Tosti A, Posati S, Rogaia D, Frassoni F, Aversa F, Martelli MF, Velardi A. Effectiveness of donor natural killer cell alloreactivity in mismatched hematopoietic transplants. *Science* 2002 ; 295 : 2097-100.
72. Heslop HE, Brenner MK, Rooney CM. Donor T cells to treat EBV-associated lymphoma. *N Engl J Med* 1994 ; 331 : 679-80.
73. Dudley ME, Rosenberg SA. Adoptive-cell-transfer therapy for the treatment of patients with cancer. *Nat Rev Cancer* 2003 ; 3 : 666-75.
74. Dudley ME, Wunderlich JR, Yang JC, *et al.* Adoptive cell transfer therapy following non-myeloablative but lymphodepleting chemotherapy for the treatment of patients with refractory metastatic melanoma. *J Clin Oncol* 2005 ; 23 : 2346-57.
75. Banchereau J, Palucka AK. Dendritic cells as therapeutic vaccines against cancer. *Nat Rev Immunol* 2005 ; 5 : 296-306.
76. Cavazzana-Calvo M, Lagresle C, Hacein-Bey-Abina S, Fischer A. Gene therapy for severe combined immunodeficiency. *Annu Rev Med* 2005 ; 56 : 585-602.

The Concept of Safety in Blood Transfusion

Jean-Hugues Trouvin

The Concept of Safety

Recourse to human blood or its components is still absolutely essential in certain clinical situations. In fact, blood and its components (called "labile blood products" or "transfusion products") make it possible to provide complex physiologic components such as red blood cells, platelets or plasma, which can compensate vital physiologic insufficiencies.

However, the use of products derived from human blood, or the use of derivatives of tissue or other biological fluids, whether of human or animal origin, involves the risk of contamination by pathogenic agents and, therefore, the potential risk of transmitting the latter to the recipients.

The risk is further increased when these products are administered using an invasive procedure, intravenous injection, which differs considerably from "natural" exposure to the same agents that are, often, part of our natural environment. In addition, these products are often given to immunocompromised patients whose natural defences are inadequate.

Use of blood products has always exposed human beings to pathogenic agents. Some of these were identified rapidly, but in some cases the pathogenic effect was harder to identify because pathology was minor or appeared at a distance from the "contact". In terms of safety, a long incubation period makes it difficult to identify the pathogenic agent. In this context, at the microbiological level, it is impossible to guarantee absolute blood safety: a new pathogen, as yet unknown, could emerge at any time. As far as these new risks are concerned, levels of knowledge vary from one situation to another; they are either fragmentary in the absence of fundamental data on the nature of the agent or the transmission mechanism (for example, the agent responsible for Creutzfeldt-Jakob disease, in its sporadic or variant forms); or complete enough but associated with technical constraints (like the West-Nile virus or the agent of Chagas disease : *T. cruzii*). The question of transfusion "safety" has to be understood in light of this reality of a permanent risk, sometimes difficult to detect, foresee and identify. In this chapter, the term "safety" is used in the larger sense of microbiological safety, that covers risk of transmission of all types of pathogenic agents, be they bacterial, fungal, parasitic, viral, or even "non conventional transmissible agents" such as the prion (agent responsible for transmissible subacute spongiform encephalopathies-TSSE).

All these microbiological "risk" agents for transfusion have the following characteristics in common:

– they can be present in blood,

– they are transmissible intravenously,

– they are deleterious for the recipient, either due to their pathogenic nature *per se* (HIV, HCV), or due to transmission to high-risk recipients (parvovirus B19, CMV, Epstein-Barr virus, toxoplasmosis…) (for a detailed discussion of diseases communicable by transfusion, see [1]).

Even if we admit that "zero risk" is not possible, we must insure that transfusion products provide "maximum" safety, and that despite a potential or specific risk, the clinical benefit of transfusion always outweighs the risk.

"Maximum" level of safety refers to the process by which all available means are used to reduce to a minimum, within the limits of current knowledge, the risk of presence of infectious agents in blood products.

To achieve this safety requirement, the concept of microbiological safety for transfusion products, like for all biological products, is founded on three essential "pillars":

– quality and mastery of the "material of origin",

– process used to prepare the desired components or derivatives, and procedures of elimination/ inactivation of pathogenic agent(s),

– control, screening and qualification tests all along the preparation chain.

However, given the original source of the material (the donor), the physical, chemical and biological characteristics of the "material of origin"[1] collected (whole blood or components), and the need to preserve intact the physiological properties of the final product to be administered to the patient (relative fragility and lability of numerous blood components), each of these safety stages has limits of application, and overall safety is achieved through the combined efforts of all those involved.

Implementing the three essential "pillars" requires the best possible knowledge of the characteristics of the risk-related infectious agent:

– its pathogenesis,

– its mode of replication,

– the kinetics of its presence in the blood and in different human tissues and fluids,

– its biological and immunological characteristics (to allow appropriate choice of diagnostic and screening tools),

– its physical and chemical characteristics and its resistance to various physical and chemical procedures that could be used.

Devising a "risk reduction" strategy for a given pathogen requires having the most complete answers possible to these questions, in order to make the most informed choice, based on the current state of knowledge, of the factors that can be influenced in view of reducing transmission risk. In matters of microbiological safety, there are no ready-made, universal solutions. A specific strategy must be developed for each pathogenic agent, and this strategy must improve with advances in knowledge concerning the pathogen, and with technical advances.

---

[1] The term "material of origin" refers to the biological product collected from the blood donor, and which is used to prepare transfusion products. This technical term is used here with all the respect due to blood donors.

This chapter presents the general principles underlying the three stages of intervention for microbiologic risk prevention in transfusion.

The concept of Microbiologic Safety in Transfusion Safety of a blood product is closely related to the procedures that can be used to reduce the presence of pathogens all along the chain leading from donor selection to administration to the recipient [2].

The organizational structure of the safety process remains the same for all transfusion products, and involves a blood donor, a collection procedure, a component separation procedure, storage of different "labile blood products", and administration to one or several recipients.

Control of the Starting Material

The first level at which microbiologic safety can be applied is that involving the starting material and its control.

In the context of blood transfusion, the "starting material" refers to blood donations (whole blood or apheresis components) obtained from blood donors.

This "starting material" is the major source of risk, since blood can contain certain pathogenic agents that are potentially transmissible. But it must be kept in mind that certain pathogens can be introduced in the blood at another stage in the chain, and can proliferate before administration to the recipient (for example, in bacterial incidents, insufficient decontamination of the skin can be a risk factor).

Therefore, the microbiological eligibility of this material must be established before use.

The process of blood donation qualification involves different screening procedures applied to the donor and to the blood collected.

Qualification of the Donor

Establishing donor suitability means looking for risk factors, both by means of a medical interview and a medical exam.

Risk factors and deferral criteria are partly specific to each pathogen, although there are common factors at the level of means of transmission and sources of contamination.

Risk factors are identified by questioning the prospective donor on life style, travel or medical history, in view of identifying elements such as previous transfusions, neurosurgical procedures or growth hormone therapy.

In this context, a recent trip to an area where a pathogen, known to be transmissible by blood, is endemic or epidemic constitutes a temporary deferral criterion, sometimes accompanied by indicative clinical signs, depending on the pathogen. Deferral of blood donation can be temporary if the contamination is acute, such as West Nile Virus infection; or permanent if the contamination is chronic, such as that caused by a prion.

For example, for Creutzfeldt-Jakob disease, a one-year cumulative stay in the British Isles during a period considered "at-risk" (in this case, 1980-1996) leads to permanent deferral, as a precaution [3].

Determining deferral criteria, whether temporary or permanent, requires in-depth knowledge of epidemiologic data that allow a better understanding of the transmission mechanisms of the pathogens concerned [4, 5].

Finally, the clinical exam should help to establish the state of health of the potential donor, and particularly to identify any symptoms indicative of infection (fever, cough, etc.), which would be factors of temporary deferral. Moreover, the donor's general good health is confirmed by laboratory blood tests performed systematically.

Thus, we can see that the medical interview and exam of the prospective donor constitute a first safety step in the process of blood collection, which starts with the deferral of subjects for whom a source of risk, potential or not, has been identified.

Of course, this medical interview/exam is not an exhaustive procedure, and other safety measures must be applied to the blood collected.

Biological Qualification of the Donation

Biological qualification of the blood donation is the second step, undertaken once the donor has successfully passed the first screening stage consisting of the medical interview/ exam.

This second step consists of serological tests that can reveal "markers" indicating current or past infection.

It is not within the scope of this chapter to present an exhaustive list of required screening tests (other chapters will do this); the objective here is to situate the logic of these screening tests in the overall context of the transfusion safety process.

We should however note, at this stage, that such screening tests only apply to a few pathogenic agents, particularly infectious agents causing chronic infections.

The example of the HIV virus illustrates the logic of conducting routine screening tests, required for qualifying each donation, whether from a "new" donor or from a more regular donor. It has been established that, in the case of HIV, the pathogen is present in the blood in the first hours following contamination, but the HIV antibodies only appear after a seroconversion period of several weeks. Investigations were undertaken to devise a means of detecting this virus. As techniques evolved, and given that this virus triggers an antibody response, the very first screening test proposed was a serological test to detect antibodies produced by the infected subject. Test kits improved with time (we speak of "generations" of the test), allowing earlier and earlier detection of serologic conversion in an infected individual. Thus, antibody kits allowed earlier identification of high-risk donors by reducing the seroconversion "window". Subsequently, technical progress made it possible to detect not only antibody response to the virus, but the virus itself, by identifying one of its surface antigens and, more recently, by recognizing its genetic material (genomic amplification technique).

This illustrates the considerable advances achieved in developing a screening test that makes it possible to identify, as early as possible, a person who could transmit an agent with known pathogenic effects, and highly transmissible by blood.

These are the steps followed when the specific objective is to reduce the risk of transmission of a major pathogen by insuring that the pathogen is actually absent (as far as it can be detected by available methods) from the donor's blood at the time of the donation. Unfortunately, there are times when this safety measure by routine screening cannot be applied in the absence of a screening method that can constitute laboratory qualification. The pathogen of Creutzfeldt-Jakob disease is a perfect illustration of the current limits of this safety procedure.

This first measure of viral safety, which follows the medical interview/exam that attempts to identify "risk factors", and the laboratory qualification of the donation that attempts to specifically identify the actual presence of a pathogen, are intended mainly to limit residual risk by selecting:

– donors with the greatest possible guarantee of "non exposure" to a risk,

– material of origin (blood) that tested negative for signs of major pathogens that can be identified by laboratory tests.

In terms of safety strategy, it is clear that these two procedures (medical interview and laboratory tests) cannot be considered exhaustive (as the saying goes, we only find what we look for) and that they are subject to the technical limits of the methods employed. These limitations include such factors as the reliability of the medical interview and the clinical diagnosis, as well as limits of detection and risks of interference (false positives and false negatives) of screening tests.

Nevertheless, these procedures represent the first link in the security chain. This link is essential because it makes it possible to reduce as much as possible the initial infection load of the material of origin, by eliminating from the collection process individuals who tested positive or who could be carriers despite testing negative.

However, and in spite of this first safety measure, it is impossible to assert absence of risk. We can only speak of risk minimization. Residual risk has to be further reduced by other safety measures in the course of the other two stages of safety implementation.

Risk Reduction Procedures and Stages

In order to take into account the residual risk of contamination of the material of origin, despite the previous risk minimization measures, the process of product preparation must include, whenever possible, stages of treatment that can eliminate or inactivate pathogenic agents.

This safety step is widely used for biological products like therapeutic plasma-derived medicinal products; for many of them, it is in fact the most important safety procedure.

However, in the case of transfusion products (labile blood products), the stages between donation and transfusion of the labile blood product do not allow the implementation of complementary measures of risk reduction. In fact, contrary to other biological products for which the preparation process includes many stages of treatment (by physical or chemical methods) of the material of origin, transfusion products, because of their nature and/or fragility, do not undergo any, or almost any, stages of transformation where elimination or inactivation of pathogens could occur.

We can cite as an example the treatment with a mixture of solvent/ detergent (SD) used for certain plasma protein fractions in the preparation of coagulation factors and immunoglobulines. This SD treatment inactivates a wide range of viruses with lipid envelopes, including HIV and certain hepatotropic viruses. (We should mention that among transfusion products there is plasma which can be virus attenuated by undergoing such SD treatment).

We could also mention the pasteurization stage to which albumin solution is submitted after plasma fractionation. These stages, whose effect on viruses can be quantified (we speak of reduction factors), can, when used in combination, significantly reduce initial residual risk to the point where this risk becomes "theoretical" for viruses that are sensitive to the agents and/or physical methods applied.

Thus, elimination/ inactivation stages can act on a range of pathogenic agents, so as to offer a broad spectrum of safety, even for pathogens that are still unknown. To illustrate, we can quote the example where, in the face of risk of emergence of a newly identified virus (West Nile Virus, SARS, avian influenza), risk analysis showed that this SD treatment, already in place, was efficacious in terms of the emerging agent, ensuring the safety of plasma-derived products.

Research should continue to develop methods of elimination/ inactivation able to act on a broader spectrum of viruses or agents. However, the application of these processes encounters technical limitations, particularly due to the relative fragility of the products submitted to treatment. In fact, the relative fragility of desirable biological products has to be contrasted with the relative resistance of some of the pathogens to be eliminated.

For example, the parvovirus is a very small virus, resistant to many physico-chemical treatments; similarly, the agent responsible for Creutzfeldt-Jakob disease (and thus, all agents responsible for transmissible spongiform encephalopathies) is known for its extreme resistance even to drastic physical and chemical treatments.

Elimination/inactivation of pathogens is, however, a very attractive and widely-used process. Each measure found to be effective against a particular infectious agent must be confirmed before it can be integrated into the global safety procedure for a given product [6]. However, elimination/inactivation has very limited applications for transfusion. In effect, in the process of transfusion, from the donor to the recipient, there is almost no stage where blood or its components may undergo "treatment" that could contribute to risk reduction.

However, it is noteworthy that in the past few years researchers have strived to develop one or several steps to be introduced in the transfusion process in view of implementing such a risk reduction strategy.

Some of these projects involved leukocyte reduction, bactericide treatment of platelet concentrates and treatment of fresh plasma for transfusion (also called therapeutic plasma).

• **Leukocyte reduction**, which consists of using a filtration step to reduce the quantity of residual leukocytes in whole blood or in blood components, was designed in the 1990s to counter the risk of transmission of intracellular pathogens that donation qualification tests did not look for. At the end of the 1990s, an additional factor reinforced the need for this measure: risk reduction for the Creutzfeldt-Jakob disease pathogen, since it had been shown that infectivity of the blood by this pathogen was divided between white blood cells and plasma. Leukocyte filtration further reduces potential infectious load present in the "starting material".

Implementation of the leukocyte reduction step requires:

– checking that the quality of derived products is not altered (particularly platelets, red blood cells or fresh plasma);

– evaluating the effectiveness of leukocyte reduction for a given filter or process, and the reproducibility of the process, in the daily course of preparation of each labile blood product.

• **Another example** is that of the different agents being developed to treat platelet concentrates and fresh frozen plasma. Exposure of platelet concentrates and plasma to a chemical photosensitizing agent, and then to UV radiation, exerts both bactericidal and virucidal action.

This inactivation capacity for certain pathogenic agents must, however, be qualified and confirmed by "validation studies" to determine the reduction ratios obtained by these different treatments, for each given pathogen. It must also be established that the treatments do not have harmful effects on the biologic properties of platelets and/or plasma, and on the proteins they contain. In the past few years, great advances have been made, and it is likely that these processes will be applied in the near future and will contribute to the increased safety of labile products.

The second safety step discussed above, which consists of using specific procedures for the elimination/ inactivation of pathogens, is a powerful concept with promising applications. Depending on the process used (filtration, chemical or physical treatment, precipitation, etc.), this step successfully achieves the elimination/inactivation of a wide range of pathogens, and even succeeds in reducing risk for emerging pathogenic agents susceptible to these treatments. In addition, this step provides a specific technical solution for each pathogen.

However, in transfusion, this step is difficult to apply, given the fragility of transfusion products. Progress has been made in the past few years in terms of trying to find solutions, case by case, in situations where the risk cannot be controlled by applying the first safety step, *i.e.* qualification of the starting material alone. We expect that, in the future, new methods (particularly of chemical treatment) that respect the intrinsic fragility of transfusion products will be found, to answer safety needs related to certain pathogens that cannot be totally controlled by the previous safety steps.

Tests during the Process

The third safety step consists of carrying out specific testing of intermediate products and/or of the finished product.

As is the case for the two previous steps, the tests to be carried out must be adapted to operating and logistical conditions. In transfusion, the path from the donor to the recipient is of relatively short duration (given the short lifetime of certain components), and it is not always possible to introduce extra screening steps or retesting of products within the limits of their holding period. Therefore, this third safety step is not generally applied in the transfusion chain. There is, however, one exception: a safety procedure can be applied to fresh frozen plasma. In this particular situation, the plasma is stored after donation and is not used until the donor has been tested again for certain specific viral markers. This *a posteriori* retesting of the donation makes it possible to confirm that the subject is still negative in terms of the viral markers targeted by the screening, and therefore to guarantee that the blood donation did not take place during the seroconversion period. The quarantine period is determined based on the best estimate of the "serological window" during which a test could be falsely negative.

In the future, it could become possible to apply this third safety procedure to check for bacterial contamination of platelet concentrates. Recent progress in the development of rapid methods of detection allows us to foresee that before they are administered to patients, platelet concentrates could be tested for bacterial sterility.

Finally, in terms of this third safety step which relies on the ability of diagnostic and screening tests to detect the presence of a pathogen, the same limitations exist as those mentioned for the first safety step in relation to testing of the starting material. Thus, due to the same limitations of detection, sensitivity and specificity, these tests have a limited scope, depending on the type of detection involved. For viruses, proposed methods are very specific, while for bacterial detection the methods used can detect a wide range of bacteria. Thus, these screening and detection methods used in the course of the process only apply to certain pathogens and cannot claim to be exhaustive.

Updating and Optimization of Safety Measures

Microbiological safety is constantly evolving, given the possible emergence, at any time, of a new pathogen (SARS, avian flu) or an epidemic situation related to a well-known pathogen (Chagas, West Nile Virus), but also given advances in scientific knowledge and in methods and techniques of detection and treatment, which now make possible certain measures and procedures not feasible only a few years ago.

Biological products, and particularly transfusion products, are constantly under surveillance. A hemovigilance program, as well as sanitary and technological surveillance programs contribute to renewed reflection and motivate the revision and updating of safety measures.

It is, in fact, thanks to the existing surveillance programs (particularly the hemovigilance and biovigilance programs) that cases of transmission of pathogenic agents can be detected.

Reporting these cases should lead to re-evaluating the safety of the product involved (or even of the entire class of products of the same type) and to proposing corrective action.

Evolution of scientific knowledge or emergence of new risks will impel health authorities to re-evaluate products and propose new measures. Microbiologic safety involves continuous assessment, surveillance, re-evaluation and introduction of corrective action, in order to keep up with advances in scientific knowledge.

Conclusion

Given their human origin, transfusion products are associated with an intrinsic risk of pathogen transmission. This risk must be controlled and held in check: this is the very foundation of the concept of safety and the idea of providing product assurance.

Microbiological safety can be achieved using three approaches (safety steps) that are complementary. None of them can guarantee, on its own, a high enough level of safety. The degree of safety provided by each step is not the same for the three stages; safety measures based on detection or screening methods have certain limitations. However, in the field of transfusion, it is important to note that the first stage, that of donor selection and biological qualification of donations, is the main safety step, and sometimes the only step that can be applied.

Thus, in terms of safety and the application of appropriate measures, the different approaches must be combined in order to reduce to a minimum the risk of pathogen transmission (viruses, bacteria, prions) when using transfusion products.

The methods that can be used vary depending on the product, on the pathogens targeted by the screening, and on the use made of the product. Safety analysis and the methods that can be applied must be evaluated one case at a time, and priority must be given to the most reliable and easily controlled approaches.

Risk analysis should lead to the proposal of prevention measures; these measures should be adapted to the risk in question and the intended use of the product. It would be inconceivable to use a biological product whose microbiological safety is doubtful, if this product is of no therapeutic interest. In the same way, it would be unacceptable to deprive a patient of a biological product that could be therapeutically beneficial, simply because an infinitesimal, or theoretical, risk of transmission of a pathogen exists.

Safety of transfusion products is a concept that attempts to maintain this delicate balance between possible risk and possible benefit.

References

1. Lefrère JJ, Rouger Ph. Maladies transmissibles par transfusion, eds. In : *Pratique nouvelle de la transfusion sanguine*, Paris : Masson, 2003 : 47-64.
2. Agut H. Le concept de sécurité virale des médicaments dérivés du sang. *Virologie* 2005 ; 9 : S3-S6.
3. Lasmezas CI. Encéphalopathies subaiguës spongiformes transmissibles et sécurité des produits sanguins. *Virologie* 2005 ; 9 : S37-S44.
4. Flahault A. La prédiction des épidémies d'origine virale. *Virologie* 2003 ; 7 : 395-9.
5. Desenclos JC, de Valk H. Les maladies infectieuses émergentes : importance en santé publique, aspects épidémiologiques, déterminants et prévention. *Méd Mal Infect* 2005 ; 35 : 49-61.
6. Flan B, Aubin JT. Évaluation de l'efficacité des procédés de purification des protéines plasmatiques à éliminer les agents transmissibles non conventionnels. *Virologie* 2005 ; 9 : S45-S52.

Residual Risks in Transfusion: a Strategic Perspective

Joliette Coste

Born at the beginning of the 20th century, blood transfusion remained a procedure performed only in exceptional circumstances until the 1940s. Starting in 1943, when it became possible to preserve blood, transfusion developed rapidly. With the increase of the number of transfusions performed, risks became apparent. Pathogens were identified and testing for them was made mandatory by a succession of government directives (*Table I*). Screening blood donations for the presence of HBsAg of the hepatitis B virus seemed to have solved the problem of transfusion-transmitted diseases. In 1983, the realization that acquired immune deficiency syndrome (AIDS) could be transmitted by transfusion was a shock for doctors and patients. From then on, transfusion safety and its relation to blood-borne diseases became the focus of sanitary monitoring, and attracted the attention of researchers, health professionals, patients and the media. In the twenty years that followed, the enormous progress accomplished in minimizing infectious risk led to an unprecedented degree of transfusion safety. However, just when blood products had never been safer, we were confronted with the fact that the fight against communicable agents was not over. New transmissible agents emerged, and they were no longer limited to viruses, but included bacteria, parasites and the infectious prion protein. We will examine these various categories of emerging risks, analyse their impact on transfusion safety and try to identify the strategic approaches likely to prevent their transmission by transfusion.

Viral Infections

Viral emergence has three major sources, although other sources exist as well:
– mutation of a known pathogen, leading to the emergence of a more virulent strain;
– transmission of an existing virus to another species, introducing the notion of zoonosis;
– wide dissemination of a virus from a small population to which it had been confined originally.

Human factors are often responsible for the emergence of infectious diseases, through growing population migrations, overdevelopment of urban areas and disturbance of the ecological system. Modern life has exacerbated these factors worldwide. Today, we are witnessing different types of viral emergence:

Table I. Entry into Effect of Directives in France.

Syphilis	1952
HBsAg	1971
Self-exclusion of populations at risk for AIDS	1983
Anti-HIV-1/2 antibodies	1985
Anti-Plasmodium antibodies	1986
Transaminases (ALAT)	1988
Anti-HBc antibodies	1988
Anti-HTLV-I/II antibodies (French West Indies)	1989
Anti-HCV antibodies	1990
Anti-HTLV-I/II antibodies (continental France)	1991
First measure of deferral of subjects at CJD risk	1992
Deferral of subjects having received previous transfusion or transplantation	1997
Leukodepletion of cellular products	1998
v-CJD: deferral of subjects with a stay of one cumulated year or longer in Great Britain	2000
Leukodepletion of all blood products	2001
Nucleic acid testing (NAT) for HCV and HIV-1	2001
WNV: 28-day quarantine for prospective donors having stayed in viral circulation zones (USA, Canada...)	2003
NAT for HBV(French West Indies)	2004
Chagas disease (continental France): temporary deferral of prospective donors, with a stay of over three consecutive months in South and Central America (excluding the Caribbean) and whose donations are intended for direct therapeutic use without inactivation treatment	2005
French Guyana: deferral of prospective resident donors	2006
Chikungunya: 21-day quarantine for prospective donors returning from an endemic zone (Reunion Island, Mauritius, Seychelles). Temporary suspension of blood donation in Reunion Island.	2006

– re-emergence of a well-known virus whose spread, is a recent phenomenon (West Nile Virus in the USA, Chikungunya in Reunion Island);

– emergence of totally new viruses causing galloping epidemics, such as Severe Acute Respiratory Syndrome (SARS) or avian influenza A(H5N1). Their responsibility in post-transfusion pathologies has not yet been clearly established;

– emergence of viruses that are probably very old but could only be identified recently thanks to new molecular biology techniques: hepatitis G virus/GBC Virus, TTV and SEN Virus.

These viruses are transfusion-transmitted but, to date, they have caused no pathologies in blood product recipients. These *sub-merging viruses* [1] must remain subject to surveillance.

- **The Human Immunodeficiency Virus (HIV)** was the unfortunate pioneer of emerging viruses. It has now been established that this virus is descendant from the SIVcpz, the simian immunodeficiency virus, transmitted to humans by the chimpanzee. The HIV was isolated for the first time in 1983 at the Pasteur Institute in France. In 1985, testing all blood donations for anti-HIV antibodies became mandatory. Today, what residual risk is there for transmission by transfusion of this virus, as well as of other major infectious agents such as the hepatitis B virus (HBV), the hepatitis C virus (HCV) and the Human T cell leukemia/lymphoma viruses (HTLV-I and HTLV-II)? In France, epidemiologic monitoring of blood donors has been described in a Report [2] which shows that over a ten-year period (1992-2002) residual risk for these four viruses has decreased considerably. Thanks to constant improvement of donor selection and to technologic progress in the screening of blood donations, labile blood products present very low viral risk today. In fact, for the last reported period (2002-2004), residual risk was estimated at 1/2,400,000 donations for HBV, 1/3,900,000 for HIV, 1/6,000,000 for HCV and close to zero for HTLV (S.Laperche, J. Pillonel, personal communication). Moreover, mandatory systematic leukodepletion of blood products has led to the elimination of leukotropic viruses like HTLV. Due to high prevalence of HBV in French overseas departments, testing for HBV DNA by Nucleic Acid Testing (NAT) has been carried out on all units donated since December 2004. At present, the contribution of NAT implementation for this virus in continental France is being studied [3]. The literature reports that epidemiological characteristics observed in donors positive for HBV, HCV or HIV reflect those of the general population. For example, for HCV, thanks to reinforcement of preventive measures among donors and in the general population, this virus no longer represents the greatest risk of infection for recipients of blood products.

- **Infection caused by the West Nile Virus (WNV)** is a zoonosis known in France since 1960, whose worldwide spread is recent. The WNV is an arbovirus of the *Flaviviridae* family, *Flavivirus* genus, which includes the dengue, yellow fever, Japanese and St. Louis encephalitis. The WNV can cause meningitis, encephalopathies and meningo-encephalopathies. Human infection is asymptomatic in 80% of cases. In 20% of cases it takes the form of a pseudo-influenzal syndrome. In one out of 150 patients, it causes neurological symptoms. The disease can be fatal in elderly or immunocompromised patients. Its life cycle involves an insect vector, a mosquito (*Culex*), and an animal reservoir, a bird, which acts as an amplifying host. The horse and man are accidental hosts in the cycle of this zoonosis, and represent epidemiological dead-ends. Until recently, the virus was only endemic in Africa, in the Middle East, in the western part of the Indian continent, and in Eastern Europe. Although micro-epidemics of this zoonosis had been reported, the virus was not classified as emergent. But, in 1999, an epidemic caused by a particularly virulent strain broke out in the United States. Initially confined to New York City, the virus subsequently spread to the entire North-American continent. In 2003, over 9,000 cases and 264 deaths were reported in forty states. The WNV is associated with brief viremia lasting two to four days, or longer in immunocompromised subjects (up to twenty-eight days). Seroconversion occurs about one week after contamination, and is marked by the presence of anti-WNV antibodies, first of the IgM type, then of the IgG type, that signal recovery and confer lasting immunity. The first case of transfusion-transmitted WNV was reported in the United States in 2002. The donor was a car-accident victim who had received sixty labile blood products [4]. The kidney, liver and heart were transplanted to four recipients who developed WNV infection one week later; one of them died as a result. Subsequently, twenty-three other transfusion-transmitted cases of WNV were reported. Therefore, systematic testing of all blood donations for RNA-WNV was introduced in the United States before the summer of 2003.

In France, the WNV was detected in 2000 in horses in the Camargue region. As a result, monitoring of human and animal viral circulation (horses, birds, mosquitoes) was instituted during the life cycle of the mosquito, from June to October. In 2003, this surveillance led to the diagnosis of seven human cases in the Var region, as well as four cases in horses. To date, no cases of transmission by transfusion have been reported. However, in July 2003, analysis of the human and equine cases concentrated in the Var, as well as the transfusion-transmitted American cases, led the French National Blood Service (EFS) to recommend a twenty-eight-day temporary deferral of all:

– potential donors having travelled to an area of viral circulation (United States, Canada...);

– subjects having travelled to overseas departments or in the Mediterranean region, and presenting clinical symptoms indicative of WNV.

In 2004, the Ministry of Health introduced additional safeguards:

– mandatory reporting to the EFS of any infectious symptoms occurring fourteen days after the donation, and deferral of the donor for twenty-eight days after the donation;

– creation of a Risk Alert Unit in charge of deciding whether additional measures are required: such as, interrupting blood collection in areas affected by the WNV and deferral of donors having travelled in these areas;

– small-scale NAT for WNV implementation until October 31, 2004 in the two blood transfusion centers (EFS) located in the Mediterranean region. In case of actual equine or human contamination, this type of testing could be performed immediately in these two establishments, to confirm donation eligibility.

• **Chikungunya virus**: since the beginning of 2005, a sizable Chikungunya virus epidemic exists in the South-Western region of the Indian Ocean, with identical epidemic foci in the Comores, in Mauritius, in Reunion Island and in the Seychelles. As of February 23, 2006, the number of cumulated cases in Reunion Island stands at 135000 infected subjects, that is, about 1 in 5 islanders. The viral agent is an arbovirus (alpha virus of the *Togaviridae* family) transmitted by an *Aedes* mosquito. The mosquito, *Aedes albopictus*, which until recently was only found in certain regions of the Far East, has now spread to many countries. Entomologists believe this to be due to mondialization of the tire trade by cargo ships which often harbor larvae beds in their water-filled hollow spaces. This mosquito, very common in Reunion Island, has replaced other species present in the region and multiplies very easily in small water containers (cups, saucers, vases..) near human habitation. The fight against this vector, an essential measure in the control of the disease, is conducted by targetted and repeated use of insecticides. Disease diagnosis is essentially serologic (no reagent is commercially available yet), based on IgM antibody detection on the 5th day following clinical signs. A home-made PCR assay exists allowing early diagnosis in the blood.

Generally, symptoms disappear spontaneously. However, previously unknown severe forms have been described, particularly in newborns, due to maternal-foetal transmission [5].In most patients, symptoms were: high fever (99.6%), articular pain (99.2%) and muscular pain (97.7%) in limb extremities, headaches (84.1%) and sometimes rash. In continental France, the EFS has taken preventive measures (January 2006) by requesting the exclusion of prospective donors having travelled to Reunion Island or Mauritius, for 21 days after their return to France. Following the progression of the Chikungunya epidemic in the French department of Reunion Island during the first two months of 2006, the EFS in Reunion Island suspended all collection of homologous whole blood on its territory as a precautionary measure. Blood units are sent by air from continental France. This measure does not apply to platelet concentrates, given that platelets are at present photochemically inactivated with amotosalen ultraviolets.

- **Severe Acute Respiratory Syndrome (SARS)** is the first serious contagious disorder to emerge in the 21st century. It is a severe febrile pneumopathy that can lead to respiratory failure. The epidemic originated in China at the end of 2002, was disseminated worldwide, contaminated over 8,000 individuals and caused over 800 deaths in thirty-three countries. The agent responsible for the disease, a coronavirus (SARS-CoV) previously unknown in man [6], was identified rapidly thanks to a genomic approach using a DNA chip. Isolated in 1937 in chickens, it crossed the species barrier by infecting certain animals, and then humans. Biological vectors are unknown. Transmission occurs through the respiratory and oro-fecal tracts. Because SARS-CoV is a respiratory disease, there is *a priori* no risk of transmission by transfusion. However, a viremic stage seems possible during the symptomatic period of the infection, given that viral RNA was detected by PCR assays in a patient whose SARS-CoV was isolated in the kidney. Tests currently being developed will be able to confirm or exclude the presence of viremia in infected donors.

In the face of this worldwide alert, and in order to safeguard the stocks of blood products, the preventive strategy used by the EFS [7] was a three-week quarantine for all potential donors who were asymptomatic but returning from an area affected by the disease, a one-month quarantine after recovery and end of treatment for potential donors suspected of having been contaminated, and a three-months quarantine when contamination is certain. Given that no cases of SARS had been reported to the WHO since June 2003, temporary deferral measures were suspended in December 2003. However, vigilance must be maintained because unknown factors still exist (reservoir, persistence of virus in the environment, possibility of seasonal outbreaks...). Moreover, no vaccine or effective treatment exists to date.

- **Avian flu** is one of more than 25 influenza A viruses that reside primarily in birds but infect humans and other mammals. An avian influenza epidemic caused by the *influenza A* virus (strain H5N1) [8] was isolated at the end of 2003 in Korea. Since then, 16 other countries were affected; among them, Vietnam, Cambodia, Indonesia and China. Recently, the epizootic has spread to Europe, including France. This extremely contagious virus can cause an acute respiratory distress syndrome, frequently with a fatal outcome. Very occasionally transmitted to humans, the virus is highly contagious in chickens, turkeys and other animals such as the pig. On February 4, 2005, a Center of Disease Control (CDC) survey in Vietnam reported that 118 subjects had been contaminated by H5N1 through direct contact with infected poultry, and that 61 had died. Genic and antigenic analysis showed that the cluster identified in the infected patients did present the specific H5N1 genes, but that mutations of the genome inducing modified antigens had led to a different variant. To date, no genetic recombination between H5N1 and human influenza viruses has been found. However, the scope of this unprecedented epizootic, and its spread to numerous countries could facilitate such a genetic recombination and modify modes of transmission, making careful epidemiologic follow-up a must. The UN considers that the epizootic has not been controlled and that it continues to spread. Several vaccines against H5N1 are being developed by Sanofi-Pasteur and Chiron, but are not yet at the commercial production stage.

- Another example of a cluster of emergent blood-borne viral infections is provided by the **family of enteroviruses.** These RNA nonenveloped viruses most often cause moderate respiratory tract infections that are seasonal (spring, summer). Transmission occurs through oro-fecal pathways, but contamination through the blood is theoretically possible, from an infected donation collected from a donor during the viremic period. In order to assess this transfusion risk, Simmonds *et al.* [9] conducted tests for twenty-two months in an unselected population of donors, using generic PCR assays for all enteroviruses. Results showed that 1/4,000 donations were positive, with greatest prevalence in the summer season (1/1,800) and lowest prevalence in winter (1/8,000). The viruses found most often were coxsackievirus A16, echoviruses 11 and 30, and enterovirus 71. This viral presence in the blood indicates the possibility that these viruses can be transfusion-transmissible.

- **Leucotropic viruses** can also be transmitted through blood. These are viruses of the *Herpes viridae* family (HHV), particularly the cytomegalovirus (CMV, HHV-5), The Epstein-Barr virus (EBV, HHV-7) and the virus associated with Kaposi's sarcoma (KSHV, HHV-8). The HHV-8 is endemic in certain African populations. However, this virus is sometimes characterized as emerging, because it is often found as an HIV coinfection, causing Kaposi's sarcoma in AIDS patients. Implementation of systematic leukodepletion of blood components in April 2001 has reduced to a very low minimum the risk of residual infection by this virus in countries applying this preventive measure. The impact of this measure was verified particularly for CMV and HHV-8.

- Conversely, we have less data on the incidence of transmission of **parvovirus B19**. This DNA nonenveloped virus of the *Parvoviridae* family causes a range of pathologies including epidemic megalerythema (fifth eruptive disease), erythroblastopenic anemia, and articular complications. We have known for several decades that it is communicable through the blood. The relatively high incidence of viremia has revived interest in this virus, and could motivate the introduction of a screening test in view of better control of the risk of transmission by transfusion. In fact, certain recipients of blood products could be vulnerable to B19 parvoviral infection, either because they are immunodeficient or because they suffer from chronic hemolysis. From its respiratory point of entry, the virus is disseminated through the system until it reaches its target cells, the erythrocytes and their precursors, as well as the megakaryocytes, the fibroblasts and the endothelial cells. The French Laboratory of Fractionation and Biotechnologies (LFB) [10] used a PCR assay for two years (March 1996 to March 1998) to test 91,563 plasma pools, representing 4.26 million donations collected from 1.25 million donors. Incidence of viremic donors was 1/5 950 on the average, and could reach 1/1420 during epidemics. Cases of transmission were also observed in haemophiliacs, through factor VIII concentrates, although all stable blood products are inactivated by treatment with solvent-detergents. The B19 parvovirus, that has no lipid envelope, resists physical-chemical treatments used to denature enveloped viruses. This is why the LFB applies NAT testing for B19 DNA. As for transmission of the B19 parvovirus through labile blood products, high prevalence of protective antibodies in both donors and recipients explains occasional transmission. Therefore, although scientific safeguards are required, systematic testing is not foreseen.

- Advances in monitoring and in molecular diagnostic techniques have made it possible to isolate **"submerging" viruses:** the so-called hepatitis G virus (HGV or GBV-C), the TT virus and related viruses, and the SEN (SEN-V). The HGV belongs to the *Flaviviridae* family, like the HCV. It was initially designated as the agent possibly responsible for non A-E hepatitis. HGV is very widespread and RNA viral seroprevalence in blood donors in continental France is as high as 4.2% [11]. Frequency of seroconverted donors (anti-E2 antibodies) attains 7.8%. In cases of coinfection with HIV, the HGV is reported to play a modulating role by slowing progression from HIV to AIDS. The TTV is a nonenveloped DNA circovirus with structural similarities to parvoviruses. Its distribution is worldwide. In the United Kingdom, prevalence in blood donors reaches 1.9%. The SEN was isolated in 1999. It is a little-known virus, but is reported to be present in 80% of patients with non A-E post-transfusion hepatitis, and in 2% of subjects who received no transfusions [12].

These three viruses, that can only be detected by NAT testing, cause no pathologies. Testing for them is not a requirement for blood screening in any country, but scientific surveys should be carried out regularly.

Bacterial Infections

We have long been aware of bacterial contamination of labile blood products. Introduction of a mini-pouch to divert out the first millilitres of blood from the blood unit, and enhanced cutaneous asepsis procedures at the time of donation, have significantly reduced bacterial risk [13]. However, despite implementation of these preventive measures, bacterial risk is not yet sufficiently controlled. Hemovigilance data for the 1999-2002 period indicate that risk of transfusional incidents by bacterial contamination from platelet concentrates is estimated at 1/25,000, for all severities of infection taken together. Thus, bacterial risk is now the major cause of post-transfusion incidents associated with an infectious agent. Reduced risk of transmission of HIV and of hepatitis viruses has revealed the emergence of bacterial contamination. Platelet concentrates are responsible for 65% of transfusional incidents by bacterial contamination, as opposed to 35% for red blood cell concentrates. In one out of three cases the consequences are serious: immediate vital threat or death of the recipient. Most (80%) of the bacteria involved are of the Gram$^+$ type, indicating contamination of the platelet concentrate by the cutaneous flora and/or the environment. However Gram$^-$ bacteria are involved in 20% of cases, creating immediate danger to life. In order to reduce the risk of bacterial contamination by platelet concentrates, introduction of detection methods applied to these concentrates is under consideration.

Other bacterial infections are transfusion-transmissible:

– syphilis (*Treponema pallidum*), which can survive three or four days in blood stored at +4 °C. However, this infection is virtually nonexistent in recipients. But serologic control remains mandatory for all blood donations;

– Lyme disease, erlichiosis and rickettsioses transmitted to humans by tick bites. The most frequent, especially in the United States, is Lyme disease, whose causative agent is a spirochete (*Borrelia burgdorferi*) transmitted by biting. The spirochete is diffused in the skin and passes into the blood. Because these bacteria are intracellular, leukodepletion has significantly reduced transmission of these organisms by transfusion.

Parasitic Infections

Some parasitic infections could constitute a transfusional risk, particularly for immunodeficient patients: malaria (*Plasmodium falciparum* transmitted by mosquitoes), Chagas (*Trypanosoma cruzii* transmitted by *Reduvüdae* insects), and more rarely, leishmaniasis. In general, these infections are endemic in tropical countries and their incidence in Europe is low. Increase in travel and tourism poses the problem of their emergence in non endemic areas. In Continental France, a survey conducted by the EFS in a sample of 164,691 prospective donors has shown that 0.29% had had a stay of over 3 consecutive months in an endemic zone, particularly in South or Central America.

Therefore, in October 2005, it was requested that blood for direct therapeutic use without pathogen inactivation treatment no longer be accepted from donors who had stayed over 3 consecutive months in South or Central America. However, prospective donors for plasma apheresis for the preparation of blood-derived therapeutic products in France could be accepted.

Screening tests expected in the near future will make it possible to select prospective donors who have been exposed to this parasitic risk, based on the same criteria as those applying to malaria. Given the high prevalence of parasitic infections (*Trypanosoma cruzii, Plasmodium falciparum*) and of other transfusion-transmissible infectious diseases, in February 2006 the EFS decided to defer all prospective donors residing in French Guyana.

Transmissible Spongiform Encephalopathies

Transmissible spongiform encephalopathies (TSE) came into the public eye in 1996, when the British government revealed possible transmission of the agent of bovine spongiform encephalopathy (BSE) to humans. BSE is part of a neurodegenerative group of disorders which, in humans, includes Creutzfeldt-Jakob disease (CJD), kuru, Gerstmann-Sträussler-Scheinker syndrome (GSS) and fatal familial insomnia (FFI). Clinically, these diseases are characterized by dementia, various motor problems and spongiform degeneration of the brain, with neuronal loss and gliosis. Also called prion diseases, these disorders are unique in that their origin is both infectious and genetic. The agent causing TSE is still controversial. The current etiological hypothesis suggests that the infectious agent is of proteinic nature. This hypothesis brings into question the classic notion that only nucleic acids are vectors of communicable information. The infectious agent is presumed to be a modified form of a normal cellular protein called prion protein, which is encoded by the PRNP gene located on chromosome 20. Disease is believed to take place through the interactions between infectious and normal prion proteins. Normal prion proteins are located on the surface of neurons and blood cells, as well as in the lymphoid system. The hypothesis holds that the buffy-coat carries a third of the infectivity, and that half of the latter is present in the plasma. Most TSEs are not considered emergent because their incidence rates have remained remarkably stable over time. Conversely, a CJD variant (v-CJD) emerged recently as an epidemic in the United Kingdom, between 1980 and 1996. The v-CJD (or "mad cow" disease) was caused by the entry of the prion protein into the food chain. In February 2006, 160 cumulated cases of v-CJD were recorded in the UK. The main identified risk factors for diet-related v-CJD are specific genotype (PRNP-129 Methionine/Methionine), relative youth and residence in the UK. In 2002, a British survey [14] reported on the follow-up of 48 patients who had received a labile blood component from donors who later became v-CJD cases. One of these recipients was identified as developing symptoms of v-CJD 6.5 years after receiving a transfusion of red cells donated by an individual,3.5 years before the donor developed symptoms of v-CJD. Interestingly, the donor and the recipient were both of the PRNP-129 Methionine/Methionine genotype. A second case was reported in July 2004, different from the first in that the patient presented no clinical symptoms indicative of CJD. The diagnosis was made based on the presence of prion proteins at autopsy. The patient's genotype was PRNP-129 Methionine/Valine.

This case raises the question of the possible existence of "silent" 129 Methionine/Valine carriers. A third case of v-CJD associated with blood transfusion has recently (February 9, 2006) been diagnosed. The patient developed symptoms about 8 years after receiving a blood transfusion from a donor who developed symptoms of v-CJD about 20 months after donating his blood. At present the patient is still alive (*www.hpa.org.uk*).However, for all these cases, contamination through food or through surgery, rather than by transfusion, could not yet be excluded. At present, risk of transfusional transmission is considered "probable" by the group of experts of the AFSSAPS [15]. Seven cases have been described in Europe (Ireland, the Netherlands and Italy), in North America (USA and Canada), in Hong-Kong and in Saudi Arabia. Four out of 7 have stayed for long times in the UK.

Sixteen cases of certain or probable v-CJD have been identified in France prior to January 31, 2006 (*www.invs.sante.fr*). Two patients are alive (who were diagnosed in 2005 and 2006), 14 have died: 7 men and 7 women. Median age at decease was 36.5 years (between 20 and 58). All were homozygotes Methionine/Methionine for the 129 codon of the PRNP gene. The 8th, 9th and 10th cases were blood donors. In France, no symptoms of v-CJD have been reported in the 26 patient cohort transfused with blood products from infected donors.

In the absence of a reliable test adapted for large scale screening for the CJD agent in the blood, the following measures have been introduced to prevent transmission by transfusion:

– deferral of blood donations from subjects presenting risk factors (family history of neuro-degenerative disease, neurosurgery, growth hormone therapy and transplantation of central nervous system tissue);

– destruction of product lots derived from fractionation of plasma pools when they contain a plasma unit from a donor found, *a posteriori*, to belong to a risk factor group;

– exclusion of previously transfused donors (1997);

– universal application of leukodepletion of cellular products (1998);

– since December 2000, exclusion of donors having resided in the UK at least one cumulated year between 1980 and 1996 (justified by the fact that during this period risk was twenty times higher in Great Britain than in France).

Finally, the absence of screening tests to detect the pathologic prion protein directly in the blood of asymptomatic carriers, and the demonstration that leukodepletion does not totally eliminate the infectious load present in the blood, have led some manufacturers to develop new generations of filters [16] that allow better retention of the infectious agent in red blood cell concentrates. National Blood Transfusion Services in Great Britain and Ireland have developed a clinical study protocol intended to check the safety of these retention filters for patients receiving units of red blood cell concentrates prepared with these new devices. If results are favorable, Health Authorities in these two countries will probably recommend routine use of these devices in the mass production of LBPs.

Although the level of risk of exposure to the v-CJD agent through blood and its components seems greatly inferior in France compared to Great Britain, the possible benefit of adding a prion reduction step in the preparation of labile blood components is being assessed in France.

Strategic Perspectives

Prevention of transfusion-transmitted infections is an essential objective of sanitary monitoring. In 2005, the EFS has reinforced its transfusion safety action plan in the areas of prevention of platelet concentrate contamination, definition of a pathogen reduction method for therapeutic plasma, and prevention of post-transfusion respiratory complications.

Investments in the optimization of transfusion safety show a far greater cost-benefit ratio than is generally expected in public health. The fact that health products have never been so safe is proof that this approach is effective.

However, preventive measures can only counter known risks, and any emerging infection not yet described can escape detection by current methods of testing and inactivation.

Thus, sanitary monitoring remains crucial in the face of new dangers. This surveillance must be applied on an international scale first, because new pathologies often emerge in developing countries and then spread to the Western world essentially through trade and travel. The Hemovigilance network keeps track of these epidemiologic trends and creates national and regional alert systems based on them. Precautionary principles will be applied in response to a possible health threat whenever an emerging or theoretical risk appears.

Technologic advances will help to reinforce sanitary safeguards. At present, innovative methods based on DNA chips allow discovery of new viruses. The human variant of the coronavirus that causes SARS was isolated thanks to this technology.

But we must keep in mind that zero risk can never be achieved, and that blood will always be a living therapeutic product associated with side effects [17].

References

1. Alter H. Blood safety 2004 onwards, EPFA and PEI NAT Workshop. Paris, May 25-26, 2004.
2. Pillonel J, Laperche S et le comité de pilotage. Surveillance épidémiologique des donneurs de sang homologues en France entre 1992 et 2002. Septembre 2004.
3. Assal AA, Coste J, Morel P, Maniez M, Rebibo D, Cornillot C, Laperche S, Pillonel J, Andreu G. Should HBV NAT be implemented in French blood donors ? *Vox Sang* 2005 ; 89 (Suppl 1): 21.
4. Iwamoto M, Jernigan DB, Guasch A, Trepka MJ, Blackmore CG, Hellinger WC et al. Transmission of West Nile virus from an organ donor to four transplant recipients. *N Engl J Med* 2003 ; 348 (22) : 2196-203.
5. Paquet C, Quatresous I, Solet JL, Sissoko D, Renault P, Pierre V, Cordel H, Lassalle C, Thiria J, Zeller H, Schuffnecker I. Epidémiologie de l'infection par le virus Chikungunya à l'Ile de la Réunion : point de la situation au 8 janvier 2006. *BEH hors série*, 2006 : 2-3.
6. Rota PA, Oberste MA, Monroe SS et al. Characterization of a novel coronavirus associated with severe acute respiratory syndrome. *Science* 2003 ; 300 : 1394-9.
7. Etablissement Français du Sang. Rapport d'activité 2003.
8. Centers for Disease Control and Prevention. Outbreaks of avian influenza A (H5N1) in Asia and interim recommendations for evaluation and reporting of suspected cases-United States, 2004. Morb Mortal Wkly Rep 2004 ; 53 : 97-100.
9. Welch J, Maclaran K, Jordan T, Simmonds P. Frequency, viral loads, and serotype identification of enterovirus infections in Scottish blood donors. *Transfusion* 2003 ; 43 : 1060-6.
10. Aubin JT, Defer C, Vidaud M, Maniez-Montreuil M, Flan B. Large-scale screening for human parvovirus B19 DNA by PCR: application to the quality control of plasma for fractionation. Vox Sang 2000 ; 78 : 7-12.
11. Loiseau P, Mariotti M, Corbi C, Ravera N, Girot R, Thauvin M. et al. Prevalence of hepatitis G virus RNA in French blood donors and recipients. *Transfusion* 1997 ; 37 : 645-50.
12. Herve P. Sécurité transfusionnelle : risques émergents ou hypothétiques.*Transfus Clin Bio*, 2000 ; 7 : 30-8.
13. Andreu G, Morel P, Forestier F, Debeir J, Rebibo D, Janvier G, Hervé P. Hemovigilance network in France : organization and analysis of immediate transfusion incident reports from 1994 to 1998. *Transfusion* 2002 ; 42 : 1356-64.
14. Llewelyn CA, Hewitt PE, Knight RS, Amar K, Cousens S, Mackenzie J, et al. Possible transmission of variant Creutzfeldt-Jakob disease by blood transfusion. *Lancet* 2004 ; 363 : 417-21.
15. Evaluation du risque v-MCJ par les produits sanguins. Réunion du groupe d'experts du 16 novembre 2004. AFSSAPS, février 2005.
16. Sowemimo-Coker S, Kascsak R, Kim A, Andrade F, Pesci S, Kascsak R, Meeker C, Carp R, Brown P. Removal of exogenous (spiked) and endogenous prion infectivity from red cells with a new prototype of leukoreduction filter. *Transfusion* 2005 ; 45 : 1839-44.
17. Toulmonde E. Le risque résiduel viral en transfusion sanguine. In: *Les virus transmissibles par le sang*. Paris: John Libbey Eurotext, 1996 : 249-57.

Toward Universal Pathogen Inactivation in Blood Cells

Jean-Pierre Cazenave

Transfusion of labile blood products: red cell concentrates and concentrates of platelets and plasma, from a donation of whole blood or produced by apheresis, is still an essential, effective and sometimes life-saving therapy, when no alternative treatment exists. Each year, in France, 2 500 0000 labile blood products are transfused to about 500,000 recipients. Transfusion of labile blood products is often indispensable for patients with serious trauma, in cardiovascular surgery, in obstetrics, after grafts and transplants during the bone marrow regeneration period, and for patients receiving heavy cancer or leukemia chemotherapy. Technologic advances in transfusion, and monitoring of donors and recipients by means of a nation-wide hemovigilance system instituted in France in 1994, have improved transfusion efficacy and, more importantly, have increased transfusion safety. Transfusion safety measures have made it possible to reduce infectious risk and, to a lesser extent, immunologic risk. These measures have a great organizational and economic impact. It is becoming increasingly clear that the notion of zero risk and the precautionary principle have certain limits, and that medical and public health decisions must be made in view of better patient care, taking into account the cost/benefit ratio of the procedure in terms of risk prevention.

Existing Measures for Transfusion Safety Improvement

Since the creation of hemovigilance, activity reports submitted by the network of blood transfusion establishments, by treatment centers and by various government agencies show constant improvement of transfusion safety, despite persistence of infectious risk. Safety of labile blood products has been increased by medical and biologic donor selection, screening tests for transfusion-transmitted viruses, systematic leukodepletion of all labile blood products as early as the preparation stage, before storage and distribution, and more recently, by genomic testing for the hepatitis C and the HIV viruses. Despite all these measures, residual risk of infection transmission persists [1, 2]. This risk varies depending on the nature of the labile blood product: bacterial with platelet concentrates stored at 22 °C [3] or parasitic (malaria, Chagas) with red blood cell concentrates.

Residual risk exists with known viruses as well because:
- screening tests applicable to transfusion are not always available;
- the pathogen is a variant of the virus;
- the test is performed during the serologic window;
- the test is not sensitive enough;
- the donor is immunosilent;
- there was human error in the laboratory- a situation aggravated by adding more tests [2].

Worldwide epidemiologic changes and travel pose the threat of new emergent viruses such as the West Nile Virus (WNV) or the coronavirus that causes avian influenza responsible for severe acute respiratory syndrome (SARS), for which there are no routine screening tests that can currently be used in transfusion [4]. Finally, the possibility of transmitting a pathological prion, the new variant of Creutzfeldt-Jakob disease (nv-CJD), by transfusion is still a potential threat against which we have neither donor screening tests nor a method of elimination from labile blood products [5, 6]. Risk of infection is even greater for recipients of labile blood products with a primary or secondary immunodeficiency syndrome [4]. Finally, certain other considerable risks are related to blood transfusion, particularly immunologic risks: red blood cell incompatibility, transfusional acute respiratory distress syndrome [7], graft-*versus*-host reaction.

Pathogen Inactivation: A New Measure to Implement?

All these considerations explain the importance of developing and implementing methods of pathogen inactivation in labile blood products [8, 9]. Current tests have limitations due to the serologic antibody window, the small number of viral copies that they can detect, the appearance of emerging viruses, and the emerging threats related to bacteria and Protozoa. This being so, inactivation of pathogenic viruses in labile blood products is a proactive procedure that has already been proven to be effective and produce no major adverse effects in the therapeutic use of plasma, and particularly plasma-derived substances (albumin, immunoglobulins, coagulation factors), an area in which inactivation has been practiced for over twenty years. Residual viral risk in transfusion after the introduction of serologic tests and genomic viral testing showed these tests to be very effective, but only for the specific viruses they targeted. For example, in 2003, according to the "Institut national de veille sanitaire" (IVS), residual risk of HIV transmission through transfusion was 1/3,150,000 donations, for HCV it was 1/10,000,000 donations, for HBV it was only 1/640,000, and for HTLV it was almost nil [10]. A risk of bacterial contamination still exists despite all the measures taken to avoid penetration of bacteria into the blood collection bag: donor selection, disinfection of phlebotomy site, diversion of the first thirty-five milliliters of blood and probable reduction of bacterial content of the bag by systematic leukodepletion by filtration. These methods have been effective, but there seems to be increased risk for platelet concentrates stored at 22 °C [11]. In 2003, the hemovigilance system reported two fatalities caused by platelet concentrate transfusion [12]. However, in 2004 there were no fatalities related to bacterial contamination of platelet or red blood cell concentrates.

The general principles of pathogen inactivation in labile blood products involve a succession of complex stages that are essential and mandatory before marketing authorization is granted by the competent regulatory authority, the "Agence française de sécurité sanitaire des produits de santé" (AFSSAPS). Research and development have identified molecules that interfere with and inactivate the nucleic acids of microbian or cellular pathogenic agents [9], have confirmed that these molecules inhibit nucleic acid replication [13, 14], and have tested their possible toxicity *in vitro* in cultures and *in vivo* in animal models [15]. Finally, phase I, II and III clinical trials will make it possible for regulatory authorities to register these molecules as "medicinal-therapeutic products". The approved substances are subjected to effective, broad-spectrum screening to identify the nucleic acids of pathogens: residual viruses, bacteria, parasites, leukocytes. The difficulty lies in obtaining highly efficient inactivation of pathogens while at the same time minimizing deleterious effects on the viability and biologic functions of platelets [16], red blood cells and plasma proteins, particularly coagulation factors and their natural inhibitors. Inactivation substances (chemicals and photo-derivatives) acting on the genome of the pathogen must not be present, at the time of labile blood product transfusion, in high enough residual concentration to constitute toxicity or genotoxicity (including mutagenicity, teratogenicity, carcinogenicity), in order to conform to regulatory norms applicable to the pharmacological industry and to transfusion [13, 14]. Moreover, the practical modes of implementation of pathogen inactivation in labile blood products must be compatible with the routine preparation procedures of these labile blood products in blood transfusion centers [17]. Finally, labile blood products subjected to pathogen inactivation must undergo therapeutic equivalence clinical trials [18] comparing them with currently used labile blood products, and must be subjected to reinforced scrutiny for possible occurrence of pharmacologic, toxic or transfusional side effects after being launched on the market.

Methods of Pathogen Inactivation

Methods of pathogen inactivation in labile blood products involve photochemical techniques for plasma and platelet concentrates, and biochemical techniques for plasma and red blood cells [19]. At present, there is no procedure that can inactivate whole blood, nor is there a single substance, except perhaps riboflavin, that can inactivate pathogens in plasma, platelets and red blood cells [20]. In general, all these methods act effectively on a large number of viruses - although nonenveloped viruses tend to be much less susceptible than enveloped viruses, as well as on Gram$^+$ and Gram$^-$ bacteria and, to a lesser extent, on spores. Some of these methods can also inactivate parasites (*Table I*).

Virus inactivation started with therapeutic plasma and could not be extended to platelet and red cell concentrated because the chemicals used destroyed cells (*Table II*). Although the therapeutic safety of fresh frozen plasma is increased by a four-month quarantine after testing, and although this measure produces plasma rich in coagulation factors and has not given rise to infectious complications to date, this plasma will inevitably be replaced by inactivated plasma. For the last dozen years, it has also been possible to inactivate therapeutic plasma by using a chemical method combining a solvent: tri-n-butyl phosphate, with a detergent: triton. This method, which is both safe and effective, is already used in France on pools of plasma from a hundred donors. It achieves a 20% to 30% reduction of coagulation factors. It is less effective on nonenveloped viruses such as the B19 parvovirus; as a result, prior screening for the B19 parvovirus by polymerase chain reaction must be carried out on the pool of plasma. Methylene blue is another plasma inactivation method, just as effective for viruses, and producing coagulation factor reduction, particularly a 20% to 30% reduction of fibrinogen. This method can be applied to units of plasma obtained by apheresis, and will be adopted in France shortly. Platelet and red blood cell concentrate inactivation is not possible by using solvent and detergent, nor by using methylene blue. New processes adapted to cellular blood products had to be found in order to achieve pathogen inactivation in all labile blood products.

Table I. Pathogen inactivation (Log10 reduction) by the different techniques available.

Routinely tested virus	Amotosalen [21, 22]	S-303	Riboflavin [20]	Inactine [35]
HBV	> 5.5			
HCV (Hutchinson)	> 4.5			
HIV-1 (cell-free)	> 6.2	> 6.5	> 4.5	> 4.8
HIV-1 (cell-associated)	> 6.1	> 6.5	> 5.9	> 5.0
HTLV-I	4.2			
HTLV-II	4.6			
Enveloped virus not routinely tested				
BVDV (HCV model)	> 6.0	> 7.3	> 5.0	> 5.0
Sindbis (HCV/togavirus)			3.2	> 5.0
CMV (cell-associated)	> 5.9			
DHBV (HBV model)	> 6.2	> 6.3		
MCMV (cell-associated, mouse)	> 3.3 - >5.1			
HSV-1		> 6.0	> 5.5	
HSV-2			> 5.5	
SARS-CoV (severe acute respiratory syndrome)	> 5.8			
Vaccina virus	> 4.7		> 5.5	
West Nile Virus	> 5.5		5.2	
Nonenveloped virus not routinely tested				
Bluetongue virus	5.6 – 5.9			> 6.5
Feline conjunctivitis virus (calcivirus)	1.7 – 2.4			
Human adenovirus 5	> 5.2			> 5.3
Parvovirus B19	3.5 - > 5.0	> 3.4 (3hrs)	> 5.0	> 6.0
Simian adenovirus 15	0.7 – 2.3			
Gram+ bacteria				
Bacillus cereus (vegetative)	> 5.5			
Corynebacterium minutissimum	> 6.3			
Listeria monocytogenes	> 6.3	> 7.0		
Staphylococcus aureus	6.6	> 5.2	> 4.0	
Staphylococcus epidermidis	> 6.6	> 6.9	> 5.0	
Streptococcus pyogenes	> 6.8			
Gram− bacteria				
Enterobacter cloacae	5.9			
Escherichia coli	> 6.4	> 7.4	> 4.3	
Klebsiella pneumoniae	> 5.6			
Pseudomonas aeruginosa	4.5	4.5	> 5.0	
Serratia marcescens	> 6.7			
Salmonella choleraesuis	> 6.2			
Yersinia enterocolitica	> 5.9	> 7.0	> 2.0	> 2.0
Anaerobic bacteria				
Bifidobacterium adolescentis	> 6.0			
Clostridium perfringens	> 6.5			
Lactobacillus spp.	> 6.4			
Propionibacterium acnes	> 6.2			

Spirochetes				
Treponema pallidum (syphilis) routinely tested	6.8 – 7.0			
Borrelia burgdorferi (Lyme disease)	> 6.9			
Parasites				
Trypanosoma cruzii (Chagas)	> 5.3	> 5.3		> 6.0
Plasmodium falciparum (malaria)	> 6	> 7.0	+	+
Leishmania mexicana (Leishmaniosis)	> 5.2	> 6		
Leukocytes				
GvHD (graft-*versus*-host reaction)	+	+	+	+
Cytokines	+	+	+	+

Pathogen Inactivation in Platelet Concentrates

The two methods currently being developed, now at the clinical trial stage, involve two photochemical agents: amotosalen hydrochlorate and riboflavin or vitamin B2.

• **Platelet concentrate inactivation with amotosalen** (Intercept® system, developed by Baxter and Cerus) involves an incubation period with the product, which forms reversible crosslinks with pathogen DNA or RNA; these crosslinks become irreversible following illumination with UVA light, forming adducts which interrupt nucleic acids at about every 83 base pairs [14]. Several major preclinical trials have shown that this treatment effectively inactivates a great number of enveloped and nonenveloped viruses, Gram+ and Gram– bacteria, parasites and spirochetes [21, 22]; it also inactivates residual leukocytes in platelet concentrates, and prevents cytokine production [23, 24]. When these residual lymphocytes are not inactivated by Gamma irradiation, they are responsible for very serious graft-*versus*-host-reaction in immunodeficient recipients. *In vitro* experimental studies and murine studies have shown treatment with amotosalen and UVA light to be more effective than Gamma irradiation in the prevention of graft *versus* host reaction [25]. This result was confirmed in humans by the euroSPRITE trial, in which inactivated platelet concentrates were not irradiated before being transfused [26]. Toxicological animal studies have shown absence of long term toxicity, of reproductive toxicity, of carcinogenicity and of neonatal toxicity [15].

Phase I and phase II clinical trials have demonstrated good recovery and life span of platelets treated after transfusion in humans [27]. Moreover, platelet functions examined *in vitro* were found to be within normal limits [16]. This method has undergone evaluation in four phase III clinical trials. Three trials were conducted in Europe on standard pooled platelet components: euroSPRITE [26], a phase III b trial and a trial on apheresis platelet concentrates [28]. The phase III SPRINT trial using apheresis platelet concentrates was conducted in 605 patients in the United States [29]. In all these clinical trials, platelet recovery in the first and the twenty-fourth hour was equivalent or slightly diminished, and clinical effectiveness on haemostasis was comparable to that of untreated platelets. CE marking of the product by the European Community and the clinical trials, particularly euroSPRITE conducted in Bristol, Rotterdam, Stockholm and Strasbourg [26], have led to marketing approval of the Intercept® system by the AFSSAPS. Of course, platelet concentrates treated with Intercept® must now be used for a greater number of transfused patients in the usual treatment settings, in order to validate the preparation method on a larger scale and

Table II. Pathogen inactivation methods for labile blood products : plasma, platelet concentrates (PC) and red cell concentrates (GRC).

	Plasma	PC	GRC
Solvent-detergent	+	−	−
Methylene blue + visible light	+	−	−
Amotosalen Hcl (S-59) + UVA	+	+	−
FRALE (S-303)			+
Inactine (PEN 110)	−	−	+
Riboflavin + UV/ visible light	+	+	+

to insure that this method actually reduces infectious risk, particularly bacterial risk; that its transfusional hemostatic effect is equivalent to that of untreated platelets; and that consumption of platelet concentrates is not, or only slightly, increased.

Amotosalen and UVA can also inactivate a wide range of infectious agents and residual leukocytes, with the same equipment that is used on platelet concentrates and for the treatment of individual therapeutic plasma, by producing a moderate reduction of coagulation factors and their natural inhibitors. Phase III clinical trials [30] have shown the efficiency of amotosalen and UVA in controlling complex bleeding syndromes (antivitamine K anticoagulant overdose, liver transplant, rare hereditary coagulation factor deficits) and especially in the treatment of thrombotic thrombocytopenic purpura by plasma transfusion, given that amatosalen does not harm the metalloproteinase ADAMTS 13 which controls the polymerisation degree of the von Willebrand factor.

• **Riboflavin methods being developed** (Mirasol®, developed by Navigant Biotechnologies and Gambro) absorb visible light and UV rays, and are a promising new technology. Riboflavin produces photolysis through electron transfer and oxidation reactions, causing DNA and RNA breaks that prevent pathogen replication [31]. Riboflavin has been used in pediatrics for neonatal jaundice phototherapy. Results of toxicology and genotoxicity studies of riboflavin and its breakdown products, lumichrome and lumiflavin, are negative. The technique is easy to use, requires little manipulation, and no removal or absorption of residual products. Pathogen inactivation studies show wide-ranging action on viruses, bacteria, parasites and residual leukocytes [20]. Enveloped viruses are much less susceptible than nonenveloped viruses. This method causes little change in platelet function *in vitro*, and produces only slight modification of recovery and survival in *in vivo* circulation [32, 33]. Phase III clinical trials on the prevention of bleeding symptoms in thrombocytopenic disorders began in France during the fourth quarter of 2005. Riboflavin can also inactivate pathogens in therapeutic plasma, and could be used with visible light to inactivate pathogens in red blood cell concentrates.

Pathogen Inactivation in Red Blood Cell Concentrates

Red blood cell concentrates represent the majority, about 75%, of transfused labile blood products. Inactivation methods use biochemical substances of the FRALE type like the S-303 (Cerus and Baxter), or disruptive agents like Inactine® PEN 110 (Vitex). These two organic chemicals have a broad spectrum inactivation effect on bacteria, viruses and parasites; they cause little change in red blood cell function *in vitro*, and in their recirculation and life span *in vivo* [34-36]. Both these methods were evaluated in phase III clinical trials temporarily interrupted by the appearance of antibodies against neoantigens linked with the inactivation technique. Antibodies without haemolysis effects developed in two patients with genetic hemoglobinopathy, chronically transfused with red cell concentrates treated with S-303. The phase III clinical protocol was interrupted as a precaution. The antibodies observed seem directed against an antigenic determinant created by the S-303. We hope to modify S-303 incubation conditions, prevent antibody development and continue S-303 trials.

Toward Universal Pathogen Inactivation in Labile Blood Products

In the 1980s, the HIV pandemic heightened awareness of the fragility of blood transfusion, and of the difficulties related to the use of safe and effective labile blood products in patient therapy [37, 38]. Transfusion specialists became obsessed with means of preventing transmission of blood-borne infections and infections communicable by blood components. Since then, we have reacted on a one-by-one basis to the emergence of each new infectious agent susceptible of posing a threat to labile blood product safety. As a result, at least seven new laboratory procedures have been introduced; they include new complex and sensitive screening tests, serologic tests and molecular biology tests, including leukodepletion by filtration. However, this ever increasing series of new technologies is reaching its limits, and is associated with increasing costs although it does not always provide real benefits in terms of efficiency [39, 40]. Introduction of genomic testing for known viruses like HIV and HCV has made it possible to reduce the serologic window. But as far as HCV is concerned, improvements can still be made in biologic control quality, which varies greatly from one manufacturer and from one country to another [41]. As far as new emerging viruses like the WNV or the SARS coronavirus or Chikungunya in the Pacific area are concerned, institution for transfusion purposes of serologic screening or screening by molecular biology is a lengthy process.

More recently, methods of bacteriologic screening in platelet concentrates, introduced in a few countries, have demonstrated a certain usefulness and many limitations [42, 43]. These methods do not generally detect anaerobic bacteria and, recently, a Dutch study showed that blood products could be transfused before positive results are known, without producing clinical symptoms indicative of a transfusional event due to bacterial contamination. The same study did not detect *Bacillus cereus* contamination before platelet concentrates were disseminated, and two out of the three patients transfused suffered serious adverse events [43]. For all these reasons, as well as the significant number of false positive results, the difficulty of application, the increased risk of expiry and high costs, further consideration is needed before deciding to adopt these screening methods in France. Moreover, bacterial risk for platelet concentrates is decreasing, hygiene and disinfection measures have been reinforced, and pathogen inactivation is an accessible alternative whose effect on pathogens is wide-ranging. It must also be remembered that parasitic infections like malaria and especially Chagas disease are not routinely detected in labile blood products, and cause serious clinical problems in certain countries, and as a result of intercontinental travel.

Introduction of pathogen inactivation methods applied to labile blood products can therefore be considered a proactive solution that would eliminate these agents before they enter transfused labile blood products. These methods exert broad spectrum inactivation of viruses, bacteria, parasites and residual leukocytes. They are proactive methods because their broad range of action on the nucleic acids of pathogens gives them the potential of eliminating risks of emerging viruses and/or risks related to population migrations. They are definitely known to eliminate a large number of bacterial stem aerobes and anaerobes. These inactivation methods present certain advantages that will be increased if the procedures can be applied to all labile blood products. Pathogen inactivation should make it possible to eliminate certain biological investigations such as tests for syphilis or for CMV; moreover, this method could make it unnecessary to introduce new tests. Prevention of transfusion induced graft *versus* host reaction is just as effective, if not more so, when leukocytes are inactivated by amotosalen, riboflavin, S-303 or Inactine®, and when the products are irradiated with gamma rays [25]. It could be possible to eliminate irradiation of products intended for patients with deficits or with immature immune systems [26]. Elimination of these stages would provide only moderate economic gain, but would facilitate the organisation of labile blood component production. These inactivation methods generally require the use of additive solutions, producing a plasma gain of about 200 ml per platelet concentrate, a quantity that can be used to produce therapeutic plasma, or for purposes of fractionation. Finally, we can consider extending the platelet concentrate conservation period to seven days.

In the long term, the logical objective is the universal introduction of pathogen inactivation methods for all labile blood products. This can only be done gradually, one step at a time: first therapeutic plasma, then platelet concentrates and red blood cell concentrates. Introduction of these methods must be evaluated in extensive, rigorously conducted clinical trials, in order not to compromise the benefits expected from these procedures by the occurrence of adverse events, either immunologic or toxic. Clinical trials are needed to insure, thanks to increased hemovigilance, the actual existence of a considerable margin of pharmacological and toxicological safety of inactivated labile blood products, when administered in single or repeated doses [15]. Finally, given the increasing number of methods of prevention, it is important to examine how well-founded they are, by carrying out in-depth analysis of their benefits in terms of efficiency and safety *versus* cost of implementation. We know that the cost of these procedures will be very high, higher than that of serologic and genomic testing methods that will continue to be used [39, 40].

Inactivation methods like the solvent-detergent procedure or methylene blue have made it possible to confer a high degree of safety to plasma-derived products; it is hard to imagine that other inactivation methods could not be used on platelet and red blood cell concentrates. Regardless of their cost, they could be very useful in countries where infectious, bacterial, viral and parasitic risks are very high and produce a risk of unacceptable post-transfusion infectious contamination. Unfortunately, these techniques do not inactivate the new vCJD prion, which cannot be detected in donors [44].

References

1. Barbara JA. The rationale for pathogen-inactivation treatment of blood components. *Int J Hematol* 2004 ; 80 : 311-6.
2. Barbara J. Why 'Safer than Ever' may not be quite safe enough. *Transfus Med Hemother* 2004 ; 31 Suppl.1 : 2-10.
3. Blajchman MA. Bacterial contamination of cellular blood components : risks, sources and control. *Vox Sang* 2004 ; 87 Suppl.1 : 98-103.
4. Allain JP, Bianco C, Blajchman MA, Brecher ME, Busch M, Leiby D, Lin L, Stramer S. Protecting the blood supply from emerging pathogens: the role of pathogen inactivation. *Transfus Med Rev* 2005 ; 19 : 110-26.

5. Blajchman MA, Goldman M, Webert KE, Vamvakas EC, Hannon J, Delage G. Proceedings of a consensus conference: the screening of blood donors for variant CJD. *Transfus Med Rev* 2004 ; 18 : 73-92.
6. Deslys JP. Prions and risks for blood transfusion: the situation in 2003. *Transfus Clin Biol* 2003 ; 10 : 113-25.
7. Goldman M, Webert KE, Arnold DM, Freedman J, Hannon J, Blajchman MA, TRALI Consensus Panel. Proceedings of a consensus conference: towards an understanding of TRALI. *Transfus Med Rev* 2005 ; 19 : 2-31.
8. AuBuchon JP. Pathogen inactivation in cellular blood components: clinical trials and implications of introduction to transfusion medicine. *Vox Sang* 2002 ; 83 Suppl. 1 : 271-5.
9. Corash L. Inactivation of viruses, bacteria, protozoa and leukocytes in platelet and red cell concentrates. *Vox Sang* 2000 ; 78 Suppl. 2 : 205-10.
10. Pillonel J, Laperche S. Trends in risk of transfusion-transmitted viral infections (HIV, HCV, HBV) in France between 1992 and 2003 and impact of nucleic acid testing (NAT). *Euro Surveill* 2005 ; 10 : 5-6.
11. Blajchman MA, Goldman M, Baeza F. Improving the bacteriological safety of platelet transfusions. *Transfus Med Rev* 2004 ; 18 : 11-24.
12. Rebibo D, Hauser L, Slimani A, Herve P, Andreu G. The French Haemovigilance System: organization and results for 2003. *Transfus Apheresis Sci* 2004 ; 31 : 145-53.
13. Wollowitz S. Fundamentals of the psoralen-based Helinx technology for inactivation of infectious pathogens and leukocytes in platelets and plasma. *Semin Hematol* 2001 ; 38 Suppl. 11 : 4-11.
14. Wollowitz S. Targeting DNA and RNA in pathogens : mode of action of amotosalen HCl. *Transfus Med Hemother* 2004 ; 31 Suppl.1 : 11-6.
15. Ciaravino V, McCullough T, Cimino G. The role of toxicology assessment in transfusion medicine. *Transfusion* 2003 ; 43 : 1481-92.
16. van Rhenen DJ, Vermeij J, Mayaudon V, Hind C, Lin L, Corash L. Functional characteristics of S-59 photochemically treated platelet concentrates derived from buffy coats. *Vox Sang* 2000 ; 79 : 206-14.
17. Janetzko K, Lin L, Eichler H, Mayaudon V, Flament J, Kluter H. Implementation of the INTERCEPT Blood System for Platelets into routine blood bank manufacturing procedures: evaluation of apheresis platelets. *Vox Sang* 2004 ; 86 : 239-45.
18. Cazenave JP, Davis K, Corash L. Design of clinical trials to evaluate the efficacy of platelet transfusion: the euroSPRITE trial for components treated with Helinx technology. *Semin Hematol* 2001 ; 38 Suppl. 11 : 46-54.
19. Corash L. Pathogen reduction technology: methods, status of clinical trials, and future prospects. *Curr Hematol Rep* 2003 ; 2 : 495-502.
20. Goodrich RP. The use of riboflavin for the inactivation of pathogens in blood products. *Vox Sang* 2000 ; 78 Suppl. 2 : 211-5.
21. Lin L, Hanson CV, Alter HJ, Jauvin V, Bernard KA, Murthy KK, Metzel P, Corash L. Inactivation of viruses in platelet concentrates by photochemical treatment with amotosalen and long-wavelength ultraviolet light. *Transfusion* 2005 ; 45 : 580-90.
22. Lin L, Dikeman R, Molini B, Lukehart SA, Lane R, Dupuis K, Metzel P, Corash L. Photochemical treatment of platelet concentrates with amotosalen and long-wavelength ultraviolet light inactivates a broad spectrum of pathogenic bacteria. *Transfusion* 2004 ; 44 : 1496-504.
23. Grass JA, Hei DJ, Metchette K, Cimino GD, Wiesehahn GP, Corash L, Lin L. Inactivation of leukocytes in platelet concentrates by photochemical treatment with psoralen plus UVA. *Blood* 1998 ; 91 : 2180-8.
24. Hei DJ, Grass J, Lin L, Corash L, Cimino G. Elimination of cytokine production in stored platelet concentrate aliquots by photochemical treatment with psoralen plus ultraviolet A light. *Transfusion* 1999 ; 39 : 239-48.
25. Grass JA, Wafa T, Reames A, Wages D, Corash L, Ferrara JL, Lin L. Prevention of transfusion-associated graft-versus-host disease by photochemical treatment. *Blood* 1999 ; 93 : 3140-7.
26. van Rhenen D, Gulliksson H, Cazenave JP, Pamphilon D, Ljungman P, Kluter H, Vermeij H, Kappers-Klunne M, de Greef G, Laforet M, Lioure B, Davis K, Marblie S, Mayaudon V,

Flament J, Conlan M, Lin L, Metzel P, Buchholz D, Corash L; euroSPRITE trial. Transfusion of pooled buffy coat platelet components prepared with photochemical pathogen inactivation treatment: the euroSPRITE trial. *Blood* 2003 ; 101 : 2426-33.
27. Snyder E, Raife T, Lin L, Cimino G, Metzel P, Rheinschmidt M, Baril L, Davis K, Buchholz DH, Corash L, Conlan MG. Recovery and life span of 111indium-radiolabeled platelets treated with pathogen inactivation with amotosalen HCl (S-59) and ultraviolet A light. *Transfusion* 2004 ; 44 : 1732-40.
28. Janetzko K, Cazenave JP, Kluter H, Kientz D, Michel M, Beris P, Lioure B, Hastka J, Marblie S, Mayaudon V, Lin L, Lin JS, Conlan MG, Flament J. Therapeutic efficacy and safety of photochemically treated aphaeresis platelets processed with an optimized integrated set. *Transfusion* 2005 ; sous presse.
29. McCullough J, Vesole DH, Benjamin RJ, Slichter SJ, Pineda A, Snyder E, Stadtmauer EA, Lopez-Plaza I, Coutre S, Strauss RG, Goodnough LT, Fridey JL, Raife T, Cable R, Murphy S, Howard F 4th, Davis K, Lin JS, Metzel P, Corash L, Koutsoukos A, Lin L, Buchholz DH, Conlan MG. Therapeutic efficacy and safety of platelets treated with a photochemical process for pathogen inactivation: the SPRINT Trial. *Blood* 2004 ; 104 : 1534-41.
30. Hambleton J, Wages D, Radu-Radulescu L, Adams M, MacKenzie M, Shafer S, Lee M, Smyers J, Wiesehahn G, Corash L. Pharmacokinetic study of FFP photochemically treated with amotosalen (S-59) and UV light compared to FFP in healthy volunteers anticoagulated with warfarin. *Transfusion* 2002 ; 42 : 1302-7.
31. Ruane PH, Edrich R, Gampp D, Keil SD, Leonard RL, Goodrich RP. Photochemical inactivation of selected viruses and bacteria in platelet concentrates using riboflavin and light. *Transfusion* 2004 ; 44 : 877-85.
32. AuBuchon JP. Pathogen reduction technologies: what are the concerns ? *Vox Sang* 2004 ; 87 Suppl. 2 : 84-9.
33. Li J, de Korte D, Woolum MD, Ruane PH, Keil SD, Lockerbie O, McLean R, Goodrich RP. Pathogen reduction of buffy coat platelet concentrates using riboflavin and light: comparisons with pathogen-reduction technology-treated apheresis platelet products. *Vox Sang* 2004 ; 87 : 82-90.
34. AuBuchon JP, Pickard CA, Herschel LH, Roger JC, Tracy JE, Purmal A, Chapman J, Ackerman S, Beach KJ. Production of pathogen-inactivated RBC concentrates using PEN110 chemistry: a phase I clinical study. *Transfusion* 2002 ; 42 : 146-52.
35. Lazo A, Tassello J, Jayarama V, Ohagen A, Gibaja V, Kramer E, Marmorato A, Billia-Shaveet D, Purmal A, Brown F, Chapman J. Broad-spectrum virus reduction in red cell concentrates using INACTINE PEN110 chemistry. *Vox Sang* 2002 ; 83 : 313-23.
36. Purmal A, Valeri CR, Dzik W, Pivacek L, Ragno G, Lazo A, Chapman J. Process for the preparation of pathogen-inactivated RBC concentrates by using PEN110 chemistry: preclinical studies. *Transfusion* 2002 ; 42 : 139-45.
37. Engelfriet CP, Reesink HW, Klein HG, AuBuchon JP, Strauss RG, Krusius T, Maki T, Rebulla P, Hogman CF, Knutson F, Letowska M, Dickmeiss E, Winter M, Henn G, Menichetti E, Mayr WR, Flanagan P, Martin-Vega C, Massuet L, Wendel S, Turek P, Lin CK, Shirato T. The future use of pathogen-inactivated platelet concentrates. *Vox Sang* 2003 ; 85 : 54-66.
38. Farrugia A. The mantra of blood safety: time for a new tune ? *Vox Sang* 2004 ; 86 : 1-7.
39. Staginnus U, Corash L. Economics of pathogen inactivation technology for platelet concentrates in Japan. *Int J Hematol* 2004 ; 80 : 317-24.
40. van Hulst M, de Wolf JT, Staginnus U, Ruitenberg EJ, Postma MJ. Pharmaco-economics of blood transfusion safety: review of the available evidence. *Vox Sang* 2002 ; 83 : 146-55.
41. Coste J, Reesink HW, Engelfriet CP, Laperche S, Brown S, Busch MP, Cuijpers HT, Elgin R, Ekermo B, Epstein JS, Flesland O, Heier HE, Henn G, Hernandez JM, Hewlett IK, Hyland C, Keller AJ, Krusius T, Levicnik-Stezina S, Levy G, Lin CK, Margaritis AR, Muylle L, Neiderhauser C, Pastila S, Pillonel J, Pineau J, van der Poel CL, Politis C, Roth WK, Sauleda S, Seed CR, Sondag-Thull D, Stramer SL, Strong M, Vamvakas EC, Velati C, Vesga MA, Zanetti A. Implementation of donor screening for infectious agents transmitted by blood by nucleic acid technology: update to 2003. *Vox Sang* 2005 ; 88 : 289-98.

42. AuBuchon JP, Cooper LK, Leach MF, Zuaro DE, Schwartzman JD. Experience with universal bacterial culturing to detect contamination of apheresis platelet units in a hospital transfusion service. *Transfusion* 2002 ; 42 : 855-61.
43. Boekhorst PA, Beckers EA, Vos MC, Vermeij H, van Rhenen DJ. Clinical significance of bacteriologic screening in platelet concentrates. *Transfusion* 2005 ; 45 : 514-9.
44. Hart J, Leier B, Nahirniak S. Informed consent for blood transfusion: should the possibility of prion risk be included ? *Transfus Med Rev* 2004 ; 18 : 177-83.

Nanotechnologies Revolutionize the Biological Qualification of Blood Donations

Moussa Hoummady, Pascal Morel

Thirty Years of Exciting Discoveries in Nanotechnology

Nanotechnologies have exerted such enormous impact and continue to exert such great fascination that strategic analysis experts consider their advent an industrial revolution comparable to that occasioned by microelectronics [1-3].

The concepts and approaches of nanosciences and nanotechnologies are new and deal with the properties of matter on a nanometric scale, that are fundamentally different from properties of matter on a larger scale. For example, on a nanometric scale, surface properties are much more important than size-related properties. Similarly, mechanical, electronic, optical and chemical dimensions are totally correlated, making possible the multifaceted approaches applied by scientific and industrial communities in the development of these new technologies.

These approaches, which look at matter as characterized by its new nanometric properties, have aroused scientific curiosity and have made this field of activity the focus of great interest.

History and Evolution of Nanotechnologies

The term "nanotechnology" was first used in 1974 in Japan, by Norio Tanigushi of the University of Tokyo, to describe building and consolidation processes on a microscopic scale.

The term was made popular in the years between 1980 and 1985 by Eric K. Drexler (Director of the Foresight Institute of Technology), when he introduced the notion of "molecular machines and manufacturing".

But it was physicist Richard Feynman (Nobel Prize winner in 1959) who was the first scientist to introduce the idea that man will soon be able to transform matter at the atomic level. In a visionary speech that has since become famous, given in December 1959 before the American Physical Society, he asserted that it would one day be possible to store the entire content of the *Encyclopedia Britannica* on the head of a pin by writing tiny letters with atoms reorganized on their surface.

This vision could not have become reality without the 1981 invention of the scanning tunnelling microscope by Gerd Bining and Heinrich Roher at the IBM laboratories in Zurich. This microscope consequently made it possible to see atoms and move them around to structure surfaces so as to endow them with properties and functions they do not possess naturally.

Other scientific advances followed, such as those introduced by Professor Lehn, winner of the 1987 Nobel Prize in chemistry, and by his work on chemical self-assembly and molecular recognition, as well as host and guest molecules. This work opened the way to the study of fundamental properties of matter, particularly self-organized forms and information transmission at the molecular level. This research was also at the origin of extended applications at the interface between chemistry, biology and engineering sciences.

In 1991, S. Jÿima of the NEC laboratory in Japan discovered carbon nanotubes with a new shape structured from carbon molecules whose physical properties could not be extrapolated from macroscopic models of matter. These properties are still being studied, but nanotubes already have a multitude of applications: nanoelectronics, plasma sheaths, hydrogen storage, capacitors.

The field of micro-electronics had to create processes for the integration and miniaturization of electronic components in order to increase the power of microprocessors and computers. As a result, the number of transistors integrated in a microprocessor is constantly increasing, doubling every eighteen months (Morre's Law, referring to the name of one of the founders of Intel). But this integration has physical limits and the micro-electronics industry is showing an ever-increasing interest in molecular electronics. The latter replaces discrete components like transistors with chemical molecules endowed with biological functions. For example, the functioning of biocomputers is based on principles governing the functioning of living matter (DNA coding), which allow calculations of unprecedented precision.

Moreover, researchers in life sciences have made considerable progress, particularly in molecular biology and sequencing of the genomes of different organisms, including the human genome. Thus, the medicine of the future can rely on the application of these discoveries to better understand the underlying mechanisms of disease (biomarkers, transcription, cellular dysfunction, etc.)

A review of the research devoted to this field clearly shows that investigation of matter on a nanometric scale has been very fruitful. Over the past three decades, major scientific and technological advances and breakthroughs have taken place, making nanotechnology a field of considerable importance.

Because of the scales involved in nanotechnologies, the latter require extensive interdisciplinary approaches (*Figure 1*). Collaboration is required with chemical and physical sciences, engineering sciences, computer science, life sciences. Thus, nanotechnologies constitute a crossroads of multidisciplinary know-how.

Nanotechnologies have repercussions for most scientific and industrial sectors, particularly health, life sciences, the automobile industry, aerospace, electronics, communications, the chemicals and materials industries, the energy sector, etc. Major repercussions for the biologic qualification of donations for blood transfusion are foreseeable.

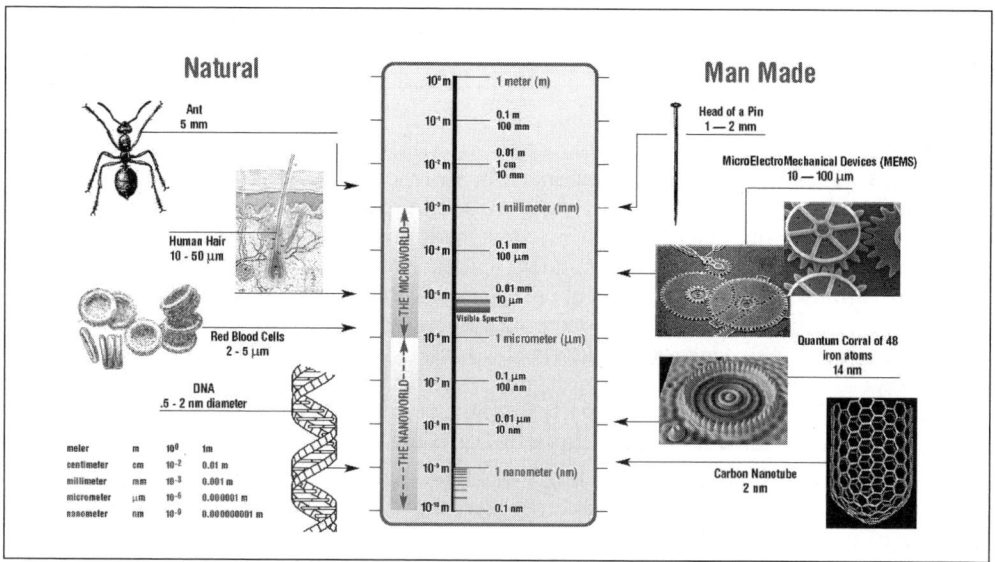

Figure 1. Size differences between natural organisms and man-made objects [2].

Biological Qualification of Donations: Limits and Development Prospects

Definitions, Present Status

Today, "biological qualification of donations" (BQD) refers to a series of biological tests carried out on a blood sample taken from a donor. Once this stage is completed, the characteristics of the donation and of the therapeutic products derived from it are defined, and it is decided whether or not this donation and these products are usable in human therapy. In terms of safety, the biological qualification of donations follows an all-or-nothing rule: conformity (possible use of the donation and of its products) is established within twenty-four hours following the donation, based on a set of legal obligations [4, 5]. A diagnosis of disease and/or infection in the donor is made during the second stage of the process, following a second series of biological tests. In this context, control of product conformity has priority over screening for communicable diseases or for biological particularities (mass testing).

Biological qualification of donations is historically associated with blood donation. In fact, it was initially created for this type of donation. Today, all other donations (organ, cell, tissue) are subjected to biological qualification and have to meet pre-established conformity criteria based on the same principle. Biological qualification of donations systematically aims to achieve three objectives :

– to define products by providing relevant information regarding the active ingredient (volume, concentration, biocompatibility);

– to guarantee the safety of the recipient(s) of therapeutic products derived from a donation; Biological qualification of donations is a complementary procedure in the context of medical selection of donors. It contributes to reduce transfusion risk, particularly viral risk [6];

– to guarantee the safety of donors. On the one hand, the tests performed for the safety of recipients allow detection of silent infections and lead to treatment of covert infections in donors. On the other hand, specific tests performed on living donors allow assessment of the consequences and tolerance of donations, and identify rare immunologic characteristics that can orient the donor toward a type of donation, or indicate precautionary measures to take if he becomes a recipient.

Today, tests performed for product characterization as well as for detection of transfusion-transmitted infections include antigen-antibody interaction tests that can detect a soluble or cellular antigen or antibody. The only exceptions are hematocrit measurement and genomic amplification. Characterization tests performed depend directly on the active ingredient (ABO typing for blood products with erythrocytes, platelet count for platelet products...) In terms of microbiological safety, current biological qualification of donations only tests regularly and systematically for six infections: syphilis, viral hepatitis B and C, HIV infections, T cell leukemia virus (HTLV), and *Plasmodium falciparum* infection (in case of exposure to risk). As far as grafts are concerned, depending on their intended use and the fragility of recipients, particularly in terms of immunosuppression, testing for other silent infections could be performed (Epstein-Barr virus, toxoplasmosis...).

Biological tests use diagnostic methods that have proven to be reliable in immunohematology, and in serological virus and parasite screening. Molecular biology procedures have been developed specifically for the biological qualification of donations, and have been adapted to large series (volume of samples, automation...). Progress has been constant over the years, as can be seen from the continuous reduction of residual risk for major viruses (HIV, HCV, HBV) [7]. These advances are related, on the one hand, to the evolution of detection strategies:

– direct markers (HBV, HIV),

– association of direct and indirect markers (HCV: ALAT+ anti-HBc),

– association of direct markers (HIV and HCV: anti-HIV/ HCV+RNA).

On the other hand, this progress is due to the efficacy of reactive test kits. HBs-Ag test kits are a good illustration of the performance improvement seen in these devices. Their sensitivity has gone from 3,000 ng/ml HBs-Ag detected by electroimmunodiffusion tests in 1970, to 0.045 ng/ml detected with ELISA in 2003.

ELISA itself has been considerably improved: for HBs antigen, first generation kits had a sensitivity of 10 to 100 times lower than that of the kits in common use today (0.36 to 1.3 *versus* 0.045 ng/ml). Finally, testing methods benefited from the creation of kits allowing simultaneous detection of two markers of the same virus [8].

Qualitative performance improvement was accompanied by an increase in the quantity of donations that can be tested. For 150,000 annual donations, a biological qualification laboratory performs about 15,000 tests, which represent over 100 million B(0.27 euro) per year. A volume of this size requires a suitable environment (automated equipment, computer systems) specifically developed to process a large number of samples in the course of the same test. Automated equipment for immunohematologic and, recently, genomic testing constitutes an unprecedented advance in clinical biology. The disadvantage of this advanced technology approach is a loss of flexibility in terms of adaptation to particular cases, introduction of new assays and requirement of highly specialized training for personnel working in this field.

Finally, the use of specialized personnel, of high-tech specialized equipment and of specifically-designed methods explains the high cost of biological qualification of donations, which is in fact the most expensive link of the transfusion chain.

Perspectives

More and more, particular patient needs constitute a priority. In transfusion medicine, it is not justified to systematically detect donors who are carriers of parvovirus B 19, but it is medically justified to prevent transmission of this virus to sickle cell anemia patients, to patients receiving bone marrow allografts, and to pregnant women. Today, it is difficult to solve this dilemma. Prevention of cytomegalovirus infection is currently the only example of "specific" processing. The method used for qualifying donations simply does not allow this type of custom-made processing. In the future, patient susceptibility will have to be taken into account to a greater extent, and the qualification/conformity of therapeutic products will have to be reconciled with recipient particularities.

Moreover, future technological developments in the biological qualification of donations should concentrate on diagnostic activities. To illustrate, we can look at the role of viral genomic diagnosis (VGD) of HIV today. Methods of mass molecular biology testing (the most sensitive) are available and unfailingly used in the biological qualification of donations, although risk for this virus is nearly one hundred times lower in the donor population than in the general population (prevalence: 0.6/10,000 new donors) [7]. A concerted effort must be made so that the effective diagnostic tools used for biological qualification of donations are made available in the future for targeted testing of exposed populations (for example, centers for free and anonymous HIV testing).

To date, adapting biological qualification of donations to safety requirements for medicinal products has led to the development of more and more efficient methods that are, at the same time, more and more constraining. Today, implementation of any new preventive measure automatically involves heavy investments and high operational costs which negatively impact cost/benefit ratios and limit further development [9]. The recent experience of the United States when faced with the West Nile Virus (WNV) pandemic has pointed out current difficulties and the efforts necessary to insure in the short term the safety of the transfused population [10]. Adaptation of current methods is the challenge of the future. Qualification of donations must be able to adapt to new microbiological safety concerns.

New methods of therapeutic product preparation (cellular expansion, tissue culture…), emergence of new communicable pathogens (prions) and increased risk associated with known pathogenic agents (WNV, bacteria) require great flexibility in terms of adaptive strategies.

We must also point out that every year about a million donors seen in transfusion centers are subjected to a series of tests to qualify their donations. It often happens that the donor population in a given region, over a given period, constitutes the "control population" in epidemiological studies: in the past, studies on the prevalence of the Puumala Hantaan-like virus, risk factors for toxocariasis, non insulin-dependent diabetes… and more recently, epidemiologic studies on the WNV [11]. It seems to be more and more important to have access to a control group in the general population in order to evaluate a public health risk or risk epidemiology. Greater adaptability of biological qualification of donations would increase its contribution to public health measures in terms of risk assessment and follow-up of relevant factors in the population.

More advanced testing procedures (generic marker identification) and the introduction of new technologies (nanotechnology) for this type of testing should guarantee the necessary adaptability.

In fact, the search for specific markers of infection (antigen/antibody genome) could be replaced in the near future by search in the donor of indirect markers of an at-risk situation for the recipient. Rather than preventing risk of a virus or a parasite, we will probably be able to prevent the risk of a whole set of communicable pathogens, thanks to biomarkers present in an infected donor. The search for new biomarkers of these at-risk situations is expanding rapidly thanks to novel proteomics techniques, and has already opened interesting perspectives pertaining to infectious risk, and particularly parasitic infections [12]. Testing strategies could become more global, while remaining based on an all-or-nothing principle. The diagnostic procedure would be carried out, as it is today, as a second step, to look for a specific pathogenic agent.

New techniques are being developed, to evaluate antigen-antibody reactions on new bases (electrical, optical modes). These methods are at the center of a new field of reference: nanotechnologies. Existing prototypes (demonstrators, for instance) can perform cell separation based on electrical and optical criteria. In the short term, these techniques should make it possible to detect bacteria in a cellular fluid. This testing model will eventually be generalized to all separation, using the same criteria, provided a repertory of expected values is available. Testing methods and methods of result management and transmission are under development. Biological qualification of donations and the field of biology in general expect these new technologies to enable them to adapt to new challenges and contribute to public health activities.

Possible Contribution of Nanotechnologies to the Biological Qualification of Donations

New approaches now available in micro and nanotechnologies allow us to foresee considerable progress in terms of operational, performance and cost flexibility. In fact, nanotechnologies could lead to great advances in transfusional biology, particularly in the area of testing method integration.

New devices can integrate, on a microscopic scale, a whole set of physical, chemical and biological functions. Miniaturization and fluid control, electronic and photonic integration are about to create a paradigm change in biological and biochemical testing. These new devices can serve different purposes: processing of biological samples, sorting of molecules and cells, mixing, dosage, specific detection, etc.

Medical biology is truly on the threshold of revolutionary changes, thanks to new technological developments, and in particular biochips and lab-on-chip technologies that go hand in hand with growing use of robotics and computer sciences in medical biology laboratories.

Biochips

The concept of biochips, which originated in the early 1990s, consists of studying and analysing biological and/or chemical affinities in a parallel manner. The reagents used are organized as a matrix, allowing multiple reactions with a single sample (*Figure 2*). Biochips rely on a series of molecular biology techniques, micro and nanotechnology, chemistry, image analysis and bioinformatics.

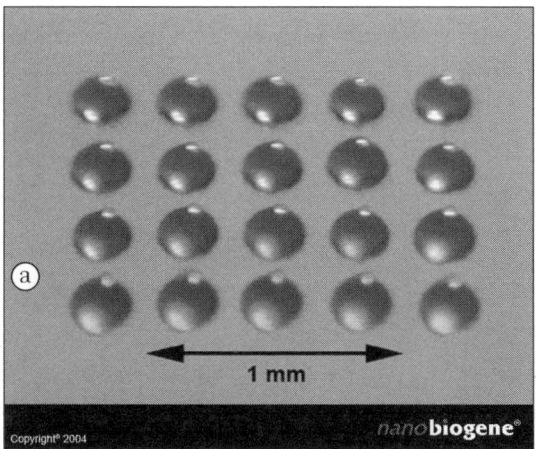 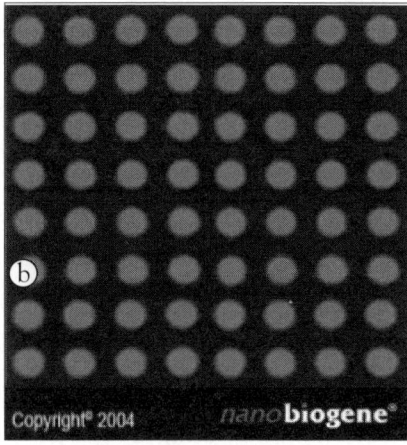

Figure 2. Typical biochip configuration : a) deposited reagents and, b) detection by fluorescent marking (research conducted by the Nanobiogene company).

Biochips consist of a very small support (a few square millimeters or centimeters) of glass, silicium or plastic, on which are synthesized or mounted thousands of probes (synthetic DNA, antibody or cell strands) in different patterns depending on the model. These probes react with the markers in the sample to be analysed, which has been magnified and stained in advance. Hybridization signals (biomolecule pairing) are generally detected by fluorescence, then analysed by a computer system.

DNA chips are the most useful for genetic signature detection, or for the study of gene transcription. Other types of biochips are starting to be produced, particularly protein and cell biochips. This revolutionary technology is much more than a trend: it is, rather, the culmination of advances made in many scientific fields, combined with the latest technological breakthroughs.

These techniques allow a better understanding of the basic mechanisms present in living organisms. They are indispensable to users who can benefit from working with thousands of biological data simultaneously. They also allow analysis output to be exponentially increased.

Biochips have applications in the biological qualification of donations. They provide answers to flexibility and updating requirements. They do away with limits on the number of analyses that can be carried out in parallel. These methods are very progressive. Depending on the pathologies studied, these devices offer custom-made probes and "characteristic marker detectors" for specific pathogens. As a result, analyses can serve to detect pathogen or contaminant signatures in labile blood products, or characteristic biomarkers of existing states (traces of infection).

These biochip techniques can now be associated with ELISA-type testing, which requires reagent manipulation systems of microscopic dimensions. ELISA techniques require several consecutive deposits in different microwells and cuplets. Reading is achieved by using optical detectors, staining or fluorescence. Several public and private laboratories are currently conducting research and development projects in the field. To illustrate the applications of these devices, *Figure 3* presents an ELISA biochip developed by Nanobiogene. This biochip can carry out nine tests on a 25 mm^2 surface. It must be noted that this possibility of performing multiple tests on a very small surface is associated with a considerable reduction of both reactant and sample volumes.

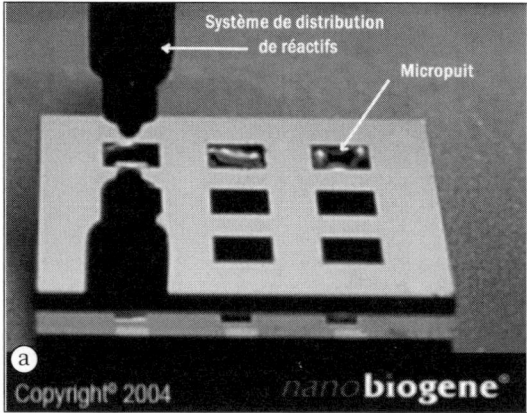 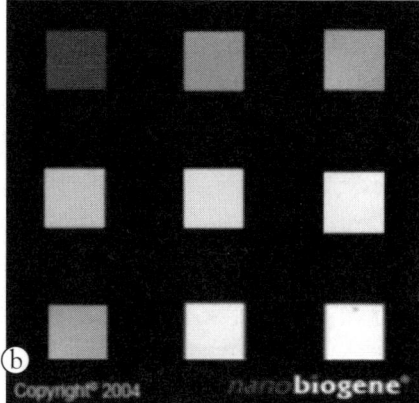

Figure 3. ELISA biochip developed by the Nanobiogene company: a) preparation and staining of reagents, b) optical reading of analysis results.

Lab-on-a-chip Technology

These devices are designed to perform simple analyses that require integration of additional functions. They are, in fact, perfectly suited to integrate, on a microscopic scale (a few cm^2), a large number of functions and components: for example, microfluidic channels, actuators, sensors or microreactors.

These devices involve multidisciplinary know-how, and require enough knowledge of microfluids to process and transport the sample to be analysed toward measurement sites, through microscopic microchannnels. This technology has revolutionized the integration of complex functions in a very reduced space.

Lab-on-chip devices offer significant advantages to the field of biology in general and the biological qualification of donations in particular. Some of these advantages are:

– the possibility of performing a large number of tests and analyses with a single device;

– the fact that the devices are portable and can be taken to the patient's bedside, or used on packs of blood or medicinal biological products;

– reduction of analysis time and reduction of technique variability decrease;

– ease of use and better management of the analysis environment;

– better response to evolving needs (epidemiologic data);

– reduction of sample and reactant volumes needed for testing;

– control and optimization of operational and infrastructure costs.

Research and development advances concerning lab-on-a-chip devices are impressive. The sensor mentioned above, endowed with the ability of sorting cells, illustrates the possibilities of this approach. The ultimate goal is to integrate the cell sorter in the therapeutic product and ask it to perform continuous fluid analysis, so that if one or several target cells are detected, it can signal their presence in real time and prevent the use of the product.

Examples of Microfluidic Devices and Lab-on-chip Devices [13]

Original articles on this subject abound in professional journals. Although industrial applications are still limited, development perspectives are great and a very wide field of application is possible. To illustrate the usefulness and concrete applications of these devices in the field of biological qualification of donations, we will provide a number of examples of projects presently in progress. The new tools presented below will turn the most ambitious dreams for donation qualification into reality. For neophytes, microchannels, integrated pumps, sorters and microneedles are present indicators of what the future holds in store.

Microfluidic Devices and Microchannel Functionalization [14]

Most lab-on-a-chip devices use microfluidic components such as microchannels, microresevoirs and micropumps. These components are the essential features of integrated laboratories. The main challenge in designing these devices concerns miniaturization and the calibration of their components. At the micro and nanoscopic scale, friction and surface forces exert considerable effect. Several teams of experts are working on minimizing these effects, so that biological functions can be integrated in very small devices. For example, the microfluidic and nanotechnological research group at the "École Normale Supérieure de Paris" has announced the possibility of physical-chemical functionalization of surfaces in channels about 100 µm wide. Surface modification inside microchannels has made it possible to suspend cells in the microchannels and therefore to produce cellular cultures in microdevices (*Figure 4*).

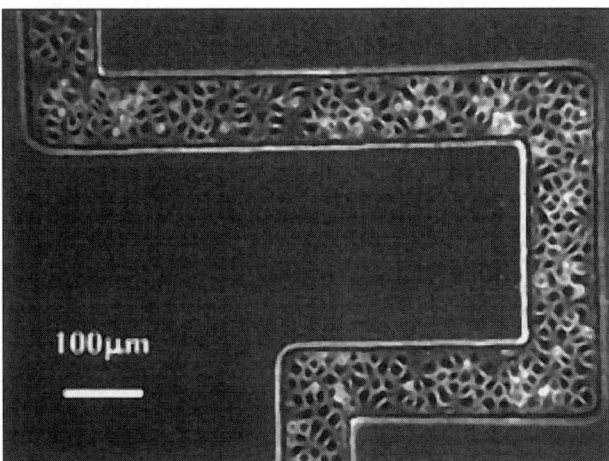

Figure 4. Microfluidic device and cell culture in fluidic microchannels (project of the Ecole Normale Supérieure de Paris).

Integrated Micropump

In order to manipulate reagents in lab-on-chip devices, several fluid activation principles are used: mechanical, electro-hydrodynamic, etc. Most microdevices require the use of operating and control systems that are quite large and cannot be integrated. One pumping device, developed by Debiotech (Switzerland) achieves considerable integration on a surface of only a few mm². Design of the device is based on manufacturing techniques taken from microelectronics (*Figure 5*).

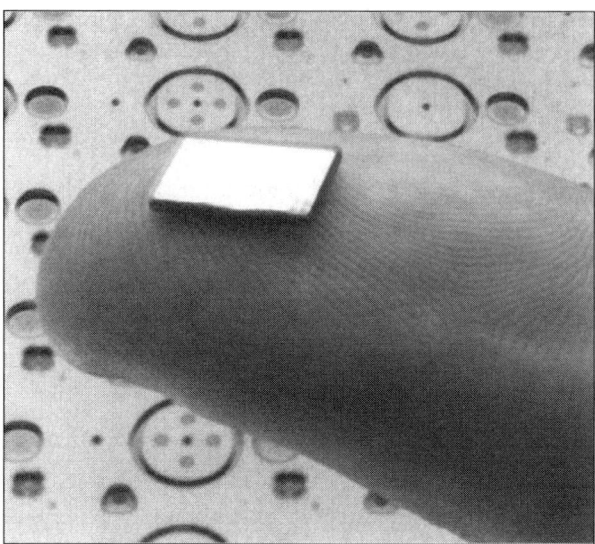

Figure 5. Integrated pump developed by Debiotech.

Microfluidic Devices for Biomolecular Separation [13]

Other, more complex, systems have been created in the past few years. These systems build nanostructures inside microfluidic microchannels. The structures take the shape of nanopillars with well-defined pillar characteristics. The purpose of these devices is to perform biomolecular separation by varying the speed of the molecules depending on their size. This can be done because smaller molecules travel faster through these nanostructures, while large molecules or cells are slowed down. Professor Yoshinobu Baba's team at the University of Tokushimla (Japan) developed these microsystems. In the long term, nanostructures will completely replace the various gels that are still commonly used in electrophoresis (*Figure 6*).

Microfluidic Devices for Cell Sorting [15]

In both cellular biology and immunology, cell characterization and sorting are commonly performed with cytometers. Integrated devices operating like flow cytometers can be produced and adapted to lab-on-a-chip scale. Professor Yong Chen's team at the "Ecole Normale Supérieure de Paris" has developed a system that integrates microfluidic components and electronic electrodes for cell characterization. Moreover, the microfluidic network makes it possible to deviate selected cells toward the appropriate microfluidic exits (*Figure 7*).

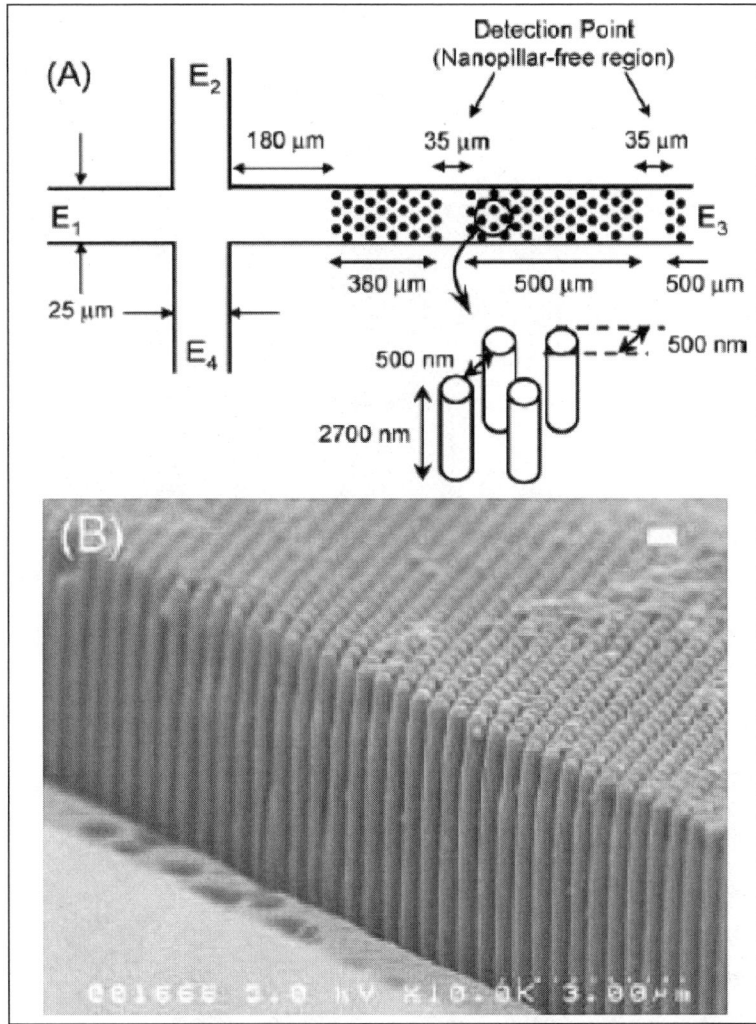

Figure 6. Biomolecular separation device with nanopillars
built inside microchannels (University of Tokushimla project, Japan).

Microneedle Array [15]

Other applications of micro and nanotechnological devices can have an impact on transfusion sectors. One of these consists of a network of microneedles fabricated collectively in the shape of a patch. The main applications of such devices include drawing blood for testing or injecting therapeutic substances through the skin without pain.

These devices are perfectly calibrated and present the potential advantage of replacing syringes, whose use is sometimes traumatizing. *Figure 8* shows a needle array developed by the Nanopass company (Israel), compared to the size of a syringe needle.

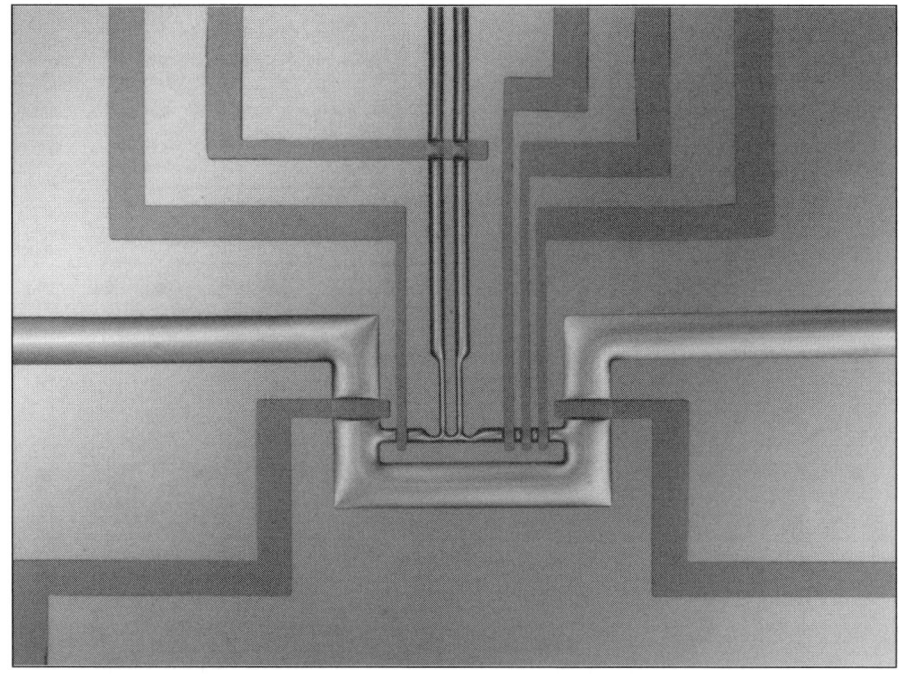

Figure 7. Cell sorting microfluidic device with microchannel network and electrical measurement (project of the Ecole Normale Supérieure de Paris).

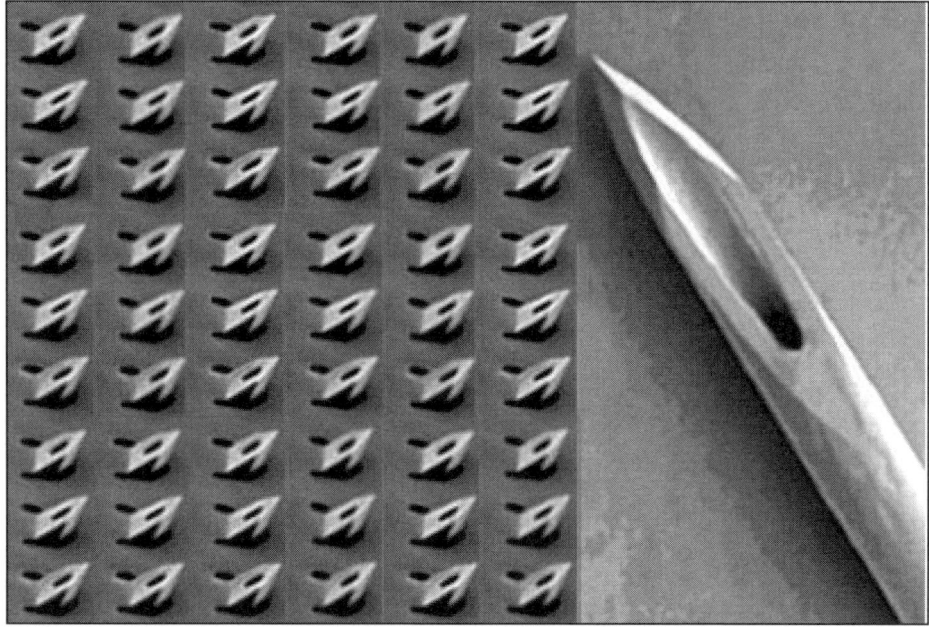

Figure 8. Needle array for drawing blood painlessly. Comparison with a syringe needle (developed by the Nanopass company).

Conclusion

In the past few years, scientific and technological developments in nanotechnologies have been spectacular. These developments will have considerable impact on all industrial sectors, and particularly on life sciences. They will contribute to the advancement of fundamental research through understanding of the mechanisms of living organisms, as well as through the development of new industrial products and methods of analysis. The sector of biological qualification of donations, at the crossroads between mass diagnostic biology and quality control, is perfectly suited to benefit very rapidly from the scientific and technological advances of nanotechnologies. Our response to the advent of cell, tissue and gene therapy involving new types of donations with a multitude of a new characterization tests, and to the difficulties raised by cellular expansion and by the absolute necessity of responding to the emergence of new infectious agents, is intimately linked to the evolution of testing methods. Progress in nanotechnologies offers the promise of total or partial integration of testing procedures in miniature devices called biochips or lab-on-chip devices. These devices will be the standard tools of biologists and biochemists of the future. A new era is about to open for the biological qualification of donations, for transfusion activities and for biology in general.

References

1. *Les nanotechnologies : la maîtrise de l'infiniment petit*. Rapport du Conseil de la Science et de la Technologie du Gouvernement du Québec, 2001.
2. « Nanotech Report », Forbes Inc. & Angstrom Publishing LCC, 2002, www.forbesnanotech.com.
3. Lorrain JL, Raoul D. *Nanosciences et progrès medical*. Rapport N° 293, Office Parlementaire d'Evaluation des Choix Scientifiques et Techniques, mai 2004.
4. Arrêté du 10 septembre 2003 portant homologation du règlement de l'Agence française de sécurité sanitaire des produits de santé définissant les principes de bonnes pratiques dont doivent se doter les établissements de transfusion sanguine.
5. Référentiel national de l'Établissement français du sang, applicable au 31/12/2004.
6. Pillonel J, Le Marrec N, Girault A, et al. Epidemiological surveillance of blood donors and residual risk of blood-borne infections in France, 2001 to 2003. *Transfus Clin Biol* 2005 ; 14 (in press).
7. Pillonel J, Laperche S. Trends in risk of transfusion-transmitted viral infections (HIV, HCV, HBV) in France between 1992 and 2003 and impact of nucleic acid testing (NAT). *Euro Surveill* 2005 ; 10 (in press).
8. Laperche S, Elghouzzi MH, Morel P, et al. Is an assay for simultaneous detection of hepatitis C virus core antigen and antibody a valuable alternative to NAT? *Transfusion* 2005 (in press).
9. Morel P, Deschaseaux M, Naegelen C, et al. Bacterial detection leading to pathogens inactivation. *Transfus Clin Biol* 2005 ; 12 : 142-9.
10. Dodd RY. Emerging infections, transfusion safety, and epidemiology. *N Engl J Med* 2003 ; 349 : 1205-6.
11. Charrel RN, de Lamballerie X, Durand JP, et al. Prevalence of antibody against West Nile virus in volunteer blood donors living in Southeastern France. *Transfusion* 2001, 41 : 1320-1.
12. Papadopoulos MC, Abel PM, Agranoff D, et al. A novel and accurate diagnostic test for human African trypanosomiasis. *Lancet* 2004 ; 363 : 1358-63.
13. Hoummady M, et al. *BioMEMS et Nanotechnologies*. Rapport SMM04-079, Ambassade de France à Tokyo, Sept. 2004.

14. Chen Y, et al. *In situ* bio functionalization and cell adhesion in microfluidic devices. *Microelectr Engineer* 2005 : 78-9.
15. Andersson H, Van Den Berg A. Microfluidic devices for cellomics : a review. *Sensors & Actuators* B 92, 2003.

Ex vivo Production of Blood Cells: the Role of Erythrocytes

Luc Douay, Marie-Catherine Giarratana

Access to additional sources of red blood cells for blood transfusion holds great interest given chronic insufficiency of supplies, lack of availability of certain phenotypes, occasional inadequacy of transfusion means, limited indication for oxygen transporters (perfluorocarbides) and the disappointing results obtained with stabilized or recombinant hemoglobins. For all these reasons, it makes ample sense to try to generate erythroid cells *in vitro* by amplification of hematopoietic stem cells originating in blood cells or placental cells.

This procedure has a double objective: first, to generate massive proliferation of hematopoietic stem cells in order to reach production levels of 1 to 4×10^{12} cells and second, to obtain complete terminal maturation, that is, a stage of mature and functional red blood cells.

The challenge also consists of establishing experimental conditions compatible with clinical requirements.

Access to Blood Stem Cells

Development of techniques for the selection of immature hematopoietic progenitors, and our knowledge of growth factors applicable specifically to certain cell lineages, have made possible *ex vivo* production of blood stem cell populations for transplantation purposes (progenitors or stem cells).

Cytapheresis allows easy harvesting of large quantities of CD34$^+$ (4 to 8×10^6 CD34$^+$/kg) progenitors through mobilisation by the granulocyte-colony-stimulating factor (G-CSF).

Umbilical cord blood has certain advantages compared to the other two sources; it is particularly rich in immature progenitors:

– blood from a single cord contains enough hematopoietic progenitors to allow graft take in children and sometimes in adults;

– these progenitors generate *in vitro* colonies of larger and larger size, and have a greater capacity for expansion.

These cells can be amplified from the proliferation of a very small number of stem cells, whether they are derived from red blood cells, marrow or placenta.

Present State of Knowledge

One of the major characteristics of the human red blood cell consists in the fact that it is the only cell with a prolonged life span (120 days) despite absence of a nucleus.

Enucleation mechanisms are presumed [1-3] but have not been formally established given the absence of experimental conditions allowing massive generalization of red blood cells *ex vivo*. Such conditions would have to satisfy three requirements:
- massive amplification of primitive hematopoietic stem cells;
- controlled induction of exclusive differentiation toward erythroid cells;
- completion of terminal maturation up to the enucleated cell stage.

Although it appears to be easy to obtain almost complete erythroid differentiation [4-7], the literature reporting on experiments conducted in different culture systems reveals either considerable cell proliferation without terminal maturation [8-10], or attainment of enucleation in nearly half the cells, but with reduced amplification [10].

Generation of Erythroid Precursors

We described earlier a protocol [11] for hematopoietic stem cell expansion from cord blood, in a conditioned medium without stroma, and with subsequent addition of growth factors. Starting with $CD34^+$ cells, the protocol achieves massive cell production (amplification up to 200,000 times); this is pure erythroid precursor production (95% to 99%) containing hemoglobin F. Contrary to what happens in these conditions *ex vivo* in the presence of growth factors alone, these progenitors/precursors injected into immunodeficient NOD-SCID mice can continue to proliferate *in vivo*, and can differentiate in four days to the terminal enucleated cell stage, with production of adult hemoglobin (HbA), confirming the major role of the microenvironment in erythroid terminal differentiation.

Hematopoiesis *in vivo* in adult humans is obtained through a dynamic process of production located in the bone marrow, starting with a small number of blood stem cells, based on a cellular hierarchy built on a pyramidal model (stem cell, progenitor, mature cell compartments) [12], in close contact with the microenvironment [13-15]. Stromal cells play a crucial role in the secretion of soluble regulation factors, and as extracellular matrix cells. Intercellular contacts and soluble factors responsible for activation or inhibition are key factors in hematopoiesis regulation [16].

Reproducing Microenvironmental Conditions

On the basis of this data, we designed a three-phase cell expansion and differentiation protocol of $CD34^+$ cells of blood cell, bone marrow and umbilical cord origin [17]:
- a first phase of cell proliferation and erythroid differentiation induction in liquid culture, with stem cell factor (SCF), interleukin -3 (IL3) and erythropoietin (Epo) [14, 18];
- a second phase, based on a microenvironment reconstitution model (stromal murine MS5 line) with Epo only;
- a third phase, with stromal cells only, without growth factors [19, 20].

Generating Enucleated Red Blood Cells

At day 15, this conditioned medium cell culture system without serum, which recapitulates *ex vivo* the existing *in vivo* environment [21], attains a mean cell amplification plateau level of 16,500 times (9,200 to 25,500) for CD34$^+$ cells from bone marrow or peripheral blood, 31,200 times (23,700 to 34,000) for cells from leukopheresis mobilised by G-CSF, and 140,000 times (93,000 to 277,000) for cells from cord blood.

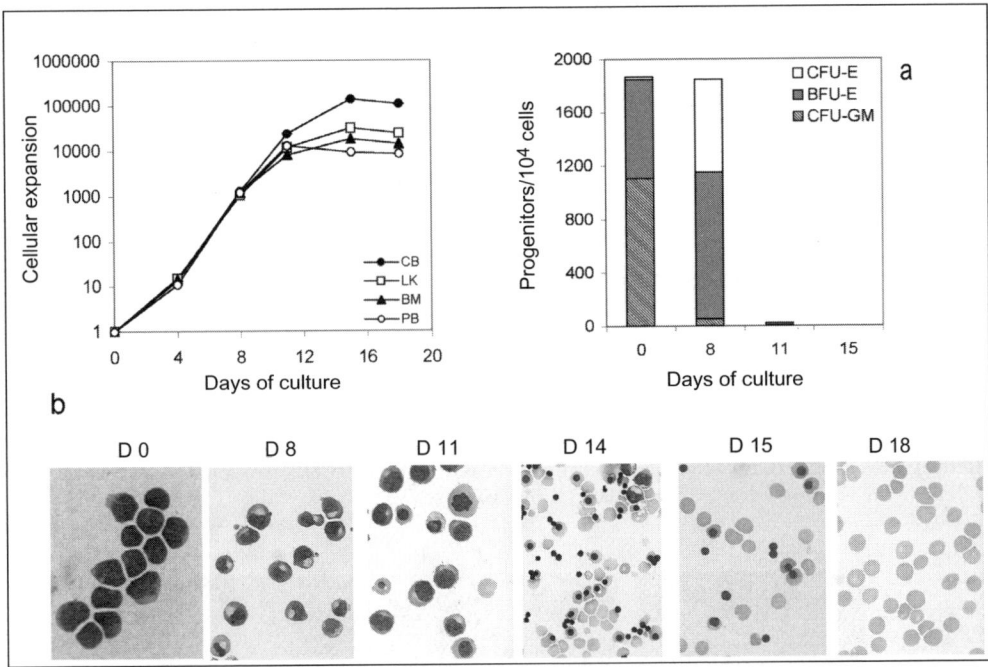

Figure 1. Erythroid proliferation and differentiation in culture: a) cells from cord blood (CB), from bone marrow (BM), from peripheral blood (PB) or from cytapheresis (LK); b) erythroid differentiation from day 0 to day 18.

Differentiation toward erythroid lineage is apparent from day 8 (95% to 98% of erythroblasts). Subsequently, terminal differentiation is rapid, as shown by the fact that the proportion of enucleated cells is 1-5% at day 11, 65-80% at day 15. At this stage, 98±1% of cells are reticulocytes, with a mean red blood cell volume of 130±5 fl, mean corpuscular hemoglobin concentration of 18±1%, and mean corpuscular hemoglobin of 23± –1pg.

Reticulocyte maturation into adult red blood cells takes place between day 15 and day 18, as demonstrated by the disappearance of nucleic material on the one hand, and progressive negativation of CD 71, receptor of transferrin and laser dye styryl on the other. At this stage, 90% to 100% of cells are enucleated (*Figure 1*).

These red blood cells have characteristics close to those of native RBCs, with a mean red blood cell volume of 113±3 fl, mean corpuscular hemoglobin of 33±2 pg, and mean corpuscular hemoglobin concentration of 29±2%. Cell production at day 18 *versus* day 15 is 77±5%, with a mean reticulocyte ratio of 18±4% (*Figures 2, 3*).

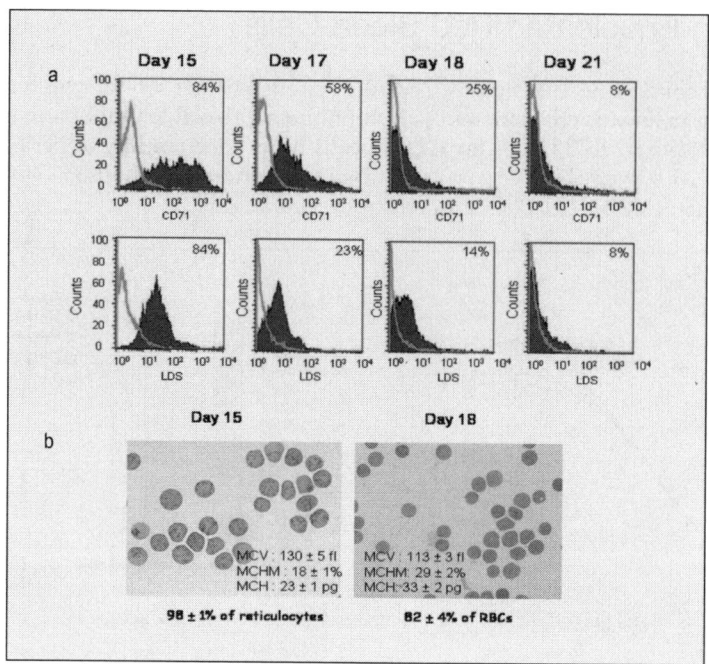

Figure 2. Maturation of red blood cell reticulocytes: a) FACScan analysis of the expression of transferrin receptor (CD71) and of staining by laser dye styril (LDS) from day 15 to day 21; b) brilliant blue staining of day 15 and day 18 reticulocytes.

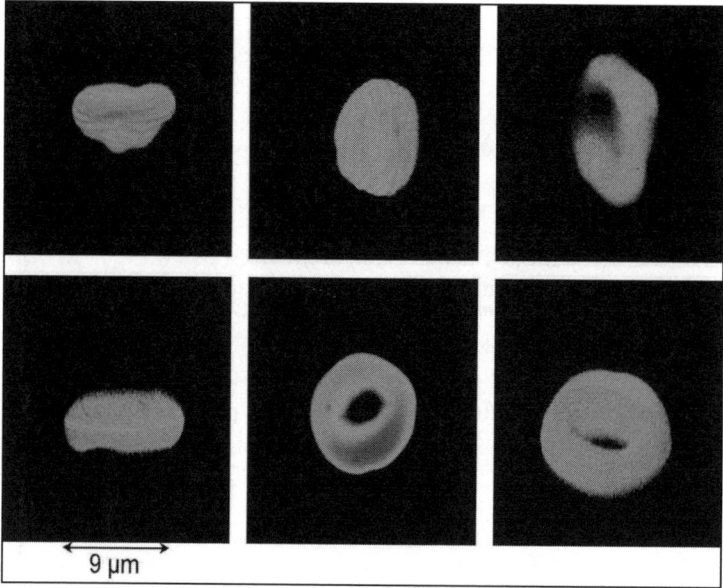

Figure 3. Confocal microscopy image after CFSE staining (carboxyfluorescein diacetate succinimidyl ester); upper row: mature reticulocytes, bottom row: mature red blood cells.

This pure and massive erythroid differentiation can certainly be attributed to targeted induction of erythroid progenitor proliferation (BFU-E and CFU-E) to the detriment of granulo-macrophagic progenitors, all of which disappear rapidly between day 8 and day 11.

The amplification level can be considerably improved if phase 1 is prolonged to day 11, to attain 1.95×10^6 times, 1.22×10^5 times or 1.04×10^5 times, for cord blood, peripheral/cytapheresis blood or bone marrow respectively, while maintaining the level of enucleation (71% to 91%).

Reticulocytes and Functional Red Blood Cells

These reticulocytes and red blood cells have, respectively, glucose-6-phosphate deshydrogenase (G6PD) content and pyruvate-kinase (PK) content of 42 ± 1.4 and 83 ± 1.8 units/g hemoglobin, reflecting the homogenous and young character of cultured cell populations [22]. This demonstrates their ability to reduce glutation and maintain ATP ratio to avoid accumulation of 2-3 diphosphoglycerate (2-3 DPG) that would reduce hemoglobin affinity.

Cell deformability, assessed by ektacytometry, is comparable to that of native red blood cells [23] (*Figure 4*).

Hemoglobin Synthesis Study Model

These culture conditions offer a study model for hemoglobin synthesis. We found that the properties of synthesized hemoglobin depend on the origin of $CD34^+$ cells and on culture conditions.

– Red blood cells produced from adult bone marrow CD34+ cells or from peripheral blood contain hemoglobin A ($95 \pm 2\%$ and $95 \pm 1\%$ respectively), with similar modulation of hemoglobin F ($\gamma A/\gamma G$ ratio: 53/47 and 52/48 respectively).

– Red blood cells produced from $CD34^+$ cord cells contain mainly fetal hemoglobin (HbF) ($64 \pm 13\%$) with partial hemoglobin F modulation (mean $\gamma A/\gamma G$ ratio: 59/41).

Functional Hemoglobin

Functional integrity of the hemoglobin of red blood cells produced *in vitro* was studied by flash photolysis. This hemoglobin behaves like tetrameric hemoglobin, as shown by the cooperation between different subunits validating its allosteric behaviour. It can bind and re-release oxygen just as native hemoglobin would do (*Figure 4*).

P_{50} of cultured red blood cells is 1.2, compared to 1.3 for control red blood cells, with a Hill coefficient of 2.28 and 2.3 respectively. This slight P_{50} difference is due to the presence of hemoglobin F in the cultured product.

Extent of P_{50} reduction in a context of diphosphyglycerate depletion is as expected. Kinetics and balance test results show normal binding capacity (*Figure 5*).

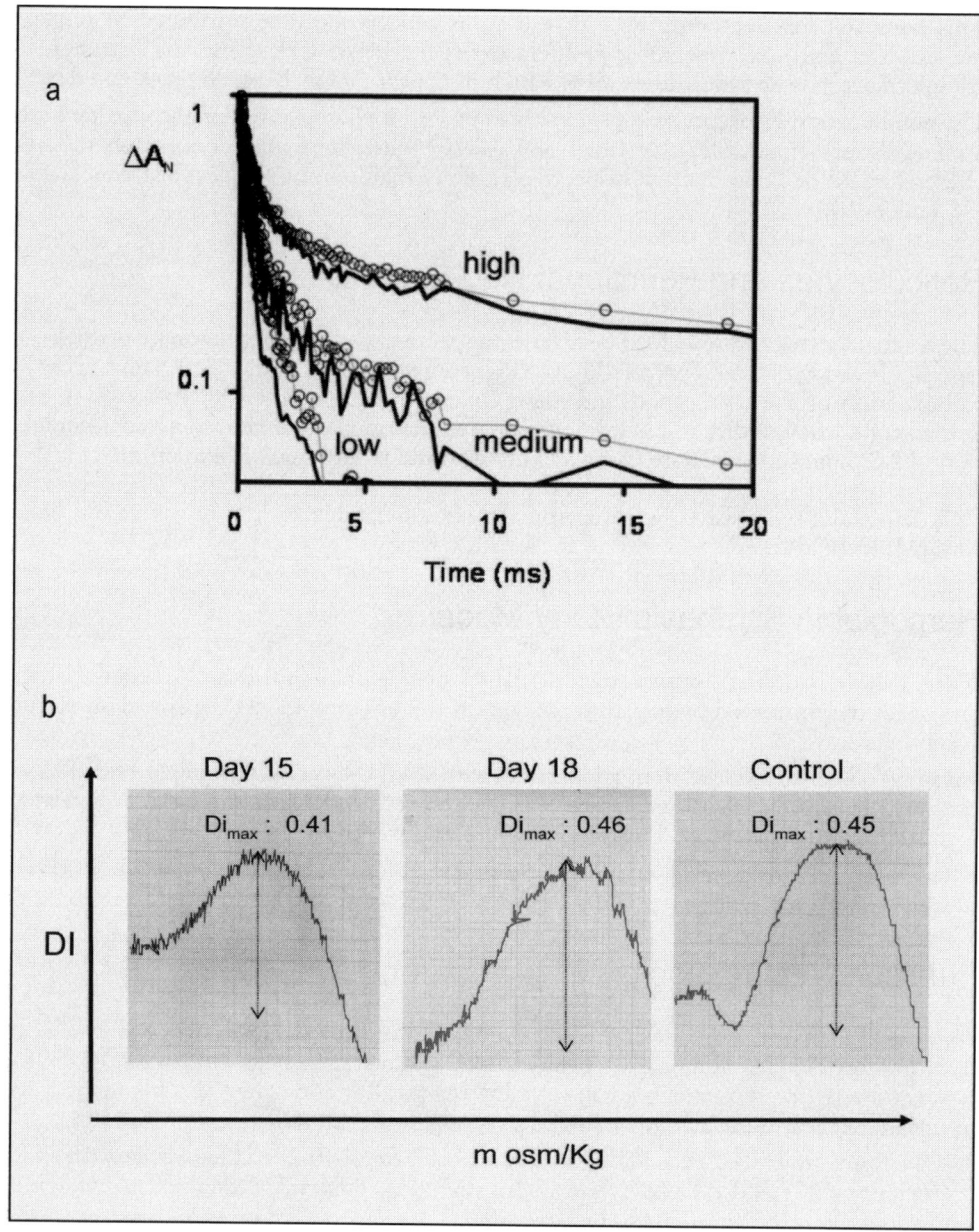

Figure 4. RBC functional integrity: CO binding curve after flash photolysis of red blood cells and of culture and control hemoglobin; b) deformability of reticulocytes studied by osmolar gradient ektacytometry in day 15 reticulocytes and day 18 red blood cells, compared to control red blood cells.

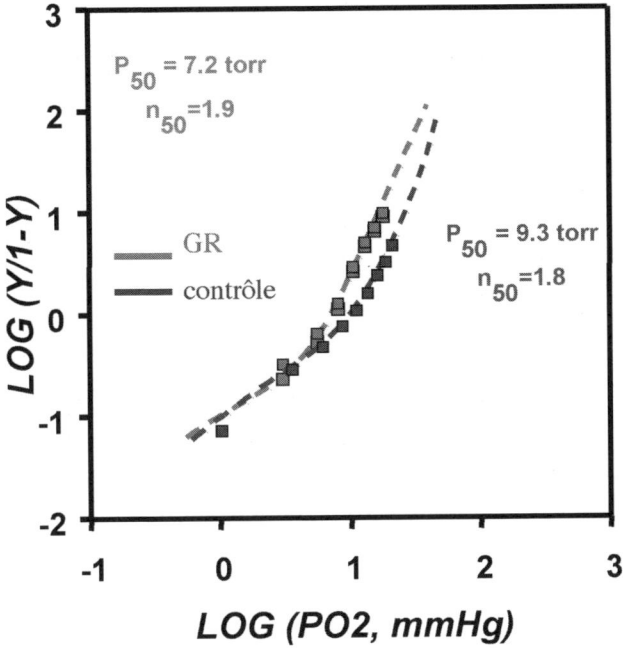

Figure 5. Oxygen dissociation curve.

Expressed Blood Type Antigens

The culture system allows observation of antigens of blood groups like ABO and Rhesus, demonstrating the normal synthesis capacity of surface immunogenic molecules (*Figure 6*).

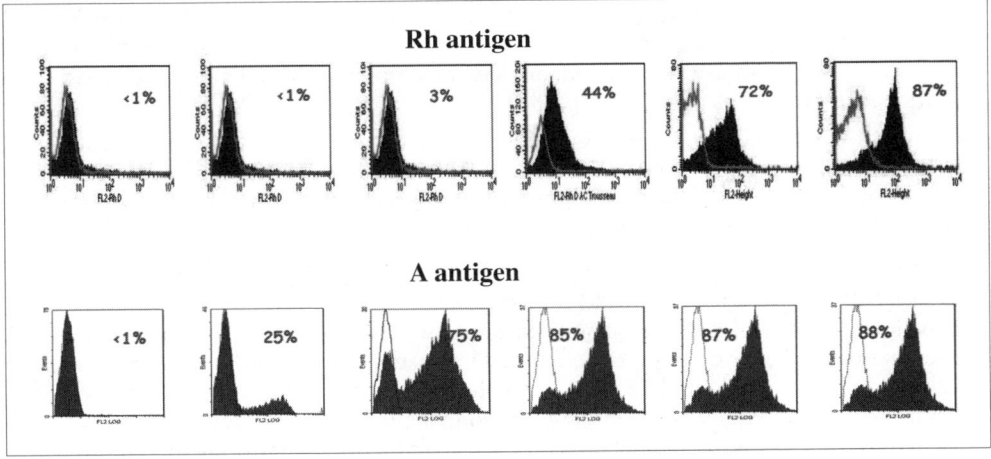

Figure 6. Study of the expression of Rh D and A antigens during erythroid differentiation in culture.

Human Red Blood Cells in NOD/SCID Mice

Reticulocytes generated *ex vivo* from cytapheresis CD34+ were stained with carboxyfluorescein diacetate succinimidyl (CFSE) and administered by intraperitoneal injection to NOD/SCID mice.

These blood cells function exactly like native human blood cells in blood circulation. CFSE+ cells are observed for three days in both cases. Reticulocytes transfused *in vivo* mature into red blood cells, as shown by the appearance of CFSE+/LDS cells: 36%±5%, 63±7% at day 1 and day 2 respectively. Remarkably, over 90% of CFSE+ cells mature into blood cells at day 3. Detection of Ag RhD at the surface of red blood cells confirms the human origin of CFSE+ cells.

Within the limits of the model, these results show normal behaviour of cultured red blood cells compared to native cells.

Thus, this protocol conducted in a conditioned medium without serum allows both massive expansion of hematopoietic CD34+ stem/progenitor cells and complete differentiation up to perfectly functional mature blood cells. These cells survive *in vivo* in NOD/SCID mice, just like human blood cells from peripheral circulation. This model opens multiple perspectives in both cognitive research on erythropoiesis and the field of clinical transfusion.

At this stage, we have to design production procedures compatible with Good Manufacturing Practice (GMP) requirements, particularly in order to escape the confines of the cellular microenvironment by reproducing its features in a conditioned acellular milieu.

Properties of a Production Model Compatible with Clinical Requirements

In order to develop such a protocol, we have identified a number of critical parameters allowing fulfilment of the two essential requirements: massive amplification of the erythroid compartment and total precursor enucleation. Observations made in different culture conditions identified three major elements indispensable for developing reproducible red blood cell production conditions:

– the target erythrocyte population must have cellular contact with the microenvironment, but this contact must be of limited duration. This suggests a mechanism based on signal transduction rather than on expulsed nucleus macrophagy, which has been considered essential until now;

– maintaining microenvironments of different origins (bone marrow, human stromal lines, murine stromal lines, autologous or allogeneic human mesenchymal cells) throughout the duration of the culture avoids apoptosis. In cultures without serum, growth factors alone cannot replace the microenvironment;

– the Epo can be removed toward the end of the culture to allow enucleation. This observation contradicts the hypothesis of the Epo as a terminal maturation factor.

We believe that it will become possible to dispense with the cellular microenvironment, while retaining the anti-apoptotic effect and the enucleation-inducing signal seen in conditions of co-culture, and to establish culture conditions allowing cell survival in a conditioned milieu. Analysis of this data should make it possible to identify the parameters involved in the process, in view of replacing the cellular microenvironment: adhesion protein(s), growth factor(s), anti-apoptotic factor(s).

Future Outlook and Potential Applications

This type of approach can have applications in several fields.

Blood Transfusion

This technology will make possible massive generation *ex vivo*, from hematopoietic stem cells, of erythroid precursors or of functional blood cells. Theoretically, blood cell production for transfusion purposes is feasible with this method: that is, quantities that could be produced are compatible with clinical requirements (a standard blood cell concentrate contains about 2×10^{12} red blood cells). Two transfusional products are possible: erythroid precursors and mature red blood cells.

Erythroid Precursor Transfusion

In addition to the fact that precursors obtained at day 10 can be frozen without losing their proliferative properties, several factors speak in favour of possible clinical use:

– 10^6 CD34$^+$ cells (the equivalent of a quarter or a third of a standard umbilical cord) can be amplified 5,000 to 10,000 times after ten days of culture, producing from 5 to 10×10^9 cells that will continue to amplify *in vivo* after transfusion, giving a final quantity of 5 to 10×10^{11} red blood cells, the equivalent of three or four red blood cell concentrates from a standard umbilical cord, harvested in conditions identical to those of graft banks (2 to 5×10^6 CD34$^+$);

– there is no concomitant amplification of contaminant parent cells; lymphocytic B CD19$^+$ or T CD3$^+$ cells are undetectable (<0.1%; only very low levels of class I HLA molecules and HLA-DR molecules are expressed by a small percentage of cells (1.4% and 3.4% respectively);

– the quantity of residual leukocytes in the amplified product at day 10 is from 3 to 50 times lower than that in a standard non leukodepleted product. In fact, if 10^6 CD34$^+$ are amplified 6,000 to 10,000 times at day 10, with a ratio of 1% to 10% of residual leukocytes, 6×10^7 to 1×10^9 leukocytes will be reinjected to the patient. Moreover, it should be noted that freezing of the final product will cause nucleated granular cell loss of the order of 2 logs, bringing the final quantity of leukocytes to a level of about 2 to 3×10^7. This quantity is to be compared to 2 to 3×10^9 residual leukocytes in a standard non leukodepleted concentrate, and to the 1×10^6 cells in a leukodepleted concentrate;

– umbilical cord blood is an easily available source of hematopoietic stem cells.

Thus, we can foresee the creation of umbilical cord blood banks for phenotypes of particular interest to transfusion, such as rare blood types.

Transfusion of Mature Red Blood Cells

Given that G-CSF mobilised cytapheresis usually produces from 4 to 8×10^6 CD34$^+$/kg and that amplification levels are 3×10^4 times, with 95% enucleation, the equivalent of several concentrates of red blood cells can be produced from a single harvesting.

Clinical Outlook for These New Labile Blood Products

These products could find their greatest usefulness in situations where transfusion can fail to provide a solution. These situations occur in two circumstances: rare erythrocytic phenotypes and anti-erythrocytic poly-immunisation.

- **A rare phenomenon** is characterized by the absence of a high frequency antigen on red blood cells. A subject with a rare phenotype can produce antibodies directed against the absent antigen of his red blood cells *via* transfusion or pregnancy. Therefore, this subject must receive concentrates of identical rare red blood cells. These red blood cell concentrates are stored frozen at the National Bank of Rare Phenotypes. However, depending on demand, reserves are not always sufficient. This is true notably for rare particularities found only in African-Caribbean populations, such as certain rare phenotypes of the Rh group (Rh: –18; Rh: –34), or blood types characterized by the absence of expression of MNS5 (U) high frequency antigen. The problem is aggravated by the fact that it occurs in populations where repeated transfusions could be necessary, especially in the course of sickle cell anemia. Therefore, it could be proposed that rare blood reserves be constituted for these patients, either from adult donors with the same rare phenotype, or from placental blood stored in a rare phenotype placental blood bank.
- **Poly-immunisation** situations in a whole population are a second application. The situation of a subject immunized for a large number of antigens is like that of rare blood types, in that units compatible with all the antibodies produced are infrequent. To solve this problem, we could produce red blood cells using the patient's own $CD34^+$ cells, given that in these cases the patient is the best prospective "donor".
- This possible new labile blood product is also promising in terms of **transfusional efficiency**. It could make it possible to transfuse blood cells homogenous in age, whose life span should be close to 120 days, compared to the 28-day average half-life of red blood cells from a donor, due to the presence of red blood cells of variable ages. This would decrease the number of transfusions and would lighten inevitable iron overload, which is a major complication in polytransfused patients.

Moreover, a red blood cell culture has no leukocytes, offering two advantages as a result:
– improvement of red blood cell storage at 4 °C without cytokines re-released by nascent leukocytes,
– reduction of residual risk of anti-HLA allo-immunization in subjects poly-transfused with cultured red blood cells.

Hemoglobinopathies

Ex vivo synthesis of hemoglobin F from umbilical cord blood is obviously related to culture conditions, since we have shown [11] that erythroblastic progenitors/precursors obtained after ten days of culture in the absence of a microenvironment produce, *in vivo*, after transfusion into NOD/SCID mice, mature blood cells containing 96% functional hemoglobin A with complete hemoglobin F modulation ($\gamma A/\gamma G$ ratio: 35/65). Therefore, our model is a new tool to decipher cellular and molecular mechanisms of hemoglobin switch.

In vitro stimulation of hemoglobin F expression in sickle cell anemia subjects is an interesting therapeutic approach. In fact, this hemoglobin F activation should reduce hemoglobin S polymerisation.

As a result, we could obtain an autologous transfusion product modified *ex vivo* so as to amplify specifically hemoglobin F synthesis.

Infectious Pathologies

This erythroid differentiation model could constitute a new, simple tool for the study of the reproductive cycle of certain infectious agents like *Plasmodium*, in order to develop new medicinal products or antimalarial vaccines [19]. The limited life span of human red blood cells injected into SCID mice requires complex preparation of the recipient model (splenectomy, irradiation, medication…) [9, 16, 21, 24]. Other teams have achieved isolation of murine reticulocytes [8] or of reticulocytes from patients with hematological pathologies [7]. This *in vitro* model is easy to set up and avoids the complexities of the *in vivo* model.

A New Drug Vector

Red blood cells naturally have ideal biodistribution and no longer divide. Properties of this kind could be utilized to transform these cells into therapeutic vectors of a new type. In fact, before erythroid differentiation induction, progenitors could be genetically manipulated to produce cytoplasmic or membrane proteins whose action would be voluntarily limited in duration, for therapeutic purposes.

Perspectives

In the near future, human embryonic stem cells, with their unlimited proliferative potential, could become an attractive alternative source for cellular engineering. At present, researchers are already reporting a rate of differentiation of human embryonic stem cells toward blood CD34$^+$ cells as high as 20%.

In vitro differentiation of embryonic stem cells toward erythroid lineage could eventually allow mass production of red blood cells.

Conclusion

We have described a method of producing large numbers of human mature red blood cells from hematopoietic stem cells of various origins, cultivated *ex vivo*.

This new concept of "cultured red blood cells" is useful for the fundamental analysis of terminal erythropoiesis mechanisms, not yet completely characterized, and for the understanding of hemoglobin synthesis, which remains a mystery.

The next step is certainly that of designing culture conditions adapted to mass production of red blood cells. Such approaches are now feasible thanks to perfusion bioreactors [25, 26] that make it possible to raise the initial concentration by a log, and to enhance the culture surface by a log, by means of microspheres.

The possibility of large scale cultivation of human mesenchymal stem cells [27] allows us to go beyond the constraints of xenogenic culture conditions and to develop GMP mass production conditions.

In conclusion, this approach is useful for the fundamental analysis of terminal erythropoiesis mechanisms and for hemoglobin synthesis. Moreover, its numerous clinical applications, particularly in transfusion, can provide considerable benefits.

References

1. Chen CY, Pajak L, Tamburlin J, Bofinger D, Koury ST. The effect of proteasome inhibitors on mammalian erythroid terminal differentiation. *Exp Hematol* 2002 ; 30 : 634-9.
2. Bessis M. Erythroblastic island, functional unity of bone marrow. *Rev Hematol* 1958 ; 13 : 8-11.
3. Lichtman MA. The ultrastructure of the hemopoietic environment of the marrow: a review. *Exp Hematol* 1981 ; 9 : 391-410.
4. Freyssinier JM, et al. Purification, amplification and characterization of a population of human erythroid progenitors. *Br J Haematol* 1999 ; 106 : 912-22.
5. Panzenbock B, Bartunek P, Mapara MY, Zenke M. Growth and differentiation of human stem cell factor/erythropoietin-dependent erythroid progenitor cells in vitro. *Blood* 1998 ; 92 : 3658-68.
6. Fibach E, Manor D, Oppenheim A, Rachmilewitz EA. Proliferation and maturation of human erythroid progenitors in liquid culture. *Blood* 1989 ; 73 : 100-3.
7. Wada H, et al. Expression of major blood group antigens on human erythroid cells in a two phase liquid culture system. *Blood* 1990 ; 75 : 505-11.
8. Von Lindern M, et al. The glucocorticoid receptor cooperates with the erythropoietin receptor and c-Kit to enhance and sustain proliferation of erythroid progenitors in vitro. *Blood* 1999 ; 94 : 550-9.
9. Sui X, et al. Erythropoietin-independent erythrocyte production: signals through gp130 and c-kit dramatically promote erythropoiesis from human CD34+ cells. *J Exp Med* 1996 ; 183 : 837-45.
10. Malik P, et al. An in vitro model of human red blood cell production from hematopoietic progenitor cells. *Blood* 1998 ; 91 : 2664-71.
11. Neildez-Nguyen TM, et al. Human erythroid cells produced ex vivo at large scale differentiate into red blood cells in vivo. *Nat Biotechnol* 2002 ; 20 : 467-72.
12. Ogawa M. Differentiation and proliferation of hematopoietic stem cells. *Blood* 1993 ; 81 : 2844-53.
13. Lemischka IR. Microenvironmental regulation of hematopoietic stem cells. *Stem Cells* 1997 ; 15 (Suppl. 1) : 63-8.
14. Koller MR, Oxender M, Jensen TC, Goltry KL, Smith AK. Direct contact between CD34+lin- cells and stroma induces a soluble activity that specifically increases primitive hematopoietic cell production. *Exp Hematol* 1999 ; 27 : 734-41.
15. Friedenstein AJ, et al. Precursors for fibroblasts in different populations of hematopoietic cells as detected by the in vitro colony assay method. *Exp Hematol* 1974 ; 2 : 83-92.
16. Verfaillie CM. Soluble factor(s) produced by human bone marrow stroma increase cytokine-induced proliferation and maturation of primitive hematopoietic progenitors while preventing their terminal differentiation. *Blood* 1993 ; 82 : 2045-53.
17. Giarratana MC, et al. Cultured human red blood cells as a new milestone in cell engineering. *In press*.
18. Zermati Y, et al. Transforming growth factor inhibits erythropoiesis by blocking proliferation and accelerating differentiation of erythroid progenitors. *Exp Hematol* 2000 ; 28 : 885-94.
19. Sato T, Maekawa T, Watanabe S, Tsuji K, Nakahata T. Erythroid progenitors differentiate and mature in response to endogenous erythropoietin. *J Clin Invest* 2000 ; 106 : 263-70.
20. Dolznig H, et al. Apoptosis protection by the Epo target Bcl-X(L) allows factor-independent differentiation of primary erythroblasts. *Curr Biol* 2002 ; 12 : 1076-85.
21. Suzuki J, Fujita J, Taniguchi S, Sugimoto K, Mori KJ. Characterization of murine hemopoietic-supportive (MS-1 and MS-5) and non-supportive (MS-K) cell lines. *Leukemia* 1992 ; 6 : 452-8.
22. Jansen G, Koenderman L, Rijksen G, Cats BP, Staal GE. Characteristics of hexokinase, pyruvate kinase, and glucose-6-phosphate dehydrogenase during adult and neonatal reticulocyte maturation. *Am J Hematol* 1985 ; 20 : 203-15.

23. Cynober T, Mohandas N, Tchernia G. Red cell abnormalities in hereditary spherocytosis: relevance to diagnosis and understanding of the variable expression of clinical severity. *J Lab Clin Med* 1996 ; 128 : 259-69.
24. Silva M, *et al*. Erythropoietin can promote erythroid progenitor survival by repressing apoptosis through Bcl-XL and Bcl-2. *Blood* 1996 ; 88 : 1576-82.
25. Koller MR, *et al*. Clinical-scale human umbilical cord blood cell expansion in a novel automated perfusion culture system. *Bone Marrow Transplant* 1998 ; 21 : 653-63.
26. Brott DA, Maher RJ, Parrish CR, Richardson RJ, Smith AK. Flow cytometric characterization of perfused human bone marrow cultures: identification of the major cell lineages and correlation with the CFU-GM assay. *Cytometry* 2003 ; 53A : 22-7.
27. Bianchi G, *et al*. Ex vivo enrichment of mesenchymal cell progenitors by fibroblast growth factor 2. *Exp Cell Res* 2003 ; 287 : 98-105.

Cytokines and Erythrocyte and/or Platelet Saving Strategy

Nahed El Kassar, Aline Schmidt-Tanguy,
Marie-Laure Bidet, Norbert Ifrah

The term cytokine refers to a set of heterogenous molecules comprising mainly the interleukins (IL), the interferons and the colony stimulating factors (CSF). These proteic or glycoproteic molecules play a major role in hemopoiesis regulation, immunity and inflammatory response. They act as ligands by binding to their specific receptors. Each cytokine can be expressed by different types of cells. At the same time, receptors can be present on different types of cells, which explains the multiple effects of their ligands. The fact that certain chains are common to several receptors explains the redundancy of some cytokines, if their respective receptors are co-expressed by the same cell.

Certain cytokines, and especially erythropoietin, have acquired an important function in therapeutic practices, where they can replace transfusions or complement them. Erythropoietin, cloned twenty years ago, is used in the treatment of anemia in chronic dialysis patients and cancer-related anemia, as well as for the prevention and treatment of anemia in the context of scheduled surgery. This treatment presents less risk and has longer lasting effects than repeated transfusions of red blood cell concentrates. It is also easier to administer to patients. The granulocyte-colony-stimulating factor (G-CSF), often used to mobilise blood stem cells for transplantation purposes, seems to actualize the beneficial effect of erythropoietin on erythroid progenitors. Thrombopoietin stimulates platelet production and reduces post-chemotherapy thrombocytopenia. Unfortunately, some incidents of immunological thrombocytopenia have slowed the development of this alternative to platelet transfusion.

Erythropoietin has clearly found its place in clinical practice. The uses of thrombopoietin, on the other hand, remain limited. In the sections that follow, we will present the advantages and limitations of these molecules in their major therapeutic applications.

Erythropoietin

Background

Erythropoietin is a glycoprotein secreted by the epithelial cells bordering the peritubular capillaries of the kidneys [1], and marginally by the liver in adults [2]. Its synthesis is regulated by hypoxia [3, 4]. In normal physiological conditions, when available functional hemoglobin rates correspond to tissue oxygen needs, erythropoietin concentrations are low. In case of hypoxia or anemic stress, its production increases considerably and its seric concentration greatly exceeds normal levels. Once it has been produced, erythropoietin is released into the circulation, where it acts exactly like a hormone. In the bone marrow, it bonds to specific erythroid receptors and acts, at a relatively late stage, on colony-forming unit erythroids (CFU-E) and on some of the burst-forming unit erythroids (BFU-E), probably the most differentiated [5]. Erythropoietin receptors belong to group I of the two receptor subgroups, and respond as homodimers to interaction with their ligands. Following this binding, there is activation of JAK tyrosine kinases preassociated with the juxtamembrane region of the cytoplasmic domain of the receptor [6], followed by activation of several signal pathways, particularly those of the STAT transcription factors (signal transducers and activators of transcription) [7]. Enhanced erythroid progenitor survival, proliferation and differentiation is the result of the activation signal and leads to hematocrit increase (HT) [8]. In the absence of erythropoietin, erythroblastic progenitors cannot differentiate into erythroblasts and die by apoptosis.

Red blood cell concentrate transfusions have long been the only option for the treatment of non deficiency anemias of central origin. However, the cloning of the erythropoietin gene in 1985 [9, 10] allowed its use as a recombinant therapy and offered an alternative. Various alfa and beta recombinant molecules are now available on the market [r-HuEPO: epoetin alfa (Eprex®) and beta (Neorecormon®, darbepoetin alfa (Aranesp®)]. Alfa and beta epoetin are produced by the cells of the Chinese hampster (CHO: Chinese ovary cells). Alfa darbepoetin has a longer terminal half-life than that of the r-HuEPO, due to its higher sialic acid content. The use of erythropoietin has made it possible to reduce the risks associated with repeated transfusion. However, certain concerns still exist and careful monitoring of these therapeutic products is a must. Possible disease aggravation has been reported in certain cancers, especially ORL. High costs constitute a public health problem in the area of chronic disorders. Moreover, modulation of doses during treatment, based on response and on thrombotic and hypertensive risk, is indispensable. In case of inadequate response, the causes of resistance to erythropoietin, and above all iron deficiency, must be carefully investigated. For all these reasons, protocols and guidelines have been published. Finally, erythropoietin is also used in the context of scheduled surgery. We will now describe in greater detail the role of erythropoietin in these different applications.

Erythropoietin and Kidney Failure

Recombinant erythropoietin was first introduced in 1989 for the treatment of chronic anemia in dialysis patients with kidney failure. Typically, the anemia is normocytic normochromic and considered the consequence of an inappropriate erythropoietin secretion; degree of anemia is proportional to that of tissue damage and therefore kidney damage [11].

Other factors contribute to the severity of the anemia: inadequate marrow production due to inflammation and aluminium overload caused by anti-acid treatments; and, most of all, iron deficiency associated with dialysis, and with hemorhhage related to telangiectasies, gastrointestinal lesions and platelet dysfunction. Because this anemia leads to left ventricular hypertrophy followed by heart failure, progression was inevitable in these disorders. Repeated transfusion of red blood cells in this setting is associated not only with the usual complications such as iron overload and risk of bacterial and viral transmission, but also with a risk of anti-HLA immunisation that could affect graft survival or the possibility of transplant in dialysis patients. This risk of immunisation and infectious transmission has been reduced by systematic leukodepletion of labile blood products in France (Feb.20, 1998 directive). Very soon after the introduction of erythropoietin, the percentage of dialysis patients receiving transfusions at least once every four months decreased from 16% in 1989 to 3.3% in 1992 [12]. Transfusion of red blood cell concentrates is now reserved for patients with severe symptomatic anemia, and for patients resistant to erythropoietin and presenting a critical hemoglobin level [13].

The first phase I-II clinical trial showing the benefits of erythropoietin treatment in kidney failure was conducted in 1987 [14]. The objective of the treatment was to reach a hematocrit level between 35% and 40%. A second phase III trial followed in 1989; its final objective was a 35% hematocrit level [15]. As a result of these two trials, the American Food and Drug Administration (FDA) approved erythropoietin treatment in June 1989, in view of maintaining hematocrit levels between 30% and 33%, a consensus followed for a long time in most countries. At present, American guidelines for hematocrit are between 33% and 36%, and for hemoglobin between 11g/dl and 12 g/dl [16]. European and Canadian guidelines recommend maintaining hematocrit levels > 33%, and hemoglobin levels > 11g/dl [13, 17]. It is estimated that if this minimum level is reached, the mean hemoglobin level for most patients will be 12 to 12.5 g/dl. Guidelines for intravenous iron administration have also been published [13, 16], given that iron deficiency is one of the causes of erythropoietin treatment failure.

The benefits of anemia control beyond 10 to 11g/dl hemoglobin levels by erythropoietin treatment have been amply demonstrated: decrease of mortality rates and hospitalization risks [18-20], reduction of left ventricular hypertrophy [21-23], improvement of quality of life [24, 25], cognitive function [26] and physiological improvement in dialysis and predialysis patients. Moreover, it has been observed that erythropoietin induces slowing of renal function deterioration in some patients [27, 28]. Two mechanisms have been invoked to explain this effect: first, that better oxygenation of ischemic tissue reduces endothelial lesions; and second, that there is suppression of angiotensin and aldosterone, both hormones being known to play a role in fibrosis and tissue lesions.

The 1999 European guidelines recommend erythropoietin doses of 50 to 150 IU/kg/week (4,000 to 8,000 IU/week) administered in three subcutaneous or intravenous injections [13]. As far as Eprex® is concerned, only intravenous administration is used for patients with kidney failure. Subcutaneous injections have been contraindicated in France since December 2002 because of the occurrence of several cases of erythroblastopenia (see Erythropoietin Treatment and Erythroblastopenia).

Erythropoietin treatment has given rise to other complications. Hypertension or destabilized blood pressure has occurred in 23% of patients [13]. The reasons are not clear, since erythropoietin does not cause hypertension in patients with normal renal function. In addition, particular care should be taken to counter the risk of arteriovenous dialysis fistula thrombosis or renal graft thrombosis. There is a 7.5% risk of this nature in these patients [16]. This risk is considered a high, but it is difficult to evaluate the risk in a similar group of patients without erythropoietin [16].

Erythropoietin in Solid Tumor and Malignant Hematopathy Management (except Myelodysplasias) and after Transplantation

In cancer patients, anemia is often of diverse origins, including chemotherapy or radiotherapy-related myelosuppression, postoperative or cancer-related hemorrhage, or chronic inflammation. However, at the physiological level, anemia is, above all, associated with inadequate erythropoietin response and inadequate iron metabolization, leading to erythropoiesis suppression.

A pilot study conducted in 1990 [29] confirmed erythropoietin efficacy in this setting through numerous hemoglobin level, transfusion requirement and, more recently, quality of life investigations. In a recent publication, these studies were reviewed and analysed in order to arrive at consensus rules applicable on a European scale [30]. Confirmed efficacy in terms of hemoglobin levels was observed in patients with anemia, whether chemotherapy induced, chronic illness related or secondary to allogeneic marrow transplant. However, these studies showed hemoglobin threshold at the start of treatment to be variable. In most cases, treatment was started at a hemoglobin level ≤ 10.5 g/dl, but no study has compared treatment benefits with initial hemoglobin levels. Similarly, no study has compared the achieved objective – a 12 to 13g/dl hemoglobin level – with clinical improvement. Transfusion requirements for patients with chemotherapy induced anemia were also reduced (20%). Patient with this type of anemia or with chronic anemia refractory to standard doses of erythropoietin responded to dose increases (8% to 18% response increase). However, no study has tested the effect of simply prolonguing treatment without changing the dose. Quality of life improvement was demonstrated in patients who responded to erythropoietin, but no conclusive results on survival were obtained. Certain studies showed that administration of darbepoetin alfa once a week to patients with postchemotherapy anemia, or to prevent cancer-related anemia, was also effective. Clinical and biological factors predictive of response to treatment were also found: low erythropoietin seric concentration (<100 mU/ml), age inferior to 60 and ≥ 9 g/dl hemoglobin were the most significant. A correlation was established between low erythropoietin seric level and clinical response for lymphomas, but not for solid tumors. The desirability of establishing fixed chemotherapy dosages from the start was reported, with maintenance doses to be determined case by case. In terms of side effects, erythroblastopenia risk did not appear to be high, but just as with renal failure, there is a slight but significant risk of thromboembolism (RR = 1.55) and hypertension increase [30].

The European guidelines adopted recommend instituting erythropoietin treatment as soon as hemoglobin levels drop below 9-10 g/dl, with or without transfusions, for four to six weeks, at fixed doses if the weight of the patient is not at one extreme or another. The goal is a 12-13 g/dl hemoglobin level, and erythropoietin administration is to be adjusted on an individual basis after the initial four-to-six week period. The dose of epoetin alfa is usually 40,000 IU/week, but can be reduced to 30,000 IU/week; the dose of darbepoetin can be reduced to 2.5 ug/kg/week. At present, there is no indication for erythropoietin as preventive treatment in these patients [30].

We should, however, note that there have been recent indications of deleterious effects of erythropoietin on the survival of patients with ORL cancer treated with radiotherapy [31], or metastatic breast cancer treated with chemotherapy [32]. In the first study, patients treated with epoetin beta had significantly increased hem oglobin levels, but also significant local disease progression and a decrease in overall survival as well as disease-free survival [31]. The second study describes increased mortality of patients treated with epoetin alfa, in the four months following the start of treatment [32]. However, the authors point out problems with study design and analysis of results.

The two studies have been examined by the American FDA and the Oncology Drugs Advisory Committee (ODAC). No definite conclusions as to the effect of erythropoietin on tumor proliferation were drawn, and new studies were requested. Nevertheless, in France, for these reasons and following critical analysis of data in the scientific literature, it has been decided that erythropoietin is not a therapeutic option for tumors treated with radiotherapy alone, and that recourse to transfusion is recommended in case of anemia [33].

Erythropoietin and Myelodysplasias

Because of its anti-apoptotic effect, erythropoietin is potentially the indication of choice for the treatment of myelodysplasic syndromes. However, a first meta-analysis of 205 patients with myelodysplasic syndromes showed a rate of response of only 17% [34]. In a randomised Italian study, 37% of patients with a low-risk myelodysplasic syndrome (patients with refractory anemia and patients without transfusion requirements) responded to erythropoietin treatment *versus* 11% in the placebo group [35]. Subsequently, Hellstrom-Lindberg *et al.* established criteria making it possible to predict response to erythropoietin. Patients with <500 U/l seric erythropoietin levels and transfusion needs of <2 red blood cell concentrates monthly had good response, patients with seric erythropoietin levels of > 500 U/l and transfusion needs of > 2 red blood cell concentrates/month had poor response, and patients with one of the two criteria had intermediary response [36]. Recent studies have shown the benefits of combining G-CSF and erythropoietin for patients with myelodysplasia [37, 38]. In a first non randomised study, patients with myelodysplasia and a <10 g/dl hemoglobin levels or anemia requiring transfusions, with good/intermediary erythropoietin response scores, were treated with a combination of G-CSF and an initial dose of 10,000 IU five times/week of epoetin beta, gradually reduced to the minimal effective dose. Forty-two percent of patients participating in the study responded to treatment; of the total number, 61% showed good response and 15% showed intermediary response. Average response duration was twenty-three months. In patients with good response, quality of life improvement was seen [38]. In the Casadevall *et al.* study, after randomisation, patients with good response to erythropoietin received epoetin alfa and G-CSF at doses of 30,000 IU three times weekly *versus* transfusions alone, for twelve weeks. At that point, G-SCF treatment was stopped and good-response patients continued to receive erythropoietin for twelve weeks. Nearly 42% of patients responded to the combination of the two cytokines. Half the patients relapsed when G-CSF treatment was stopped, but all patients responded to the reintroduction of treatment. Contrary to the previous study, there was no quality of life improvement in patients responding to treatment, but it was not possible to collect over half the data at the end of the study. Cost of treatment tripled for patients treated with cytokines [37]. Darbepoetin alfa also proved to be effective when administered by injection once a week to patients with myelodysplasia [39].

Despite the proven efficacy of G-CSF, particular attention must be paid to the recently described risk of thrombopenia induced by this treatment, particularly because myelodysplasia is responsible for pancytopenia. In effect, in a retrospective study comparing two G-CSF molecules, filgrastim and lenograstim, in healthy donors subjected to peripheral stem cell mobilisation, transient 90×10^9/l trombopenia was observed in all donors [40].

Preoperative Homologous Blood Saving Strategy and Erythropoietin Strategy in a Perisurgical Setting

At present, we estimate that 20% of moderately anemic patients are scheduled for surgery involving sufficient blood loss to require a transfusion. When estimated transfusion needs are two or three units of blood, as is the case for orthopedic surgery, preoperative hemoglobin count determines the need for transfusion. Preplanned autologous transfusion is one of the main techniques of saving homologous blood. Preplanned autologous transfusion is effective because it reduces homologous transfusion, even though it increases overall transfusion risk (autologous and homologous taken together), as confirmed by the meta-analysis performed by Forgie [41]. This type of transfusion is also beneficial to the patient because it produces three or four times less undesirable effects than homologous blood transfusion. However, preplanned autologous transfusion increases the risk of preoperative anemia and therefore the need of perioperative or postoperative transfusion. Preplanned autologous transfusion also causes serious iron deficiency, since 1 ml of red blood cells corresponds to 1 mg of iron. The advantages of erythropoietin treatment in surgical transfusion practice have been demonstrated both in the presence and absence of preplanned autologous transfusion. In the Goodnough et al. study, administration of a dose of 600 IU/kg/week of erythropoietin for two to three weeks before surgery, to non anemic patients registered in a preplanned autologous transfusion program, made it possible to increase the number of units and the volume of autologous red blood cell concentrates collected [42]. However, in other studies, including the previous trial, erythropoietin treatment did not succeed in reducing the percentage of patients exposed to homologous transfusion [42-44]. In 1996, a large multicentric trial demonstrated the benefits of erythropoietin in a group of patients with hemoglobin levels between 10 and 13 g/dl, registered in a preplanned autologous transfusion program [45]. Twenty-eight percent of these patients received homologous blood in the placebo group, as opposed to 14% in the erythropoietin group, placing patients with initial hemoglobin levels between 10 and 13 g/dl in the same situation as patients with initial hemoglobin levels of ≥ 13 g/dl. Conversely, erythropoietin proved to be insufficient to limit exposure to homologous blood in patients with hemoglobin levels of ≤ 10 g/dl [45]. Other studies without preplanned autologous transfusion programs confirmed the existence of an ideal hemoglobin range for erythropoietin action [46].

The action of a weekly dose of erythropoietin started three weeks before the surgery, and a dose on the day of surgery (2,400 IU/kg total subcutaneous dose) has proven as effective as daily injections from D-10 to D+5 (4,500 IU/kg total subcutaneous dose) [47]. Each erythropoietin injection increases hematocrit by 2%. However, red blood cell regeneration is much more significant after the third injection, because marrow production is slowed compared to the first injections. None of these studies showed increased risk of hypertension or of thrombo-embolic complications in patients treated with erythropoietin [48]. At present, only the marketing of Eprex® is approved for orthopedic perioperative use, for patients with hemoglobin levels between 10 and 13 g/dl, without iron deficiency, administered subcutaneously at doses of 40,000 IU weekly. Two to four injections maximum are administered, starting three weeks before surgery, not exceeding a 15 g/dl hemoglobin level, and accompanied by 200 mg/day orally administered iron [48]. Planned autologous transfusion will be performed if needed, depending on the patient's preoperative hematocrit and on foreseeable blood loss. Given that some patients will no longer need planned autologous transfusion, erythropoietin injections will not be more costly than a preplanned autologous transfusion program (427 euros/40,000 IU), patients will not have to make medical visits or undergo serologic testing, and will not be exposed to the risks of autologous transfusion (assignment errors, infection). For patients with <10 g/dl hemoglobin levels, and who need five or six units of blood, erythropoietin is not sufficient to avoid exposure to homologous blood. Finally, other alternatives to transfusion exist: erythro-apheresis when hemoglobin levels are above 13 g/dl; and perioperative blood recovery.

Erythropoietin Treatment and Erythroblastopenia

Between 1988 and 1998, immune origin erythroblastopenia was reported in three patients receiving epoetin [49, 50]. Between 1998 and 2004, 175 new cases related to Eprex® treatment, eleven cases related to Neocormon® treatment and five cases related to Epogen® (epoetin alfa) were reported [51-53]. In almost all cases, the indication for erythropoietin treatment was renal failure, and administration was subcutaneous. Most cases were described in Canada, with a peak of incidence in 2002. In France, Spain and England incidence peak occurred in 2001. Since then, incidence has decreased by 83%. Immunogenicity of the product has been attributed to several factors, including the conservation agent, storage and mode of administration. In 1998, due to the risk of transmission of the Creutzfelt-Jakob variant, human serum albumin was replaced, as an epoetin alfa conservation agent, by a new, presumably more immunogenic agent - which could explain the increased incidence of erythroblastopenia after this date. Subcutaneous administration was also blamed. Absence of this complication in cancer patients could be due to their immunosuppression status and perhaps to shorter exposure to the medication. Presence of anti-erythroblast antibodies was shown in 25% of cases in the same laboratory. Erythroblastopenia was responsible for a rapid drop in hemoglobin, making transfusions necessary. Most patients responded to corticosteroid, endoxan, ciclosporin or intravenous immunoglobulin treatment. In a number of cases, epoetin treatment was repeated successfully and it was even possible to perform a kidney transplant in twenty of these patients. Therefore, present guidelines recommend intravenous administration of epoetin alfa when the conservation agent is not human serum albumin, and when anemia is due to kidney failure [51]. Moreover, a group of international hematology experts has established a set of criteria for diagnosing erythroblastopenia associated with erythropoietin [54].

Thrombopoietin

Background

A common abnormality, thrombopenia can occur in very diverse settings such as cancer or malignant hemopathy, following chemotherapy or blood stem cell transplantation, hepatopathy, idiopathic thrombopenic purpura, or HIV infection. Platelet transfusion, the only current emergency treatment, can cause allo-immunisation that can, in turn, be responsible for unsuccessful transfusion; or produce post-transfusion reactions and infectious agent contamination. The quantity of available blood products can also be a limiting factor. For all these reasons, the use of platelet growth factors is very appealing.

In the past twenty years, certain growth factors endowed with thrombopoietic activity have been isolated. Among them, GM-CSF, the stem cell factor (c-kit ligand or steel factor), IL-1, IL-3, IL-6, IL-11 and thrombopoietin. IL-1 or alpha, IL-6 and IL-11 have shown their efficacy in patients with post-chemotherapy thrombopenia [55-60].

However, due to their pleiotropic effect, interleukins have induced dissuasive secondary toxic symptoms (fever, headache, skin rash, fatigue related or unrelated to rapid onset anemia, hyperbilirubinemia...).

Biological Effects and Thrombopoietin Regulation

Contrary to interleukins, thrombopoietin exerts relatively specific action on megakaryocyte lines. This ligand of the c-Mpl was identified and cloned simultaneously by different laboratories [61-64] and, as a result, it was also called megapoietin, c-Mpl ligand and megakaryocyte growth and development factor (MGDF). Thrombopoietin is synthesized by the liver on a constitutive level, and is eliminated by c-Mpl receptors on platelet surfaces. Therefore, platelet transfusion to thrombopenic humans or animals causes breakdown of seric thrombopoietin [63-65]. Thrombopoietin increases the size, ploidy and number of megakarocytes, and stimulates expression of specific platelet markers [63, 66, 67]. In addition, thrombopoietin synergizes with erythropoietin and the stem cell factor on myeloid precursors and erythroids [68-70].

Recombinant Thrombopoietin Molecules and Preclinical Studies

Two recombinant thrombopoietin molecules were evaluated in clinical and preclinical studies: rh TPO and PEG-rHuMGDF. The first, identical to endogenous thrombopoietin produced by the cells of mammals, undergoes glycolisis. The second, consisting only of the portion of the molecule that binds to the receptor, is produced by *E.coli* and is conjugated with polyethylene glycol to increase its half-life. The two recombinant molecules have similar pharmacological effects [71, 72]. Administration of these molecules to non human primates increases the size, ploidy and number of megakaryocytes, and the level of circulating platelets is multiplied by five. In murine models, thrombopenia induced by chemotherapy or radiotherapy improves with daily administration of thrombopoietin [73, 74].

Recombinant Thrombopoietin Molecules and Clinical Studies

Efficacy of rh TPO and PEG rHuMGDF has been clearly demonstrated in patients treated with conventional chemotherapy. PEG-rHuMGDF, the most widely studied molecule, showed a dose-dependent response in randomised studies involving advanced cancer and moderate thrombopenia patients after chemotherapy [75-77]. The group receiving this medication after carboplatin chemotherapy had less severe thrombopenia (188×10^9/l) of shorter duration than the control group receiving a placebo (14 days *versus* > 21 days) [77]. A more recent study showed the same beneficial effect on thrombopenia severity reduction. No improvement was seen when PEG-rHuMGDF was administered before chemotherapy [76]. As for rhTPO, it was shown to be effective in patients with sarcoma or genital area cancer, when administered before chemotherapy [78] or after chemotherapy [79].

However, neither of these two recombinant molecules produced significant improvement of severe thrombopenia such as that associated with acute leukemia, or occurring after hematopoietic stem cell transplantation [80-82]. Platelet increase was moderate, and did not reduce trombopenic duration or transfusion requirements.

Other than their use as chemotherapy consolidation therapy, injections of PEG-rHuMGDF administered to thrombopenic patients with myelodysplasia doubled platelet levels in a third of these patients after five or six weeks, according to a preliminary study [83].

As a thrombopenia treatment, recombinant thrombopoietin molecules have been used successfully in patients with idiopathic thrombopoienic purpura, infection caused by the AIDS virus, liver disease, or in patients undergoing surgery [84]. In transfusion medicine, three other applications are feasible: hematopoietic stem cell mobilisation in association with other mobilisation factors like G-CSF, to increase reception of $CD34^+$ cells; *ex vivo* expansion of stem cells derived from bone marrow or cord (in addition to Flt3); and increased quantity of platelets from healthy donors [84].

Limits of Recombinant Thrombopoietin Molecule Uses

Repeated injections of PEG-rHuMGDF have caused the appearance of neutralizing antibodies in patients and healthy volunteers [85, 86]. These IgG-type antibodies neutralize both recombinant and endogenous thrombopoietin, by inducing thrombopenia. The latter occurred in 4/665 patients and 2/210 healthy volunteers after two injections, and in 11/124 healthy volunteers after three injections. A single injection did not lead to neutralizing antibody development. In two patients, thrombopenia was associated with anemia and neutropenia, which indicates an effect on hematopoietic stem cells [84, 86]. The PEG-rhuMGDF molecule has been off the market since 1998 in the United States.

Conclusions and Future Outlook

Development of recombinant erythropoietin constitutes an important advance in terms of saving labile blood products. Complications related to immune thrombopenia occurrence have decreased considerably thanks to better storage and more appropriate use of these products. Indications have become more precise, given that we know the clinical and biological criteria for identifying patients likely to have good response. Cost is still high but will soon decrease thanks to dose reduction and reduction of injection frequency. Recombinant thrombopoietin has not reached the stage of actual clinical development. But pharmaceutical companies are conducting research projects on the development of mimetic molecules, both peptidyl and nonpeptidyl [87, 88].

References

1. Jacobson LO, Goldwasser E, Fried W, Plzak L. Role of the kidney in erythropoiesis. *Nature* 1957 ; 179 : 633-4.
2. Lacombe C, Da Silva JL, Bruneval P, Casadevall N, Camilleri JP, Bariety J, Tambourin P, Varet B. Erythropoietin : sites of synthesis and regulation of secretion. *Am J Kidney Dis* 1991 ; 18 : 14-9.
3. Koury ST, Bondurant MC, Koury MJ. Localization of erythropoietin synthesizing cells in murine kidneys by in situ hybridization. *Blood* 1988 ; 71 : 524-7.
4. Lacombe C, Da Silva JL, Bruneval P, Fournier JG, Wendling F, Casadevall N, Camilleri JP, Bariety J, Varet B, Tambourin P. Peritubular cells are the site of erythropoietin synthesis in the murine hypoxic kidney. *J Clin Invest* 1988 ; 81 : 620-3.
5. Donahue RE, Emerson SG, Wang EA, Wong GG, Clark SC, Nathan DG. Demonstration of burst-promoting activity of recombinant human GM-CSF on circulating erythroid progenitors using an assay involving the delayed addition of erythropoietin. *Blood* 1985 ; 66 : 1479-81.
6. Huang LJ, Constantinescu SN, Lodish HF. The N-terminal domain of Janus kinase 2 is required for Golgi processing and cell surface expression of erythropoietin receptor. *Mol Cell* 2001 ; 8 : 1327-38.
7. Levy De, Darnell JE Jr. STATs : transcriptional control and biological impact. *Nat Rev Mol Cell Biol* 2002 ; 3 : 651-62.
8. Egrie JC, Browne JK. Development and characterization of novel erythropoiesis stimulating protein (NESP). *Br J Cancer* 2001 ; 84 (Suppl. 1) : 3-10.
9. Egrie JC, Browne J, Lai P, Lin FK. Characterization of recombinant monkey and human erythropoietin. *Prog Clin Biol Res* 1985 ; 191 : 339-50.

10. Jacobs K, Shoemaker C, Rudersdorf R, Neill SD, Kaufman RJ, Mufson A, Seehra J, Jones SS, Hewick R, Fritsch EF, Kawakita M, Shimizut T, Miyake T. Isolation and characterization of genomic and cDNA clones of human erythropoietin. *Nature* 1985 ; 313 : 806-10.

11. Eschbach JW. The anemia of chronic renal failure : pathophysiology and the effects of recombinant erythropoietin. *Kidney Int* 1989 ; 35 : 134-48.

12. US Renal Data System : USRDS Annual Data Report, treatment modalities. *Am J Kidney Dis* 1994 ; 24 : S57-S75 (Suppl. 2).

13. European Best Practice Guidelines for the management of anaemia in patients with chronic renal failure. *Nephrol Dial Transplant* 1999 ; 14 : S1-S50 (Suppl. 5).

14. Eschbach JW, Egrie JC, Downing MR, Browne JK, Adamson JW. Correction of the anemia of end-stage renal disease with recombinant human erythropoietin: results of a combined phase I and II clinical trial. *N Engl J Med* 1987 ; 316 : 73-8.

15. Eschbach JW, Abdulhadi MH, Browne JK, Delano BG, Downing MR, Egrie JC, Evans RW, Friedman EA, Graber SE, Haley NR, Korbet S, Krantz SB, Lundin AP, Nissenson AR, Ogden DA, Paganini EP, Rader B, Rutsky EA, Stivelman J, Stone AJ, Teschan P, Van Stone JC, Van Wyck DB, Zuckerman K, Adamson JW. Recombinant human erythropoietin in anemic patients with end-stage renal disease. Results of a phase III multicenter clinical trial. *Ann Intern Med* 1989 ; 111 : 992-1000.

16. NKF-K/DOQI Clinical Practice Guidelines for Anemia of Chronic Kidney Disease : Update 2000. *Am J Kidney Dis* 2001 ; 37 : S182-238.

17. Barrett BJ, Fenton SS, Ferguson B, Halligan P, Langlois S, Mccready WG, Muirhead N, Weir RV. Clinical practice guidelines for the management of anemia coexistent with chronic renal failure. *J Am Soc Nephrol* 1999 ; 10 : S292-S296 (Suppl. 13).

18. Locatelli F, Pisoni RL, Akizawa T, Cruz JM, DeOreo PB, Lameire NH, Held PJ. Anemia management for hemodialysis patients: Kidney Disease Outcomes Quality Initiative (K/DOQI) guidelines and Dialysis Outcomes and Practice Patterns Study (DOPPS) findings. *Am J Kidney Dis* 2004 ; 44 : 27-33 (Suppl. 3).

19. Ma JZ, Ebben J, Xia H, Collins AJ. Hematocrit level and associated mortality in hemodialysis patients. *J Am Soc Nephrol* 1999 ; 10 : 610-9.

20. Xia H, Ebben J, Ma JZ, Collins AJ. Hematocrit levels and hospitalization risks in hemodialysis patients. *J Am Soc Nephrol* 1999 ; 10 : 1309-16.

21. Foley RN, Parfrey PS, Harnett JD, Kent GM, Murray DC, Barre PE. The impact of anemia on cardiomyopathy, morbidity, and mortality in end-stage renal disease. *Am J Kidney Dis* 1996 ; 28 : 53-61.

22. Levin A, Thompson CR, Ethier J, Carlisle EJ, Tobe S, Mendelssohn D, Burgess E, Jindal K, Barrett B, Singer J, Djurdjev O. Left ventricular mass index increase in early renal disease: impact of decline in hemoglobin. *Am J Kidney Dis* 1999 ; 34 : 125-34.

23. O'Riordan E, Foley RN. Effects of anaemia on cardiovascular status. *Nephrol Dial Transplant* 2000 ; 15 : 19-22 (Suppl. 3).

24. Valderrabano F. Erythropoietin in chronic renal failure. *Kidney Int* 1996 ; 50 : 1373-91.

25. Walls J. Haemoglobin-is more better? *Nephrol Dial Transplant*. 1995 ; 10 : 56-61 (Suppl. 2).

26. Nissenson AR. Epoetin and cognitive function. *Am J Kidney Dis* 1992 ; 20 : 21-4 (Suppl. 1).

27. Jungers P, Choukroun G, Oualim Z, Robino C, Nguyen AT, Man NK. Beneficial influence of recombinant human erythropoietin therapy on the rate of progression of chronic renal failure in predialysis patients. *Nephrol Dial Transplant* 2001 ; 16 : 307-12.

28. Tapolyai M, Kadomatsu S, Perera-Chong M. r.hu-erythropoietin (EPO) treatment of pre-ESRD patients slows the rate of progression of renal decline. *BMC Nephrol* 2003 ; 4 : 3-6.

29. Ludwig H, Fritz E, Kotzmann H, Hocker P, Gisslinger H, Barnas U. Erythropoietin treatment of anemia associated with multiple myeloma. *N Engl J Med* 1990 ; 322 : 1693-9.

30. Bokemeyer C, Aapro MS, Courdi A, Foubert J, Link H, Osterborg A, Repetto L, Soubeyran P. EORTC guidelines for the use of erythropoietic proteins in anaemic patients with cancer. *Eur J Cancer* 2004 ; 40 : 2201-16.
31. Henke M, Laszig R, Rube C, Schafer U, Haase KD, Schilcher B, Mose S, Beer KT, Burger U, Dougherty C, Frommhold H. Erythropoietin to treat head and neck cancer patients with anaemia undergoing radiotherapy : randomised, double-blind, placebo-controlled trial. *Lancet* 2003 ; 362 : 1255-60.
32. Leyland-Jones B ; BEST Investigators and Study Group. Breast cancer trial with erythropoietin terminated unexpectedly. *Lancet Oncol* 2003 ; 4 : 459-60.
33. Marchal C, Spaeth D, Casadevall N, Daouphars M, Marec-Berard P, Fabre N, Haugh M ; Comite d'organisation des Standards, Options and Recommendations. [Standards, options and recommendations for the use of recombinant erythropoietin (epoietin alpha and beta darbepoietin-alpha, EPO) in the management of anaemia in oncology for patient undergoing radiotherapy-update 2003]. *Cancer Radiother* 2004 ; 8 : 197-206.
34. Hellstrom-Lindberg E. Efficacy of erythropoietin in the myelodysplastic syndromes: a meta-analysis of 205 patients from 17 studies. *Br J Haematol* 1995 ; 89 : 67-71.
35. Italian cooperative study group for rHuEpo in myelodysplastic syndromes. A randomized double-blind placebo-controlled study with subcutaneous recombinant human erythropoietin in patients with low-risk myelodysplastic syndromes *Br J Haematol* 1998 ; 103 : 1070-4.
36. Hellstrom-Lindberg E, Negrin R, Stein R, Krantz S, Lindberg G, Vardiman J, Ost A, Greenberg P. Erythroid response to treatment with G-CSF plus erythropoietin for the anaemia of patients with myelodysplastic syndromes : proposal for a predictive model. *Br J Haematol* 1997 ; 99 : 344-51.
37. Casadevall N, Durieux P, Dubois S, Hemery F, Lepage E, Quarre MC, Damaj G, Giraudier S, Guerci A, Laurent G, Dombret H, Chomienne C, Ribrag V, Stamatoullas A, Marie JP, Vekhoff A, Maloisel F, Navarro R, Dreyfus F, Fenaux P. Health, economic, and quality-of-life effects of erythropoietin and granulocyte colony-stimulating factor for the treatment of myelodyplastic syndromes : a randomized, controlled trial. *Blood* 2004 ; 104 : 321-7.
38. Hellstrom-Lindberg E, Gulbrandsen N, Lindberg G, Ahlgren T, Dahl IM, Dybedal I, Grimfors G, Hesse-Sundin E, Hjorth M, Kanter-Lewensohn L, Linder O, Luthman M, Lofvenberg E, Oberg G, Porwit-MacDonald A, Radlund A, Samuelsson J, Tangen JM, Winquist I, Wisloff F. A validated decision model for treating the anaemia of myelodysplastic syndromes with erythropoietin + granulocyte colony-stimulating factor : significant effects on quality of life. *Br J Haematol* 2003 ; 120 : 1037-46.
39. Musto P, Falcone A, Sanpaolo G, Bodenizza C, La Sala A, Perla G, Carella AM. Efficacy of a single, weekly dose of recombinant erythropoietin in myelodysplastic syndromes. *Br J Haematol* 2003 ; 122 : 269-71.
40. Martino M, Console G, Irrera G, Callea I, Condemi A, Dattola A, Messina G, Pontari A, Pucci G, Furlo G, Bresolin G, Iacopino P, Morabito F. Harvesting peripheral blood progenitor cells from healthy donors: retrospective comparison of filgrastim and lenograstim. *J Clin Apheresis* 2005 ; 12 mai (sous presse).
41. Forgie M, Wells P, Laupacis A, Fergusson D. Preoperative autologous donation decreases allogeneic transfusion but increases exposure to all red blood cell transfusion : results of a meta-analysis. International Study of Perioperative Transfusion (ISPOT) Investigators. *Arch Intern Med* 1998 ; 158 : 610-6.
42. Goodnough LT, Rudnick S, Price TH, Ballas SK, Collins ML, Crowley JP, Kosmin M, Kruskall MS, Lenes BA, Menitove JE, et al. Increased preoperative collection of autologous blood with recombinant human erythropoietin therapy. *N Engl J Med* 1989 ; 321 : 1163-8.
43. de Pree C, Mermillod B, Hoffmeyer P, Beris P. Recombinant human erythropoietin as adjuvant treatment for autologous blood donation in elective surgery with large blood needs (> or = 5 units): a randomized study. *Transfusion* 1997 ; 37 : 708-14.

44. Walpoth B, Galliker B, Spirig P, Haeberli A, Rosenmund A, Althaus U, Nydegger UE. Use of epoetin alfa in autologous blood donation programs for patients scheduled for elective cardiac surgery. *Semin Hematol* 1996 ; 33 : 75-7; (Suppl. 2).
45. Price TH, Goodnough LT, Vogler WR, Sacher RA, Hellman RM, Johnston MF, Bolgiano DC, Abels RI. Improving the efficacy of preoperative autologous blood donation in patients with low hematocrit: a randomized, double-blind, controlled trial of recombinant human erythropoietin. *Am J Med* 1996 ; 101 : 22S-27S.
46. Canadian, Orthopedic, Perioperative, Erythropoietin, Group S. Effectiveness of perioperative recombinant human erythropoietin in elective hip replacement. *Lancet* 1993 ; 341 : 1227-32.
47. Goldberg MA. Perioperative epoetin alfa increases red blood cell mass and reduces exposure to transfusions: results of randomized clinical trials. *Semin Hematol* 1997 ; 34 : 41-7 (Suppl. 2).
48. Rosencher N, Ozier Y. Peri-operative use of EPO. *Transfus Clin Biol* 2003 ; 10 : 159-64.
49. Peces R, de la Torre M, Alcazar R, Urra JM. Antibodies against recombinant human erythropoietin in a patient with erythropoietin-resistant anemia. *N Engl J Med* 1996 ; 335 : 523-4.
50. Prabhakar SS, Muhlfelder T. Antibodies to recombinant human erythropoietin causing pure red cell aplasia. *Clin Nephrol* 1997 ; 47 : 331-5.
51. Bennett CL, Luminari S, Nissenson AR, Tallman MS, Klinge SA, McWilliams N, McKoy JM, Kim B, Lyons EA, Trifilio SM, Raisch DW, Evens AM, Kuzel TM, Schumock GT, Belknap SM, Locatelli F, Rossert J, Casadevall N. Pure red-cell aplasia and epoetin therapy. *N Engl J Med* 2004 ; 351 : 1403-8.
52. Casadevall N, Nataf J, Viron B, Kolta A, Kiladjian JJ, Martin-Dupont P, Michaud P, Papo T, Ugo V, Teyssandier I, Varet B, Mayeux P. Pure red cell aplasia and antierythropoietin antibodies in patients treated with recombinant erythropoietin. *N Engl J Med* 2002 ; 346 : 469-75.
53. Gershon SK, Luksenburg H, Cote TR, Braun MM. Pure red-cell aplasia and recombinant erythropoietin. *N Engl J Med* 2002 ; 347 : 1584-6.
54. Casadevall N, Cournoyer D, Marsh J, Messner H, Pallister C, Parker-Williams J, Rossert J. Recommendations on haematological criteria for the diagnosis of epoetin-induced pure red cell aplasia. *Eur J Haematol* 2004 ; 73 : 389-96.
55. D'Hondt V, Humblet Y, Guillaume T, D'Hondt V, Humblet Y, Guillaume T, Baatout S, Chatelain C, Berliere M, Longueville J, Feyens AM, de Greve J, Van Oosterom A. Thrombopoietic effects and toxicity of interleukin-6 in patients with ovarian cancer before and after chemotherapy : a multicentric placebo-controlled, randomized phase Ib study. *Blood* 1995 ; 85 : 2347-53.
56. Gordon MS, McCaskill-Stevens WJ, Battiato LA, Loewy J, Loesch D, Breeden E, Hoffman R, Beach KJ, Kuca B, Kaye J, Sledge GW Jr. A phase 1 trial of recombinant human interleukin-11 (neumega rhIL-11 growth factor) in women with breast cancer receiving chemotherapy. *Blood* 1996 ; 87 : 3615-24.
57. Smith JWD, Longo DL, Alvord WG, Janik JE, Sharfman WH, Gause BL, Curti BD, Creekmore SP, Holmlund JT, Fenton RG, Sznol M, Miller L, Shimizu M, Oppenheim J, Fiem S, Hursey J, Powers G, Urba W. The effects of treatment with interleukin-1 alpha on platelet recovery after high-dose carboplatin. *N Engl J Med* 1993 ; 328 : 756-61.
58. Tepler I, Elias L, Smith JW, *et al.* A randomized placebo-controlled trial of recombinant human interleukin-11 in cancer patients with severe thrombocytopenia due to chemotherapy. *Blood* 1996 ; 87 : 3607-14.
59. Vadhan-Raj S, Kudelka AP, Garrison L, Gano J, Edwards CL, Freedman RS, Kavanagh JJ. Effects of interleukin-1 alpha on carboplatin-induced thrombocytopenia in patients with recurrent ovarian cancer. *J Clin Oncol* 1994 ; 12 : 707-14.
60. Vredenburgh JJ, Hussein A, Fisher D, Hoffman M, Elkordy M, Rubin P, Gilbert C, Kaye JA, Dykstra K, Loewy J, Peters WP. A randomized trial of recombinant human interleukin-11 following autologous bone marrow transplantation with peripheral blood progenitor cell support in patients with breast cancer. *Biol Blood Marrow Transplant* 1998 ; 4 : 134-41.

61. Bartley TD, Bogenberger J, Hunt P, Li YS, Lu HS, Martin F, Chang MS, Samal B, Nichol JL, Swift S, Johnson R, Hsu Y, Parker P, Suggs S, Skrine JD, Merewether LA, Clogston C, Hsu E, Hokom MM, Hornkohl A, Choi E, Pangelinan M, Sun Y, Trollinger D, Sieu L, Padilla D, Trail G, Elliott G, Izumi R, Covey T, Crouse J, Garcia A, Xu W, Del Castillo J, Biron J, Cole S, Hu MCT, Pacifici R, Ponting I, Saris C, Wen D, Yung YP, Lind H, Rosselmann RA. Identification and cloning of a megakaryocyte growth and development factor that is a ligand for the cytokine receptor Mpl. *Cell* 1994 ; 77 : 1117-24.

62. de Sauvage FJ, Hass PE, Spencer SD, Malloy BE, Gurney AL, Spencer SA, Darbonne WC, Henzel WJ, Wong SC, Kuang WJ, Oles KJ, Hultgren B, Solberg Jr LA, Goeddel DV, Eaton DL. Stimulation of megakaryocytopoiesis and thrombopoiesis by the c-Mpl ligand. *Nature* 1994 ; 369 : 533-8.

63. Kuter DJ, Beeler DL, Rosenberg RD. The purification of megapoietin : a physiological regulator of megakaryocyte growth and platelet production. *Proc Natl Acad Sci USA* 1994 ; 91 : 11104-8.

64. Lok S, Kaushansky K, Holly RD, Kuijper JL, Lofton-Day CE, Oort PJ, Grant FJ, Heipel MD, Burkhead SK, Kramer JM, Bell LA, Sprecher CA, Blumerg H, Johnson R, Prunkard D, Ching AFT, Mathewes SL, Bailey MC, Forstrom JW, Buddle M, Osborn SG, Evans SJ, Sheppard PO, Presnell S, O'Hara P, Hagen F, Roth G, Foster D. Cloning and expression of murine thrombopoietin cDNA and stimulation of platelet production in vivo. *Nature* 1994 ; 369 : 565-8.

65. Scheding S, Bergmann M, Shimosaka A, Wolff P, Driessen C, Rathke G, Jaschonek K, Brugger W, Kanz L. Human plasma thrombopoietin levels are regulated by binding to platelet thrombopoietin receptors in vivo. *Transfusion* 2002 ; 42 : 321-7.

66. Broudy VC, Lin NL, Kaushansky K. Thrombopoietin (c-mpl ligand) acts synergistically with erythropoietin, stem cell factor, and interleukin-11 to enhance murine megakaryocyte colony growth and increases megakaryocyte ploidy in vitro. *Blood* 1995 ; 85 : 1719-26.

67. Kaushansky K, Lok S, Holly RD, Broudy VC, Lin N, Bailey MC, Forstrom JW, Buddle M, Oort PJ, Hagen FS, Roth GJ, Papayannopoulou T, Foster DC. Promotion of megakaryocyte progenitor expansion and differentiation by the c-Mpl ligand thrombopoietin. *Nature* 1994 ; 369 : 568-71.

68. Ku H, Yonemura Y, Kaushansky K, Ogawa M. Thrombopoietin, the ligand for the Mpl receptor, synergizes with steel factor and other early acting cytokines in supporting proliferation of primitive hematopoietic progenitors of mice. *Blood* 1996 ; 87 : 4544-51.

69. Rasko JE, O'Flaherty E, Begley CG. Mpl ligand (MGDF) alone and in combination with stem cell factors (SCF) promotes proliferation and survival of human megakaryocyte, erythroid and granulocyte/macrophage progenitors. *Stem Cells* 1997 ; 15 : 33-42.

70. Sitnicka E, Lin N, Priestley GV, Fox N, Broudy VC, Wolf NS, Kaushansky K. The effect of thrombopoietin on the proliferation and differentiation of murine hematopoietic stem cells. *Blood* 1996 ; 87 : 4998-5005.

71. Begley CG, Basser RL. Biologic and structural differences of thrombopoietic growth factors. *Semin Hematol* 2000 ; 37 : 19-27.

72. Sheridan WP, Kuter DJ. Mechanism of action and clinical trials of Mpl ligand. *Curr Opin Hematol* 1997 ; 4 : 312-6.

73. Hokom MM, Lacey D, Kinstler OB, Choi E, Kaufman S, Faust J, Rowan C, Dwyer E, Nichol Jl, Grasel T. Pegylated megakaryocyte growth and development factor abrogates the lethal thrombocytopenia associated with carboplatin and irradiation in mice. *Blood* 1995 ; 86 : 4486-92.

74. Ulich TR, del Castillo J, Yin S, Swift S, Padilla D, Senaldi G, Bennett L, Shutter J, Bogenberger J, Sun D. Megakaryocyte growth and development factor ameliorates carboplatin-induced thrombocytopenia in mice. *Blood* 1995 ; 86 : 971-6.

75. Basser RL, Rasko JE, Clarke K, Cebon J, Green MD, Hussein S, Alt C, Menchaca D, Tomita D, Marty J, Fox RM, Begley CG. Thrombopoietic effects of pegylated recombinant human megakaryocyte growth and development factor (PEG-rHuMGDF) in patients with advanced cancer. *Lancet* 1996 ; 348 : 1279-81.

76. Basser RL, Underhill C, Davis I, Green MD, Cebon J, Zalcberg J, MacMillan J, Cohen B, Marty J, Fox RM, Begley CG. Enhancement of platelet recovery after myelosuppressive chemotherapy by recombinant human megakaryocyte growth and development factor in patients with advanced cancer. *J Clin Oncol* 2000 ; 18 : 2852-61.
77. Fanucchi M, Glaspy J, Crawford J, Garst J, Figlin R, Sheridan W, Menchaca D, Tomita D, Ozer H, Harker L. Effects of polyethylene glycol-conjugated recombinant human megakaryocyte growth and development factor on platelet counts after chemotherapy for lung cancer. *N Engl J Med* 1997 ; 336 : 404-9.
78. Vahdan-Raj S, Murray LJ, Bueso-Ramos C, Patel S, Reddy SP, Hoots WK, Johnston T, Papadopolous NE, Hittelman WN, Johnston DA, Yang TA, Paton VE, Cohen RL, Hellmann SD, Benjamin RS, Broxmeyer HE. Stimulation of megakaryocyte and platelet production by a single dose of recombinant human thrombopoietin in patients with cancer. *Ann Intern Med* 1997 ; 126 : 673-81.
79. Vadhan-Raj S, Verschraegen CF, Bueso-Ramos C, Broxmeyer HE, Kudelka AP, Freedman RS, Edwards CL, Gershenson D, Jones D, Ashby M, Kavanagh JJ. Recombinant human thrombopoietin attenuates carboplatin-induced severe thrombocytopenia and the need for platelet transfusion in patients with gynecologic cancer. *Ann Intern Med* 2000 ; 132 : 364-8.
80. Archimaud E, Ottman OG, Yin JA, Lechner K, Dombret H, Sanz MA, Heil G, Fenaux P, Brugger W, Barge A, O'Brien-Ewen C, Matcham J, Hoelzer D. A randomized, double-blind, placebo-controlled study with pegylated recombinant human megakaryocyte growth and development factor (PEG-rHuMGDF) as an adjunct to chemotherapy for adults with de novo acute myeloid leukemia. *Blood* 1999 ; 94 : 3694-701.
81. Nash RA, Kurzock R, DipPersio J, Vose J, Linker C, Maharaj D, Nademanee AP, Negrin R, Nimer S, Shulman H, Ashby M, Jones D, Appelbaum FR, Champlin R. A phase I trial of recombinant human thrombopoietin in patients with delayed platelet recovery after hematopoietic stem cell transplantation. *Biol Blood Marrow Transplant* 2000 ; 6 : 25-34.
82. Schiffer CA, Miller K, Larson RA, Amrein PC, Antin JH, Zani VJ, Stone RM. A double-blind, placebo-controlled trial of pegylated recombinant human megakaryocyte growth and development factor as an adjunct to induction and consolidation therapy for patients with acute myeloid leukemia. *Blood* 2000 ; 95 : 2530-5.
83. Nichol JL. Thrombopoietin levels after chemotherapy and in naturally occurring human diseases. *Curr Opin Hematol* 1998 ; 5 : 203-8.
84. Kuter DJ, Begley CG. Recombinant human thrombopoietin: basic biology and evaluation of clinical studies. *Blood* 2002 ; 100 : 3457-69.
85. Basser RL, O'Flaherty E, Green M, Edmonds M, Nichol J, Menchaca DM, Cohen B, Begley CG. Development of pancytopenia with neutralizing antibodies to thrombopoietin after multicycle chemotherapy supported by megakaryocyte growth and development factor. *Blood* 2002 ; 99 : 2599-609.
86. Li J, Yang C, Xia Y, Bertino A, Glaspy J, Roberts M, Kuter DJ. Thrombocytopenia caused by the development of antibodies to thrombopoietin. *Blood* 2001 ; 98 : 3241-8.
87. Cwirla SE, Balasubramanian P, Duffin DJ, Wagstrom CR, Gates CM, Singer SC, Davis AM, Tansik RL, Mattheakis LC, Boytos CM, Schatz PJ, Baccanari DP, Wrighton NC, Barrett RW, Dower WJ. Peptide agonist of the thrombopoietin receptor as potent as the natural cytokine. *Science* 1997 ; 276 : 1696-9.
88. Erickson-Miller CL, DeLorme E, Tian SS, Hopson CB, Stark K, Giampa L, Valoret EI, Duffy KJ, Luengo JL, Rosen J, Miller SG, Dillon SB, Lamb P. Discovery and characterization of a selective, nonpeptidyl thrombopoietin receptor agonist. *Exp Hematol* 2005 ; 33 : 85-93.

Reducing Immunogenicity of Labile Blood Products and Creating Universal Erythrocytes

Jean-Yves Muller, Jacques Chiaroni

Injecting blood cells from one person to another can, on the one hand, stimulate the recipient's immune system through mechanisms still partly unknown and, on the other hand, trigger a reaction with preexisting antibodies, either naturally developed with no identifiable immunisation, or acquired following previous immunisation through pregnancy or transfusion. This can result in serious transfusion reactions, including hemolytic shock, anaphylactic shock, post-transfusion acute respiratory distress syndrome, and febrile non hemolytic reactions. Allo-immunisation, which has made the object of numerous research studies and preventive strategies, still causes many transfusion-related accidents whose analysis shows that despite rigorous application of donor-recipient compatibility rules, they cannot be prevented in every case. Two alternatives to compatibilisation, not mutually exclusive, exist: the first is to reduce reactivity of injected cells to preexisting antibodies, the second is to reduce their immunogenicity. The first alternative has led to the concept of universal erythrocytes, a false concept, since given the present state of knowledge, these erythrocytes could only be universal in terms of their compatibility in the ABO system. Essentially, this alternative constitutes ABO haemolytic accident prevention, and would increase availability of O erythrocytes, solving the problem of emergency stock creation and composition, as well as the problem of rarer phenotype transfusion.

The second alternative, that can also prevent allo-immunisation development and extension by transfusion, involves all antigenic systems normally exposed on blood cells.

Some of these methods are already in use: for example, leukodepletion that is relatively effective in preventing primary anti-HLA allo-immunisation. The other methods are still being examined in fundamental and developmental studies that have not yet led to extensive clinical use. A and B erythrocyte deglycosylation in view of transformation into O erythrocytes is the subject of the first part of the present chapter. The second part of the chapter deals with immuno-camouflage consisting of masking antigenic motifs by grafting methoxypoly chains (ethylene glycol) (mPEG) on erythrocyte surfaces.

A, B or AB Erythrocytes Enzymatically Converted to Group O

This first solution consists of manipulating the biochemical properties of ABO blood group antigens. In fact, at the start of the 1950s, Morgan and Watkins demonstrated that antigens of the ABO system were represented by terminal sugars of the lateral glucidic glycoprotein or glycolipid chains (*Figure 1*). At that time, these authors reported that bacterial origin exoglycosidases could eliminate immunodominant sugars of A and B antigens represented respectively by N-acetylgalactosamine (GalNAc) and galactose (Gal). It was not until thirty years later that this concept was proposed as a basis for the production of O erythrocytes for therapeutic use [1].

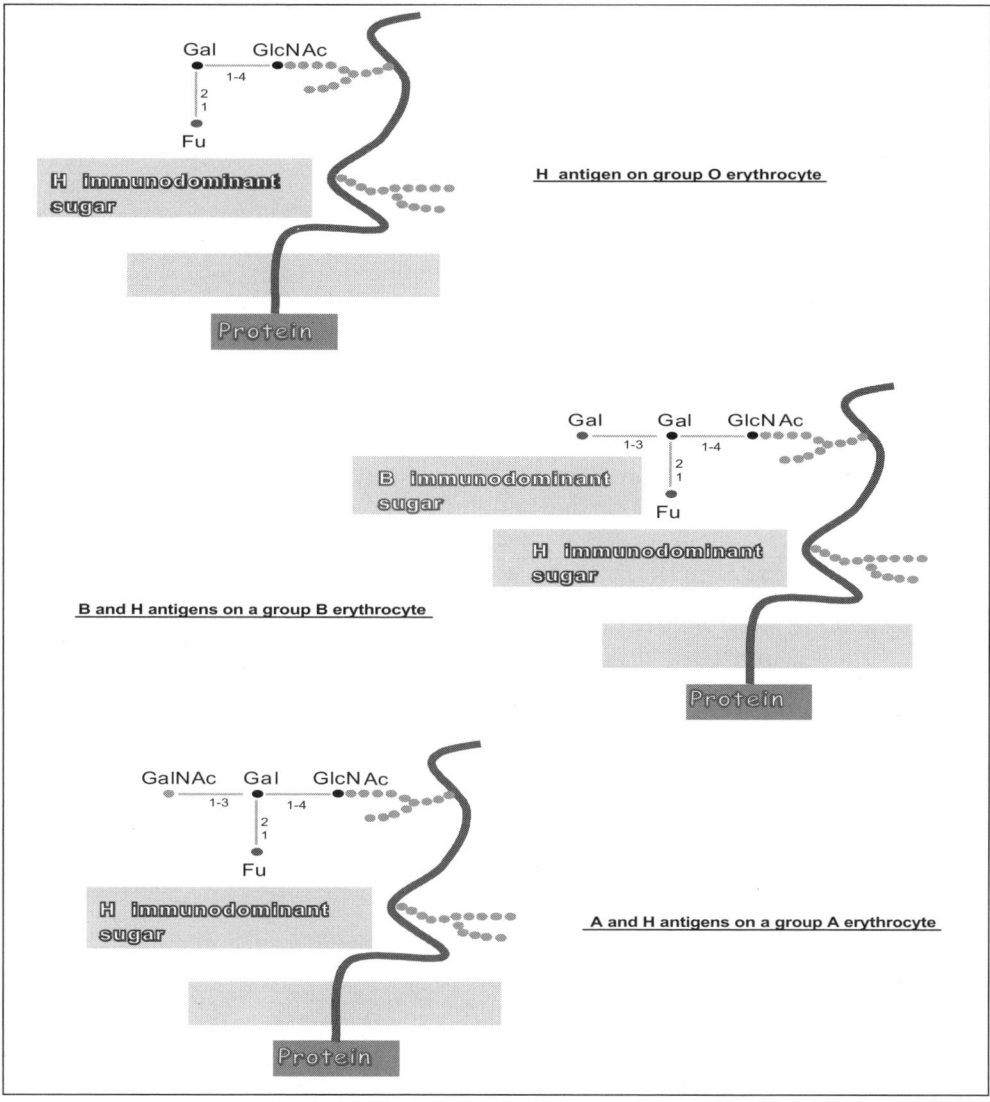

Figure 1. Biochemical structure of A, B and H antigens.

Conversion of B Erythrocytes to O (B-ECO: B enzyme converted to O)

The first reported conversion was that of B erythrocytes to O, with alpha galactosidase purified from coffee beans [2]. The very first *in vitro* and *in vivo* experiments were conducted with a small quantity of gibbon erythrocytes initially, then with human erythrocytes. After treatment, the erythrocytes obtained tested normal for osmotic fragility, for physiological ATP concentrations and for 2,3-DPG, and showed minimal production of methemoglobin, unchanged hemoglobin affinity for oxygen, as well as normal life span in A, B or O recipients. The only change consisted in loss of antigen P1 whose immunodominant sugar is the same as that of antigen B.

Subsequently, all studies were conducted in humans; injected B-ECO erythrocytes presented normal life span, with no transfusion reactions. These clinical trials started with injections of small quantities of treated erythrocytes given to group A and O volunteer participants (initial 2 ml injection followed two weeks later by another 2 ml injection, then a 1 ml injection labeled with Cr51 two weeks later [3]. In addition, these volunteers did not present increases of anti-B and their serum had not agglutinated B-ECO erythrocytes seven weeks after transfusion.

At a later time, a whole unit of B erythrocytes treated with the same galactosidase was injected to three group A and four group O patients [4]. A preliminary immunohaematologic assay showed absence of agglutination of these erythrocytes in anti-A and anti-B antibodies registered with the Food and Drug Administration (FDA) and used in conventional technical conditions. In any case, normal erythrocyte life span and absence of transfusion reactions were observed once again. Finally, two other units were transfused to the four initial group O patients. Only an increase of anti-B was observed in one of them, but still without transfusion reaction and with normal erythrocyte life span [5, 6]. In summary, it appeared that this enzyme, used at pH 5.5 with a 6 mg/ml concentration of globular sediment, was effective and non immunogenic, since no specific antibody to this molecule was detected after transfusion. However, the quantity of enzyme needed is still an economic hinderance to routine use of this enzyme in transfusion center laboratories.

Subsequently, phase II clinical trials produced successful outcomes [7]. In 2000, Kruskall transfused twenty-one A and O group subjects with erythrocytes of this type. No transfusion reactions occurred and hemoglobin levels were as expected. Only an increase in the anti-B titre and slight erythrocyte agglutination at indirect antiglobulin test were reported in certain individuals. In fact, all compatibility indirect antiglobulin tests on A, B and AB sera produced negative results, including tests using Liss or PEG methods. A certain number of group O sera tested positive, but they had no impact on the clinical picture, nor on erythrocyte life span. Moreover, as in the initial studies, ELISA antigalactosidase antibody assays conducted four weeks after transfusion were negative.

Conversion of A Erythrocytes to O (A-ECO: A Enzyme Converted to O)

A to O conversion took longer to achieve due to lack of suitable glycosidases and the more complex character of the A antigen.

Thus, although the first experiments [3], using an enzyme extracted from chicken liver, achieved complete conversion of group A2 erythrocytes, conversion of group A1 erythrocytes was only partial. Moreover, the conditions of use of this enzyme (3.65 pH and 3 mg/ml erythrocyte ratio) seem incompatible with large-scale production.

This partial failure is due to the existence of a type 3 A antigen on A1 phenotype erythrocytes, and not on A2 phenotypes [8, 9]. In fact, an A group erythrocyte expresses two types of H substrates: H type 2 and H type 3, the latter called repetitive. Although the two enzymes can convert from H type 2 to A type 2, only enzyme A1 can convert from H type 3 to A type 3 (*Figure 2*). Where phenotype A1 erythrocytes are concerned, elimination of type 2 A antigens, deeply embedded in the molecule, is made more difficult by this accessibility problem. Only suitable glycosydases, which eliminate external and internal determinants, can achieve complete conversion of A1 phenotype erythrocytes.

Discovery of new glycosidases in the course of the NYBC project in cooperation with Zymequest Inc. (Beverly, MA, USA) [10, 11] has provided a partial solution to this problem. New enzymes able to eliminate A and B antigens have been characterized and cloned. Conversion assays have proven effective (with negative reactions to anti-A, anti-B and anti-AB monoclonal reagents) on complete group A and B units. Conditions for the use of these enzymes seem altogether compatible with large-scale technological transfer, since they can be used at ambient temperature and neutral pH.

A new recombinant alpha-N-acetyl-galactosaminidase has proven to be effective for A_1 and A_2 erythrocyte conversion (negative reaction with anti-A and anti-AB). In addition, the quantities necessary for this conversion are smaller than those previously needed (20 mg/erythrocyte concentrate) [10, 11]. As for clinical trials, phase I trials were conducted successfully and phase II trials are planned for the near future.

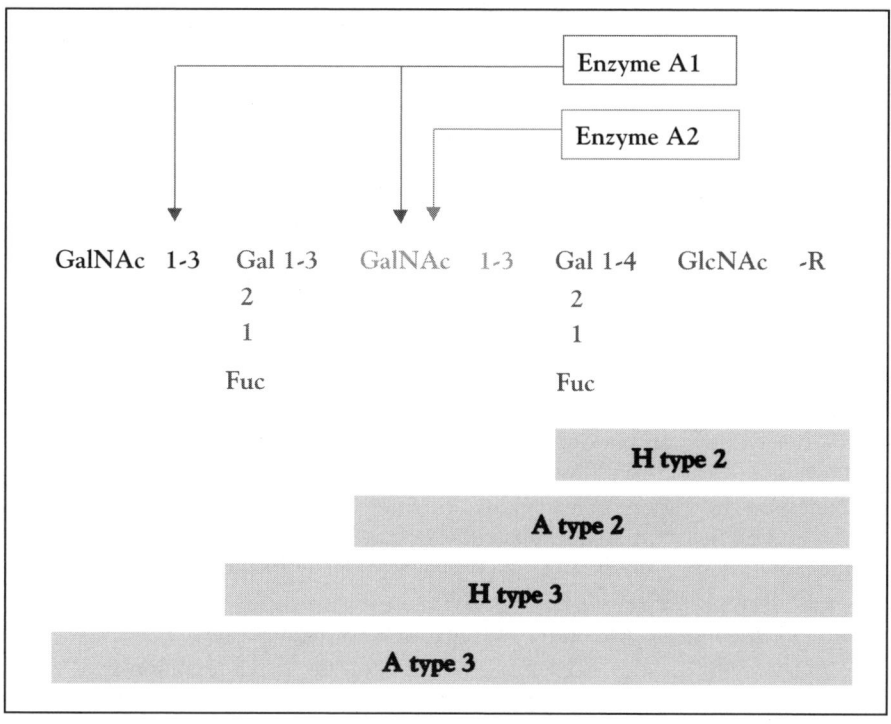

Figure 2. Type 2 and 3 A antigens and action of A1 and A2 enzymes.

In summary, production of enzyme-converted erythrocytes is well advanced; the first phase II clinical trials have been completed, with B erythrocytes transformed to O, and phase III trials should be planned. If the new A enzymes are promising, phase II clinical trials should be conducted. However, technical improvements are still needed before these procedures can be used routinely in transfusion centers. Finally, Clausen [8, 9] and Olsson [10] have described the production of new glucidic hydrolases that can be used for both A and B antigens [10, 11]. These enzymes have been cloned and used at neutral pH and ambient temperature to transform complete A and B group units.

Possible Attenuation or Elimination of Human Blood Cell Immunogenicity

The idea of masking foreign substances by using polyethylene glycol (PEG) is not new and has been applied since 1977 [12, 13] to reduce albumin immunogenicity and bovine hepatic catalase, in order to improve biocompatibility of proteins, biomaterials and, more recently, cells. As far as transfused erythrocytes are concerned, this concept has developed particularly since the advent of techniques allowing membrane structures to be hidden under a family of biologically neutral substances, the PEGs. The method developed at the same time as the terms "pegylation" and "pegylated". These terms designate a multitude of applications and techniques leading to different outcomes, and likely to influence the camouflage effect. A clear definition of terms is important. Pegylation is associated with problems of different types: biochemical, biophysical and immunologic, that are related to the technique and can be solved by one of the various pegylation methods. Finally, the concept of "stealth cell" involves several immunology notions that must be analysed in order to define the various objectives that can be attained using this method, as well as the various applications that extend beyond the sphere of transfusion and include the protection of functional molecules, as well as allogenous and even heterologous cell grafting.

Biochemical Possibilities of Pegylation

The basic facts involved in the pegylation of blood cells are not difficult to understand, and some fundamental notions taken from specialized articles should be sufficient. PEGs are a family of neutral polyethers with a common identical basic structure: $HO-(CH_2-CH_2)n-CH_2-CH_2-OH$.

PEGs are not charged and are water soluble thanks to hydrogen bonding which attaches three molecules of water to each oxyethylene unit.

This significant hydration considerably modifies the physical properties of pegylated molecules and particles. In an aqueous milieu, each PEG molecule and, by extension, each pegylated structure, is surrounded by a coccus of water molecules bonded to PEG, modifying accessibility to biomolecules and to cells.

Variability of pegylations depends essentially on three factors:

– molecular weight of the derivative, related to the variable number of responsible oxyethylenes, with molecular weight between 8 and 100 g/mol. In practice, PEG erythrocytes between 2.5 and 20 KDa are used for pegylation;

– spatial structure with three main forms: linear, branched and star-shaped;

– mode of coupling with proteins.

The combination of these three factors produces an infinite number of possible composites which, despite identical biochemical composition, will have very different spatial structure and biological properties. Molecular weight being equal, the branched forms are distinct from the linear forms by their different densities and by different spatial exclusion volumes. This is particularly relevant in terms of the distancing of certain erythrocytic antigenic determinants from the lipid bilayer of the red blood cell membrane (*Figure 3*). Linear PEGs are methylated at one end, creating methoxy PEGs (mPEG), which allow association with a coupling agent that insures bonding of the PEG with the target molecule. Three main coupling agents are used:

– cyanide chloride, which produces C-mPEG;

– benzotriazole carbonate, which supplies BTC-mPEGs;

– N-hydroxysuccinimidyl, a propionic acid ester, source of SPA-mPEGs.

These three coupling agents insure covalent attachments, primarily linkage with _ amine lysine groups, and secondarily linkage with amine end groups. Two other coupling factors have to be taken into account: concentration of the PEG derivative used in the reaction, varying normally between 0 and 7.5 mmol/l; and concentration of the erythrocyte suspension in a serum milieu, or NaCl suspension of washed erythrocytes.

So far, studies of the characteristics of compounds obtained with different coupling agents have not shown very significant differences in results and biological effects.

Biochemical Pegylation Criteria

Physical properties considered indicative of pegylation are: modification of electrophoretic mobility of pegylated particles, formation of stacks of erythrocytes and separation in the aqueous form [14].

• **Separation in the aqueous form** is made possible by the fact that the two liquid polymers, PEG and dextran, are immiscible. Because pegylated erythrocytes have great affinity with PEG, efficacy of pegylation in different technical conditions can be assessed based on erythrocyte separation in this two-phase system. Erythrocytes that are only slightly or not at all pegylated will remain in the dextran, while considerably pegylated erythrocytes will segregate into the PEG. This method allows evaluation of pegylation homogeneity, and separation of pegylated erythrocytes from the rest.

• **Reduced mobility** of erythrocytes in an electrical field constitutes a measure of the masking of surface erythrocyte charges by PEG. Technical differences can also be evaluated by this criterion.

• **In vitro stack formation** produced by dextran-type macromolecules, or sedimentation speed measuring an analogous parameter, is decreased with pegylated erythrocytes. This criterion provides another measure of the degree of erythrocyte pegylation.

These different criteria used to evaluate the effectiveness of coupling agents and the influence of molecular weight have shown that the three coupling agents mentioned above have similar efficacy, with slightly more rapid kinetics for cyanide chloride. Molecular concentration being equal, 20 KDa polymers reduce electrophoretic mobility and stack formation the most, while producing an optimal percentage of pegylated erythrocytes at phase separation testing.

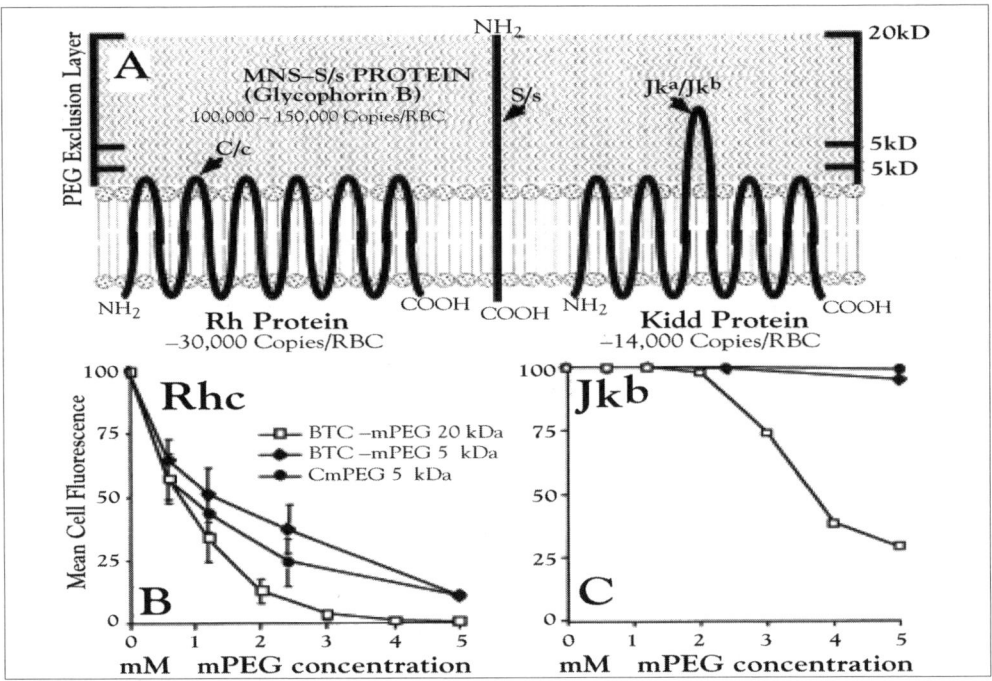

Figure 3. Immunocamouflage of membrane antigens depends on the biochemical coupling procedure, the size of the polymer and its surface density.

(A) Graphic representation of erythrocyte membrane and topographic distribution of antigens of group Rh (Cc), Kidd (Jk $^{a/b}$) and MNSs. The PEG exclusion layer is the physical entity responsible for immunocamouflage of membrane antigens. The effectiveness of the exclusion layer, highly hydrated and with neutral charge, depends on the length and density of highly mobile PEG polymers which produce (by serum inhibition) a cloud filling the space around the cell. In fact, the exclusion layer attached to PEG acts like a molecule-size filter that lets small molecules (for example, O^2 and glucose) and small proteins enter, while excluding larger proteins like antibodies. In the same way, the masking of surface electrical charges by the neutral PEG layer plays an important role by preventing antigen-antibody interactions as well as cellular interactions. Here, exclusion zones of 2.5, 5 and 20 KDa polymers are shown.

(B) Rh antigens are located near the membrane surface; as a result, even relatively short polymers (5 KDa) can mask these sites effectively. The masking of the Rhc antigen shown here depends on decrease of cellular fluorescence. As indicated, each 5 KDa polymer masks the Rhc antigen in an identical manner. Although increased polymer length (20 KDa) augments immunocamouflage of Rh antigens, the difference is moderate.

(C) Contrary to Rh antigens, polymer length is a crucial factor for immunocamouflage of MNS and Kidd blood group antigens. As shown, no 5 KDa polymer masks Jk ^{b} antigens. However, 20 KDa polymers are starting to produce effective masking of Jk ^{b}.

(Based on Bradley et al. [14] with permission).

Biological Quality Criteria [15]

Attachment of mPEG on erythrocytes does not seem to show significant physiologic effects in the course of normal use, based on a set of experimental criteria.

- **Morphological modifications:** different research teams noted no significant modifications in the erythrocytes observed using an optical or electronic microscope, in a very wide range of mPEG concentrations.

- **Viability modifications:** until now, survival of pegylated erythrocytes has been tested in animal models. In mice, pegylated erythrocytes with BTC-mPEG 20 KDa concentrations between 0 and 2.0 mmol/L did not produce significant survival modifications when they were reinjected intravenously or administered by IP injection.

- **Oxygen transport:** oxygen transport functions of pegylated erythrocytes, as well as their permeability function, their anion and cation transport functions and their osmotic resistance are entirely preserved [16].

Objectives

Immunological objectives of pegylation camouflage of antigenic structures at the surface of erythrocytes can have several types of impact on immune response; each one of them can disrupt this response at different levels. Represented graphically, PEG can:

– affect the afferent phase of the immune response by inhibiting or attenuating interaction of immune cells with their specific antigens, producing various effects: ignoring of the antigenic motif by the immune system, resulting in absence of response; or modification of immune response. PEG intervention can induce a peripheral tolerance reaction toward certain antigens;

– intervene in the effector phase by protecting antigenic motifs and the structures that support them from aggression by effector cytotoxic or phagocitic antibodies or cells.

In vivo studies on prevention of graft-*versus*-host reaction and on *in vitro* lymphocyte reaction in mixed culture have contributed to showing the effect of PEG treatment on immune stimulation [17]. The proliferative response in mixed lymphocyte culture, evaluated by incorporation of 3H-thymidine, decreases in direct proportion to the PEG concentration used to treat mononuclear peripheral blood cells. This loss of proliferation is not caused by an anergic state, nor by loss of viability, since cells remained responsive to stimulation by phytohemagglutinin. Flux cytometry studies with mononuclear heterologous antibodies showed reduced reactivity of T cells with anti-CD3, CD4, CD8, CD28, CD11a and CD62L; while cells with the antibody showed reduced reactivity with CD80, CD58 and CD62L. This data suggests that PEG acts by limiting accessibility to these functional surface molecules, reducing as a result the interaction of adhesion molecules and the stimulation and co-stimulation signals indispensable to the activation of these cells.

The protective effect of immunocamouflage vis-à-vis post-transfusion graft-*versus*-host reaction is demonstrated in an experimental murine model in which irradiated $H2K^d$ mice receive allogeneic $H2K^b$ spleen cells, modified by mPEG and not modified. In these circumstances, comparison of survival in the two groups of mice shows that the group which received mPEG treated cells has significantly higher survival rates than the other group, according to assessment of dates or rates of survival beyond 50%. The authors [18] draw the conclusion that treatment with mPEG confers protection vis-à-vis graft-*versus*-host reaction. This conclusion is based on the observation of reduced proliferative power of injected cells in mice receiving mPEG treated cells.

The same research team made another interesting observation concerning secondary lymphocyte response in mixed culture. When the cells used for initial stimulation of target cells are treated with mPEG, response is abolished even if the cells used in the second stimulation are not pegylated. This is considered to be due to a state of active tolerance induced by the low stimulating power of pegylated cells, since the proliferative power of the cells rendered tolerant is controlled by their proliferative response to mitogens, which is not at all abolished.

The capacity to protect islet of Langerhans cells against rejection reaction while preserving their glucoregulator potential has also been demonstrated, opening new perspectives in the field of cellular pegylation [19].

In any case, PEG is presumed to be immunologically neutral, meaning that it is not supposed to provoke an immune reaction, nor be able to react with specific antibodies. But observation of the facts raises two questions [20]:

- The first concerns **passive absorption of plasmatic proteins by PEG** which, in this situation, could become carriers of antigenic motifs. This was reported by a team [21] which showed that pegylated erythrocytes could, in this case, be reactive and sensitive to adhesion and to experimental phagocytosis on a monolayer of monocytes. These researchers consider this finding equivalent to the clinical importance of antibody action against blood group antigens [22]. The author suggests that this absorption and phagocytosis possibility could explain the shortened survival of pegylated erythrocytes observed by two other research teams [16, 23].

- The second concerns the possible existence of antibodies reacting with the PEG itself, likely to be involved in positive serologic reactions, if not to cause clinical reactions outright. This introduces ambiguity in the laboratory evaluation of antigen site accessibility of pegylated erythrocytes [19, 24]. Several observations support this argument: blood from certain normal donors agglutinates pegylated erythrocytes, while cord blood never does. Pretreatment of these samples with mercapto-ethanol abolishes this agglutination. Spontaneous existence of anti-PEG antibodies has been described in 3.3% of allergic patients and 0.2% of normal subjects. After desensibilization with allergens modified by mPEG, 50% of patients produce anti-PEG antibodies with titer distribution between 32 and 512 [25].

Immunohematologic Objectives

- **Transfusion objectives of stealth erythrocytes:** these objectives are of two types.

  – The first is **alloimmunisation prevention.** This is particularly crucial for subjects with abnormal phenotypes likely to develop anti-public antibodies, making it impossible for them to receive transfusions other than autologous. This prevention is also essential for all patients receiving repetitive transfusions. At present, there is no proof that pegylated erythrocytes are effective in these settings, although their attenuated immunogenicity makes them good candidates for these applications.

  – The second is **transfusion of immunized patients,** be it by natural or irregular allo-antibodies, or by autoantibodies. A *priori*, hemolitic autoimmune anemias requiring transfusions seem to be the best candidates, but the inability of pegylated erythrocytes to prevent erythrocyte membrane access to the complement should temper hopes founded on this indication. For allo-immunized subjects, the problem is more complex because access to antigenic structures varies according to the system involved. Moreover, risk of immediate severe hemolysis associated with this type of antibody makes it difficult to test the efficacy of this application in clinical studies.

- **Problems encountered in transfusion practice**

Studies and experiments: the first studies on human red blood cell antigenicity were conducted in 1996. They showed that erythrocytes treated with 5 KDa C-mPEG had reduced anti-A, anti-B and anti-D reactivity at direct agglutination, which was the only technique used in this research. However, these erythrocytes maintained normal morphology and attached oxygen normally [26].

Subsequently, another team using PEG with different molecular weight (3.4 KDa) and a different coupling agent (propionyl-N-hydrosuccinimide, SPA-mPEG) showed that with PEG >20% concentrates it is possible to obtain an anti-A titer reduction of 2048 to 2-32, and negativation of the reaction with anti-D in concentrates starting at PEG ≥ 10 mmol/L. However, this method was associated with a very significant life cycle reduction in rats [27].

Later, the same team used 3.4 KDa second generation PEG (x-PEG) attached to albumin and was able to completely abolish erythrocyte reactivity with anti-A, -B, -D, -C, -c, -E, -e, -Fya, -Fyb, -Jka, -Jkb, while maintaining low-level reactivity with anti-A and anti-B [27]. This procedure allowed better survival in mice: half-life rose from twelve hours to 5 days; in control mice, the normal equivalent figure was 9 days.

A third team working at about the same time presented results for 5 KDa CN-PEG; the use of an agregometry technique showed absence of reactivity with anti-A and anti-B. This research showed that sheep erythrocytes treated in this manner had reduced human monocyte phagocytosis. Similarly, these PEG-sheep erythrocytes injected to mice had prolonged survival in mice whose heterophile antibodies usually shorten their recirculation [28]. The longest survival observed by this team was related to weaker PEG concentration. Murine erythrocytes are relatively sensitive to strong concentrations of PEG [16], and their survival is shortened by the 1 to 5 mM concentrations necessary to mask human antigenic erythrocytes. Using standard laboratory methods, this team showed an agglutination decrease of 2 or 3 $^+$ with PEG, 1.2 mM with anti-C, -c, -E, -e, -K, -S, -s, and reduced anti-A titers. Finally, the only immune reaction study available concerns a project conducted by this team, which showed that mPEG sheep erythrocytes injected to mice provoke attenuated response, with about 90% reduction in antibodies produced, compared to the number in control mice injected with untreated erythrocytes [29].

A fourth team studied different mPEGs with 5 KDa, 15 KDa ad 18.5 KDa molecular weight, in a 1.3 mM concentration. At this concentration, the 18.5 K/Da CN-PEG completely inhibits agglutination by different anti-D, -c, -C, -E, -Le^b, -Jka, -Jkb, -P1, -N antibodies and causes a 256 to 4 drop in the agglutinating titer of anti A-/B, and a 128 to 16 drop in titers of anti-I. The 5 mM CN-PEG prevents agglutination much less effectively. The three derivatives, whatever their molecular weight, retain their ability to attach anti-D detected by an indirect technique to antiglobulin, and to D$^+$ erythrocytes by flux cytometry, while D-erythrocytes remain completely negative [30]. The same team has recently shown that better results for antigen masking can be obtained by using PEG mixtures of the three molecular weights [20]. In a different context, this team suggested that coating erythrocytes with PEG considerably reduces their viscosity to low shear forces, and that this could be of considerable interest in the treatment of venous-occlusive diseases or myocardial infarction [31].

Overall, all these projects show that even in optimal conditions it is at best possible to inhibit direct agglutination of erythrocytes by the specific antibodies of blood group antigens, but that indirect tests using an antiglobulin remained for the most part positive, particularly with anti-D, anti-A and anti-B. The study of complement activation by pegylated erythrocytes can provide additional data shedding light on their clinical applications. In fact, it was important to ensure that pegylation does not cause direct activation of the complement, especially through an alternative pathway, and does not interfere with regulatory proteins like CD55 (decay accelerating factor, DAF) and CD59 (membrane inhibitor of reactive lysis, MIRL).

The work of the Albany team shows that erythrocytes coupled with 5 KDa CmPEG at concentrations of 0, 1, 2, 4 and 5 mM do not produce any activation [32]. Residual activity of the complement of a serum incubated with pegylated or control erythrocytes remains normal after decantation. This residual activity is tested for the classic pathway by activation using aggregated IgGs, and for the alternate pathway by using insulin. Moreover, the generation of C3a in these sera, in contact with CMPEG erythrocytes, remains identical with that of controls incubated with normal erythrocytes.

These experiments clearly show that pegylated erythrocytes alone produce no activation of the complementary system. By contrast, incubation of pegylated erythrocytes (≥ 1.2 mM) with incompatible serum in the ABO system leads to increased lysis compared to that of non pegylated control erythrocytes placed in the same ABO incompatibility conditions in a serum milieu or in soluble PEG. This shows that it is the attached PEG itself which contributes to increased hemolysis. The latter is completely dependent and does not occur with decomplemented sera. It is the classic pathway that is involved, since its blockage by EGTA in the presence of Mg^{2+} abolishes this hemolysis while preserving activability of the alternate pathway. Analysis of complement protein membrane attachment on pegylated erythrocytes compared to control erythrocytes shows very significant increase of the attachment of the different C3 α and β chains when pegylated erythrocytes are placed in ABO incompatible serum, while in compatible or autologous serum there is no attachment. Complement activation in these circumstances goes as far as activation of C9 which, in pegylated erythrocytes, is attached in greater quantity than the quantity of non pegylated controls. This proves that classic pathway activation, for pegylated erythrocytes, goes as far as activation of the membrane attack complex, and that pegylation facilitates this activation. This raises the question of blockage of the regulatory proteins of the complement by the pegylation process.

The studies conducted by this team have shown that where neither CD55 whose activity can be tested by sensitivity to lysis in an acid milieu, nor CD59 whose activity can be tested by activation with cobra venom factor (CVF), are blocked, while C3 and C5 convertases are blocked (by EDTA), lysis of pegylated erythrocytes is not superior to that of control erythrocytes. Pegylated erythrocyte lysis is a direct effect of attachment of class IgM antibodies, in this case very likely anti-As and anti-Bs. This is shown by the addition of an anti-IgM blocking the Fc fragment which, in this experiment, leads to dose-dependent reduction and then abolition of hemolysis of both pegylated and control erythrocytes.

The conclusions of this work constitute one of the current bases of reflection on use of pegylated erythrocytes. In fact, pegylation creates a zone of exclusion around erythrocytes likely to mask antigenic sites near the cellular membrane, such as antigens of the Rh system. However, the effect of PEG on more distant antigens is less clear; for the ABO system in any case, this effect does not prevent interaction of "natural" IgMs with their molecular target. This interaction is responsible for lysis which involves classic pathway activation of the complement, and conditions for complement attachment are facilitated by pegylation. This observation implies that the role of PEG vis-à-vis the erythrocyte surface should be understood to be that of a molecular filter likely to stop large proteinic molecules, but not less heavy molecules. The IgM is prevented from entering the exclusion zone on the surface of pegylated erythrocytes. Once inside the exclusion zone, PEG can facilitate molecular interactions [33]; this could explain its enabling effect in the complement-dependent lysis related to anti-As and anti-Bs.

However, this accessibility of pegylated erythrocyte membranes to complement proteins poses interpretation problems that cannot be analyzed simply by reference to molecular weight. In fact, the molecular weight of complex C1 approaches 800 KDa, which is not very far from IgMs, and the molecular weight of C4 (200 KDa) and C3 (180 KDa) is not lower than that of IgG. Thus, we have to conceive that attachment of an IgM disturbs a PEG layer sufficiently to allow access of the membrane to the different proteins of the classic path of the complement.

Future Outlook

Erythrocyte pegylation is still in its infancy and a synthesis of its possibilities and perspectives is necessarily incomplete, inasmuch as all aspects of the question are not yet understood. But present state of knowledge provides us with a few key elements that shed some light on the future of this procedure.

It is clear that the totality of biochemical data to consider in defining the diversity of possible types of pegylation is immense. Molecular weight and concentration are two basic factors; moreover, the first must take the molecular shape prescribed, linear or branched. Chain length is an important factor because it can make possible the masking of the antigenic elements located the farthest away from the membrane. Concentration has a direct effect on surface PEG density. It acts on the compactness of the exclusion zone, and it seems to be a crucial factor of fragilisation of erythrocytes and their viability, as shown by murine erythrocytes.

In addition to the various coupling agents, modes of attachment to surface reactive molecules are important. Bifunctional PEGs that can couple at both ends have been associated with an increase of sensitivity to agglutination. PEGs associated with other biomolecules, like the X-PEGs of the University of Alabama in Birmingham, link a 3.4 kDa bifunctional PEG with an albumin molecule; this reduces reactivity with antierythrocitic alloantibodies, very significantly improving viability in mice.

This example illustrates the great diversity of biochemical solutions available for solving the bio-efficiency problems of pegylated erythrocytes.

Nevertheless, the objective of producing universal erythrocytes, sometimes invoked in support of the procedure, is still utopian. In fact, attainable objectives should be set, and future possibilities should be assessed accordingly. At this time, it seems unrealistic to imagine that pegylation will solve ABO compatibility problems, and the risk of the other IgM antibodies should be evaluated with precision no matter what the objective. In this context, it should be noted that the Albany Medical College team has shown that PEG not only does not hinder classic pathway attachment of the complement activated by anti-A or anti-B IgMs, but that it enhances it, increasing consecutive erythrocyte lysis. This observation brings into question the usefulness of this technology for solving the transfusion problems of patients with dangerous natural or acquired hemolysis producing antibodies.

The objective of preventing or decreasing the probability of occurrence of alloimmunisation against minor blood group antigens seems more realistic, and pegylation could find an interesting clinical application in repeated transfusions of blood cell concentrates for subjects with hemoglobinopathy, who are known to be susceptible to progressive occurrence of alloimmunisation, which will affect nearly 35% of them. This application depends on the fulfilment of two preliminary conditions: the non-toxicity of the PEG attached to erythrocytes must be carefully proven, although several studies assert the absence of toxicity of this polymer. The role of anti-PEG antibodies has to be clarified. That they in fact exist seems certain, but their pathogenic effect remains to be established. However, in the laboratory, they are likely to produce direct or indirect agglutination reactions to positive antiglobulin.

Transfusion therapy to treat autoimmune hemolitic anemias is another area where pegylated erythrocytes could be of interest. The latter could favourably influence outcome and survival of blood cells transfused to a patient with anti-erythrocytic antibodies, and prevent the development of alloimmunisation whose frequency and danger are known in these circumstances. However, enhanced attachment of the complement to this type of erythrocyte should incite to great caution in regard to this application. Is it possible that only the cases where the antibodies do not attach the complement could be good candidates?

We have not discussed the problem of pegylation of blood cells other than erythrocytes. It would be tempting to do so, but experimental data is too fragmented to allow us to draw any conclusions. Reduction of reactivity in mixed lymphocytic culture is interesting. It has been said that this reactivity reproduces *in vitro* the immunologic conditions of graft *versus* host reaction. But transplantation of pegylated progenitors will produce other progenitors and non pegylated daughter cells; it is not likely that the low reactivity of immunocompetent pegylated cells will be perpetuated from one cell generation to another. As far as preventing post-transfusion graft-*versus*-host reaction is concerned, it is a problem which remains outside the scope of this technique.

As for fields where tissue transplant is not associated with immunologically competent cell transfer, such as Langerhans islets cell transplant, pegylation would be an interesting possibility if its "tolerance producing" character is confirmed.

The role of pegylation in the immuno-modification of transfusion products should also be considered from a technological point of view, in order to assess the possibility of integrating this procedure in a safe production chain, introducing at the same time pegylation quality control. We have mentioned different methods used by the research teams working in this field, including phase separation and electrophoretic migration of particles, as well as the crucial immuno-hematologic exam required for correct evaluation of the masking of antigenic motifs by antibodies, and the most relevant methods of performing this evaluation. Could pegylated erythrocytes constitute a means of assessing cross compatibility reaction? Will it be necessary to neutralize possible anti-PEG antibodies? These questions are still unanswered. Abolition or, at least, reduction of the agglutinability of pegylated erythrocytes should, in any case, be taken into account when conducting the final compatibility test at the patient's bedside, particularly because in this setting a negative result could lead to a false conclusion of ABO compatibility, revealed by a hemolysis reaction.

Could Lublin [34] be right to say that a futuristic vision of blood cell concentrate preparation would insert erythrocyte pegylation in an automated chain, after white blood cell reduction, pathogen inactivation, enzyme conversion and maybe even irradiation? We have chosen not to discuss the economic problems created by such industrial-scale production of safe erythrocytes, but we can imagine that at the end of the production chain and the multiplication of safety controls the number of erythrocytes will diminish and production costs per unit will grow exponentially. Another way of looking at the problem is to ask ourselves if this growth curve will not at some point cross that of erythrocytes cultured from stem cells, whose production costs could, on the contrary, decrease with the quantity of industrially produced erythrocytes.

References

1. Goldstein J, Siviglia G, Hurst R, Lenny L. Group B erythrocytes enzymatically converted to group O survive normally in A, B and O individuals. *Science* 1982 ; 215 : 168-70.
2. Lenny L, Goldstein J. Enzymatic removal of blood group B antigen from gibbon erythrocytes (abstract). *Transfusion* 1980 ; 20 : 618.
3. Goldstein J. Conversion of ABO blood groups. *Transfus Med Rev* 1989 ; 3 : 206-12.
4. Lenny LL, Hurst R, Goldstein J, Benjamin LJ, Jones RL. Single-unit transfusions of RBC enzymatically converted from group B to group O to A and O normal volunteers. *Blood* 1991 ; 77 : 1383-8.
5. Lenny LL, Hurst R, Goldstein J, Galbraith RA. Transfusions to group O subjects of 2 units of red cells enzymatically converted from group B to group O. *Transfusion* 1994 ; 34 : 209-14.
6. Lenny LL, Hurst R, Zhu A, Goldstein J, Galbraith RA. Multiple-unit and second transfusions of red cells enzymatically converted from group B to group O: report on the end of phase 1 trials. *Transfusion* 1995 ; 35 : 899-902.
7. Kruskall MS, AuBuchon JP, Anthony KY, Herschel L, Pickard C, Biehl R, et al. Transfusion to blood group A and O patients of group B RBCs that have been enzymatically converted to group O. *Transfusion* 2000 ; 40 : 1290-8.
8. Clausen H, Levery SB, Nudelman E, Tsuchiya S, Hakomori S. Repetitive A epitope (type 3 chain A) defined by blood group A1-specific monoclonal antibody TH-1: chemical basis of qualitative A1 and A2 distinction. *Proc Natl Acad Sci USA* 1985 ; 82 : 1199-203.
9. Clausen H, Holmes E, Hakomori S. Novel blood group H glycolipid antigens exclusively expressed in blood group A and AB erythrocytes (type 3 chain H). II. Differential conversion of different H substrates by A1 and A2 enzymes, and type 3 chain H expression in relation to secretor status. *J Biol Chem* 1986 ; 261 : 1388-92.
10. Olsson ML, Hill CA, de la Vega H, Liu QP, Stroud MR, Valdinocci J, et al. Universal red blood cells—enzymatic conversion of blood group A and B antigens. *Transfus Clin Biol* 2004 ; 11 : 33-9.
11. Olsson ML. New developments in immunohaematology. *Vox Sang* 2004 ; 87 Suppl. 2 : 66-71.
12. Aubuchowski A, van Es T, Palczuck NC, Davis FF. Alteration of immunological properties of bovine serum albumin by covalent attachement of polyethylene glycol. *J Biol Chem* 1977 ; 252 : 3578-81.
13. Aubuchowski A, McCoy JR, Palczuck NC, van Es T, Davis FF. Effect of covalent attachement of polyethylene glycol on immunogenicity and circulating life of bovine liver catalase. *J Biol Chem* 1977 ; 252 : 3582-6.
14. Bradley AJ, Murad KL, Regan KL, Scott MD. Biophysical consequences of linker chemistry and polymer size on stealth erythrocytes: size does matter. *Biochim Biophys Acta - Biomembranes* 2002 ; 1561 : 147-58.
15. Scott MD, Murad KL, Koumpouras F, Talbot M, Eaton JW. Chemical camouflage of antigenic determinants: stealth erythrocytes. *Proc Natl Acad Sci USA* 1997 ; 94 : 7566-71.
16. Murad KL, Mahany KL, Brugnara C, Kuypers FA, Eaton JW, Scott MD. Structural and functional consequences of antigenic modulation of red blood cells with methoxypoly(ethylene glycol). *Blood* 1999 ; 93 : 2121-7.
17. Murad KL, Gosselin EJ, Eaton JW, Scott MD. Stealth cells: prevention of major histocompatibility complex class II-mediated T-cell activation by cell surface modification. *Blood* 1999 ; 94 : 2135-41.
18. Chen AM, Scott MD. Immunocamouflage: prevention of transfusion-induced graft-versus-host disease via polymer grafting of donor cells. *J Biomed Mater Res* 2003 ; 67A : 626-36.

19. Chen AM, Scott MD. Current and future applications of immunological attenuation via pegylation of cells and tissue. *BioDrugs* 2001 ; 15 : 833-47.
20. Garratty G. Will stealth RBCs replace blood donors of rare types? *Vox Sang* 2002 ; 83 Suppl. 1 : 101-4.
21. Garratty G, Leger R, Arndt P, Armstrong JK, Meiselman HJ, Fisher TC. Polyethylene treatment can mask blood group antigens, but also cause non-specific protein uptake. *Blood* 1997 ; 90 : 473a.
22. Garratty G. Evaluating the clinical significance of blood group alloantibodies that are causing problems in pretransfusion testing. *Vox Sang* 1998 ; 74 (S2) : 285-90.
23. Hortin GL, Lok HT, Huang ST. Progress toward preparation of universal donor red cells. *Artif Cells Blood Substit Immobil Biotechnol* 1997 ; 25 : 487-91.
24. Garratty G. Stealth erythrocytes: a possible transfusion product for the new century? *Vox Sang* 2000 ; 78 Suppl. 2 : 143-7.
25. Richter AW, Akerblom E. Polyethylene glycol reactive antibodies in man: titer distribution in allergic patients treated with monomethoxy propylene glycol modified allergens or placebo, and in healthy blood donors. *Int Archs Allergy Appl Immun* 1984 ; 74 : 36-9.
26. Jeong ST, Byun SM. Decreased agglutinability of methoxy-polyethylene glycol attached red blood cells: significance as a blood substitute. *Artif Cells Blood Substit Immobil Biotechnol* 1996 ; 24 : 503-11.
27. Huang ST, Hortin GL, Huang Z. Coating of red blood cells with crosslinked polyethylene glycol(XPEG) inhibits agglutination and shows favourable red cells survival. *Transfusion* 1998 ; 38 : 62S.
28. Murad K, Kompouras F, Talbot M, Eaton J, Scott MD. Molecular camouflage of antigenic determinants on intact mamalian cells: possible applications to transfusion medecine. *Blood* 1996 ; 88 : 444a.
29. Scott MD, Murad KL. Cellular camouflage: fooling the immune system with polymers. *Curr Pharm Des* 1998 ; 4 : 423-38.
30. Fischer TC, Armstrong JK, Meiselman HJ, Leger RM, Arndt PA, Garratty G. Polyethylene glycol coating of red blood cells strongly inhibits agglutination but does noy produce cells that are antigenically "silent". *Transfusion* 1997 ; 37 : 88S.
31. Armstrong JK, Meiselman HJ, Fisher TC. Covalent binding of poly(ethylene glycol) (PEG) to the surface of red blood cells inhibits aggregation and reduces low shear blood viscosity. *Am J Hematol* 1997 ; 56 : 26-8.
32. Bradley AJ, Test ST, Murad KL, Mitsuyoshi J, Scott MD. Interactions of IgM ABO antibodies and complement with methoxy-PEG-modified human RBCs. *Transfusion* 2001 ; 41 : 1225-33.
33. Tardi DH, Ingham KC. Mechanism of precipitaiton by polyethylene glycols. Analysis in terms of excluded volume. *J Biol Chem* 1981 ; 256 : 12108-17.
34. Lublin DM. Universal RBCs. *Transfusion* 2000 ; 40 : 1285-9.

Contribution of New Technologies to Blood Cell Collection and Preparation

Georges Andreu, Anne Chabanel, Bertrand Pelletier

Modern transfusion was born in the early 1940s, when the first methods of storing whole blood in satisfactory conditions were perfected [1]. However, transfusion really entered a stage of rapid development when whole blood collection in plastic bags became the common procedure, and cell separators started to be used. These two innovations that came about in the late 1960s made it possible to prepare, and therefore to transfuse to patients, labile blood products adapted to their needs, be it red blood cell concentrates, platelet concentrates or therapeutic plasma. Plastic software contributed to the development of sophisticated techniques for the separation of blood components, making it possible to preserve the functional qualities of blood cells in the best possible manner. Platelets made the object of the most significant advances, particularly through the development of methods of separation applied to the leuko-thrombocytic layer [2].

Starting in the 1980s, apheresis collection techniques, which had been entirely manual until then, gradually became more and more automated, first in the actual separation process [3], then in the prediction of platelet quantities collected, allowing results to be more easily reproduced and paving the way to standardization of labile blood product preparation. At the same time, leukocyte reduction techniques, by filtration [4] or by other physical methods like the surge technique [5], reached performance levels that made it possible to establish more and more rigorous quality standards for red blood cell concentrates, platelet concentrates and plasma [6-8].

This chapter deals with more recent developments in the field of labile blood product collection and preparation, perfected in the past ten years, some of which have not yet been introduced in our daily practice. For each of them, we will discuss impact on quality and/or safety improvement of labile blood products, on donor and transfusion center personnel safety, and on the organization of donations.

New Collection Procedures

Collection of Whole Blood

Derivation of the First Millimeters of Drawn Blood

This procedure has been in common use in France since the year 2000, for whole blood collection devices. Its installation on all apheresis collection devices was instituted in 2004. Its introduction was justified by the rigorous demonstration that eliminating the first 35 millimeters of drawn blood significantly reduces (3-fold reduction) the frequency of bacterial contamination of whole blood by germs of the cutaneous flora [9]. In current accepted practice, these 35 millimeters are not eliminated, but are used, rather, as samples for the biological qualification of donations. This development is mentioned in the present chapter because, despite the simplicity of its application, recognition of its efficacy by the scientific community and its moderate cost, very few countries have adopted it to date.

Needle Protectors and Tube Guides

Safety systems for collection devices were introduced in 1998, have been generalized in France since 2001 for whole blood collection devices, and since the end of 2004 for apheresis devices. They consist of full-proof needle protectors, easily handled as soon as the needle is withdrawn from the arm of the donor, and tube guides for sample collection, connected directly to the predonation sample pocket. These devices, which do not affect the quality or safety of labile blood products given to patients, play a crucial role in improving prevention of accidental exposure of the collection personnel to blood.

Control of Anticoagulant/Whole Blood Ratio

At present, whole blood is drawn directly into a bag containing a fixed volume of anticoagulant. Thus, it is not possible to ensure a perfectly controlled anticoagulant/whole blood (AC/WB) ratio. In practice, given the present accepted limits for whole blood donation (between 400 and 500 ml), and a fixed anticoagulant volume of 63 ml, the AC/WB ratio varies between 0.13 and 0.16, with an average of 0.14. A project currently in progress will develop a procedure ensuring a constant AC/WB ratio of 0.14. This procedure allows easier reproduction of the anticoagulant mixture and of the whole blood, reducing the risk of initiating coagulation during the drawing of the blood. This procedure can therefore improve the quality of red blood cell concentrates, of platelet concentrates and of plasma, and can reduce rejection of a small percentage of labile blood products during the production process. Finally, if we take into account the variability of hematocrit in blood donors, the anticoagulant/plasma ratio (AC/PL) after separation of the red blood cell concentrate varies between 0.2 and 0.35. Controlling for a constant AC/WB ratio in whole blood collection reduces by half the variability of the AC/PL ratio; this is undeniably an improvement of plasma standardization, whether plasma is intended for fractionation or for direct therapeutic use.

This procedure is in the first stages of evaluation. Therefore, its application is not expected unless required improvements, particularly decrease of clots in the collected blood, are demonstrated and rigorously quantified.

Whole Blood Collected in a Blood Bag

The immense contribution of plastic software has consisted in the production of devices with several transfer packs, even integrated filters, making it possible to separate blood components in a closed system. However, the complexity of the devices used today introduces new obstacles to efficient preparation of labile blood products by requiring the handling of awkward devices, poorly adapted to the collection environment, particularly collection by mobile teams, as well as certain labile blood product preparation stages such as centrifugation. Moreover, these devices are very costly if all the applications they allow are not utilized.

This difficulty could be overcome if whole blood was collected in a standard blood bag and if, in the labile blood products preparation laboratory, a sterile connection of the bag to the appropriate complementary device was made. The reliability and efficacy of the new sterile connection devices [10] make it possible to foresee such a strategy change, which will also facilitate the creation of more complex closed systems, allowing better automation of labile blood products preparation techniques.

Collection by Apheresis

Collection of Red Blood Cell Concentrates by Apheresis

The first attempts to perform separation of red blood cell concentrates directly in the apheresis devices were made over ten years ago [11]. However, it has only been in the last few years that these procedures became more developed and their impact better understood.

- **Collection of two concentrates of red blood cells.** Today, many donor cell separators make it possible to collect two red blood cell concentrates from the same donor, with leukodepletion by integrated filter.

Some of these separators are devices already used for other apheresis collections (Compas model made by Fresenius, Trima made by Gambro, MCS+ made by Haemonetics), while others are used strictly for the collection of two blood cell concentrates (Alyx model by Baxter, Cymbal by Haemonetics) [12].

Collecting two red blood cell concentrates at once during blood donation has the following advantages :

– for patients, when the two red blood cell concentrates are collected together, this method reduces the number of donors required for the same course of treatment. This is particularly useful when treating immunized patients; when there are few compatible donors; in cases of transfusion of rare blood group red blood cell concentrates; in the treatment of patients receiving repeated transfusions for life, such as carriers of major thalasemia or sickle-cell anemia patients; or in certain pediatric protocols. Moreover, this type of collection allows better standardization of red blood cell concentrates in terms of hemoglobin content, given that the latter can be easily controlled;

– for blood transfusion centers, this method makes it possible to prepare two red blood cell concentrates with a single biological qualification, and to considerably reduce the stages of red blood cell concentrate preparation, so that the concentrates are ready to be labelled immediately after collection. This can be a useful alternative in case of supply shortages.

The disadvantages and limitations of this type of collection are :

– for volunteer blood donors, the blood donation has a duration of about thirty minutes, a period of intermediary length between a whole blood donation and a classic apheresis plasma donation. It is essential to respect much more rigorous criteria than those applying to whole blood donations; in Europe, the criterion is a volume of blood estimated at over five liters – a condition generally fulfilled by a non obese person whose weight is > 70 kg, predonation hemoglobin concentrate over 140 g/L, and collection conditions guaranteeing a hemoglobin concentration equal to or above 110 g/L at the end of the donation [8]. These conditions considerably reduce the number of eligible donors;

– for blood transfusion centers, in addition to the high cost of collection devices and the need for available separators, prolonged duration of the donation and the complex eligibility criteria constitute obstacles to widespread use of this technique. Finally, despite the claims of certain manufacturers, these techniques are not really adapted to collection by mobile teams, which represents nearly 85% of total blood collection in France.

In conclusion, in France this type of collection cannot involve more than 3% to 5% of donations intended for red blood cell concentrate production.

In France, the place of this type of collection of two red blood cell concentrates by standard apheresis remains to be determined, since the procedure has only recently been authorized.

In the United States, only a small number of transfusion centers have adopted this procedure on a significant scale. This method is perhaps better suited to the different characteristics of the European population in terms of height and weight, and to conditions at fixed collection sites. Nevertheless, this type of donation requires very strict control of iron levels in volunteer blood donors, and iron supplementation has proved to be necessary to maintain these levels [13].

- **Collection of red blood cell concentrate in conjunction with another blood component.** Most cell separators used for platelet collection (Amicus by Baxter, Compas by Fresenius, Trima by Gambro, MCS+ by Haemonetics) are adapted to concurrent collection of a red blood cell concentrate and an apheresis platelet concentrate or plasma [14].

Contrary to collection of two red blood cell concentrates, this type of collection does not require particular selection criteria in terms of hemoglobin concentration (normal value equal to or over 125 g/L for women and 135 g/L for men), of blood volume (provided weight is superior or equal to 50 kg), and platelet concentration superior to 150 g/L, on condition that recommendations concerning total volume collected from a donor are strictly respected, knowing that this volume must not exceed 600 milliliters, not including the anticoagulant.

This combined collection has the same advantages for recipients and transfusion centers as collection of two red blood cell concentrates. In addition, this procedure could contribute to regulate red blood cell concentrate supplies. Moreover, today, collection centers often hesitate to solicit apheresis platelet donations from O RH-1 blood group blood donors; the possibility of combined platelet and red blood cell donations should lead to increasing the ratio of group O RH-1 apheresis donors.

Disadvantages and limitations are less considerable :

– for patients, this type of collection can limit the quantity of platelets present in apheresis platelet concentrates, at least in the absence of collection methods that include platelet storage media; this disadvantage will be controlled when cell separators will be adapted to the collection of very concentrated platelets, of the order of $3,10^6/\mu L$;

– for volunteer blood donors, the duration of the collection remains almost unchanged, lasting at most two hours; this duration corresponds to usual practices in France.

In France, the place of this type of combined apheresis collection has not yet been defined, given that their authorization is recent. In any case, their contribution to red blood cell concentrate supplies will remain within the limits of apheresis platelet collection, which have been set at under 7% of total supply of red blood cell concentrates.

Innovations in Labile Blood Product Preparation

Developments Applying to Red Blood Cell Concentrates

Integrated Filters

Leukodepletion filters were first integrated in whole blood collection devices at the end of the 1990s. In principle, this integration guarantees that the entire preparation process takes place in a closed system. Implementation of this development met with some difficulties, particularly in the case of devices exposed to centrifugation before leukodepletion, where the filter required to withstand centrifugal force must satisfy very strict quality criteria.

This was one of the reasons (the other being reduced loss of hemoglobin) that motivated the development of collection systems in which leukodepletion of whole blood by filtration takes place before centrifugation. Although leukodepletion performance is slightly inferior to that of red blood cell concentrate filtration, it satisfies French and European requirements (less than 10^6 residual leukocytes per red blood cell concentrate), as shown at Table I, based on the national data base for norms of quality control of labile blood products, set by blood transfusion establishments.

We must point out that this procedure, in general use in France today, has only been implemented by a minority of countries, including those that perform systematic leukodepletion.

Table I. Residual leukocyte content (x 10^6 residual leukocytes per red blood cell concentrate) with the technique of red blood cell concentrate preparation (2003).

	Control number	Lower quartile	Mean	Upper quartile
WB filtration	14,816	0.032	0.073	0.153
RBC filtration with integrated filter	5,550	0.012	0.014	0.048
RBC filtration with connectable filter	484	0.012	0.013	0.044

Developments Applying to Platelet Concentrates

Automation of Platelet Concentrate Mixture Preparation from Buffy-Coats

Preparation of platelet concentrate mixtures from buffy-coats, as it was first developed [2], is a complex succession of various operations that include centrifugation, extraction, mixing and filtration. These platelet concentrates have very satisfactory functional qualities [15, 16].

The Orbisac procedure created by Gambro has introduced a level of automation that has improved result reproducibility. One study [17] compares this automated technique of platelet concentrate preparation from a mixture of four leuko-thrombocytic layers extracted from whole blood with a recognized manual procedure. The study reports statistically significant performance improvement in platelet recovery (74+/-4% *versus* 56+/-14%), as well as better reproducibility of platelet content of the platelet concentrate obtained (VC 14% *versus* 19%) with the automated method.

Platelet Storage Media

The first media for platelet storage were developed at the end of the 1980s. Available media are presented at *Table II*. Recent developments indicate that their use will be generalized in the years to come [18].

Table II. Composition (mmol/L) of the most common platelet storage media.

	Plasmalyte A	PAS-II	PAS-III	PAS-IIIM	Composol
NaCl	90	115.5	77	69	90
KCl	5			5	5
MgCl2	3			1.5	1.5
Citrate Na3		10	10	10	10
NaH2PO4			26	26	
Acetate Na	27	30	33	30	27
Gluconate Na	23				23

The advantages of storage media can be resumed as follows :

– reduction of transfusion-related incidents such as allergic reactions and chills-and-fever [19, 20]; in a cohort of 36 patients (109 transfusion episodes), frequency of transfusion reactions to platelets was reduced by one third in recipients of leukodepleted platelet concentrates suspended in PAS-1 storage medium, compared to recipients of non leukodepleted platelets; allergic reactions were divided by 2, and febrile reactions by 5 [19]. In a prospective, randomized study with rigorous methodology comparing leukodepleted platelet concentrates from buffy-coats suspended in plasma with concentrates suspended in PAS-2 storage medium, marketed under the name T-Sol, overall frequency of reactions drops from 12% to 5.3%, allergic reactions drop from 5.2% to 0%, but febrile reactions remain unchanged, at 4.6% and 4.2% [20];

– although it has not been demonstrated in the scientific literature to date, reduction of TRALI-type incidents (transfusion-related Acute Lung Injury) is also expected; as an indication, in 2003 the French Hemovigilance System confirmed that nine of the fifteen cases of TRALI designated as strongly suggestive were due to platelet concentrates, leading to three fatalities [21];

– these storage media are a required preliminary step to at least one viral inactivation technique [22];

– finally, the use of these media makes it possible to obtain more plasma for fractionation and therefore, for the preparation of blood-derived therapeutic products.

The disadvantages of platelet storage media can be resumed as follows :

– all cell separators are not able to collect sufficiently concentrated platelets in one operation, requiring additional processing for certain apheresis platelet concentrates; however, all cell separators will be adapted, in the medium term, to the collection of highly concentrated platelets (concentration over $3 \times 10^6/\mu L$);

– storage lesions in platelet concentrates are more significant than those produced by storage in plasma, leading to considerably less effective recirculation of transfused platelets [18, 20, 23]; however, here again, better control of these lesions will be achieved with the introduction of media containing magnesium and phosphates, whose *in vitro* performances are more satisfactory [24], but for which we do not yet have clinical data.

Storage of Platelet Concentrates at 4 °C

Storing platelets at 22 °C is indispensable for limiting their activation *in vitro* and therefore preserving their aggregation capacity *in vivo*. In usual preparation conditions, when platelet concentrates are stored at 4 °C, there is almost total absence of recirculation *in vivo* after transfusion; the mechanism responsible for this phenomenon is not yet completely clear. Some of the reasons that have been suggested include activation of P-selectin (CD62p, or GMP-140) [25], as well as reorganization on the platelet surface of Willebrand factor receptors which might form clusters at 4 °C [26].

The first study described on the subject reported that inhibiting this reorganization on the Willebrand factor receptor surface [27] by enzyme glycosylation in the presence of UDP-galactose allowed effective platelet recirculation in mice. Another method [28], metabolic suppression induced by the addition of antimycin-A in a storage medium without glucose, allowed prolonged storage of human platelets for 72 hours at 4 °C, without major changes in *in vitro* function after resuspension in a storage medium with glucose at room temperature.

This data does not allow us to foresee, at present, platelet storage at 4 °C in our daily practice; but it shows that new approaches are possible and that they could certainly reduce bacterial risk associated with platelet concentrates stored at 22 °C, which is now greatly superior to that of red blood cell concentrates stored at 4 °C [29].

Developments Related to Preparation Activities in General

Automation of Whole Blood Component Separation

The separation of whole blood components comprises several stages : filtration, centrifugation and separation by extraction. To illustrate, filtration can precede centrifugation (whole blood filtration) or, on the contrary, it can follow it (filtration of red blood cell concentrate); speed of centrifugation can be high or low; extraction can be from the top (plasma) or from the top and the bottom (plasma and red blood cells respectively), with the buffy-coat stored in the main bag at the end of the separation process. At present, none of these stages is completely automated and manual intervention is always necessary between the stages.

New methods are currently being developed for regrouping, automating and standardizing the centrifugation and extraction stages. However, the filtration stage remains separate, taking place either before the other two (whole blood filtration), or after them (red blood cell concentrate filtration). These techniques are based on two very different preparation strategies: one enabling blood component separation at the time of collection, illustrated mainly by Baxter's Alyx device [12]; the other serving to build integrated technical preparation systems, illustrated mainly by the Atreus device made by Gambro, a device based on the Orbisac system mentioned above [17]. Because the first system is heavy and difficult to use at the collection site, particularly by mobile teams (given that in France 85% of whole blood is collected by mobile teams, while in Sweden this system is practically unknown, since whole blood is almost always collected at fixed locations), the second system is by far the one preferred in France.

Virus Inactivation

Virus inactivation techniques were first developed for plasma-derived medicinal products, and later for plasma. To date, two main techniques are available for plasma: the solvent-detergent method, that requires mixing plasmas (several thousand in the original technique [30] and one hundred in the method adopted in France) and acts on enveloped viruses; and methylene-blue [31], that can be used on individual plasmas from whole blood or apheresis, and acts on enveloped viruses and certain naked viruses.

Important developments concerning platelets are in progress. One method, based on the effect produced by a psoralen activated by UV-A rays on nucleic acids, is in an advanced stage of development, with EC values, and about to be authorized in France [22, 32, 33]. Another method, also based on forming covalent links between riboflavin and nucleic acids after visible light and UV activation, is being developed and is at the beginning stage of phase β III clinical trials [34].

However, at present there are no short or medium term projects planned for the development of pathogen inactivation techniques suitable for red blood cells.

All these techniques are described in greater detail in another chapter of this book, but they should be mentioned here given the important role they are likely to play in the future in improving microbiological transfusion safety, at least in terms of platelets and plasma.

In Vitro Blood Cell Production

Increased knowledge of hematopoietic stem cells, and the ability to control their expansion and orient their differentiation toward a particular blood cell line, have been used to prepare, from hematopoietic stem cells of various origins (placental blood and bone marrow), large quantities of red blood cells suitable for clinical use [35]. Initially, numerous obstacles had to be overcome, particularly an absence of understanding of the final red blood cell maturation phase, enucleation. A French team [35] which reproduced a medullar microenvironment *in vitro* by using cytokines and stromal cells was able to obtain CD34+ hematopoietic stem cell amplification by a factor of 2 million, with differentiation totally oriented to the production of mature red blood cells functional *in vivo*. The life cycle of these red blood cells, after transfusion to tolerant mice, is comparable to that of human red blood cells obtained from standard blood collection.

The data obtained from this research so far indicate that starting with collected placental blood it is possible to prepare a quantity of red blood cells equivalent to that of a classic unit of red blood cell concentrate, with an approximate hemoglobin content of about 50 grams. Of course, present methods of culture must be adapted to ensure the safety of such production volumes and to improve performance, but this approach will certainly become a reality. Clinical applications will probably be limited at first, and could be reserved to a few patients whose exceptional blood groups constitute a real therapeutic impasse. In immediate terms, this culture tool can improve our understanding of red blood cell physiology, particularly the mechanism of enucleation, and can also serve as a model for the study of interactions between red blood cells and parasites, or between red blood cells and medications.

Conclusion

During the past decade, numerous advances were made in the field of volunteer donor blood collection and the preparation of labile blood products.

These advances inevitably brought about improvements in the quality and safety of labile blood products, but, as we have seen, improvements have not been simultaneous in these two areas. Safety improvements (platelet storage media, viral inactivation techniques, etc.) often lead to modifications in the functional quality of blood cells and/or of plasma proteins. Therefore, reasonable decisions leading to the implementation of a new technique must take all these factors into account.

We can now expect important advances in the standardization of labile blood product preparation. For example, in red blood cell concentrates, distribution of hemoglobin content still covers a very wide range : quality control data from the national data base of the French National Blood Service (*Table III*) show a mean hemoglobin content variation between 50 and 56 grams, depending on the preparation technique, with standard deviation of the order of 6, and extreme values between 36 and 74 grams.

Table III. Hemoglobin content of red blood cell concentrates prepared in France in 2001, 2002 and 2003, depending on preparation technique.

	WB Filtration			RBC Filtration, top and bottom extraction			RBC Filtration, top extraction		
Year	2001	2002	2003	2001	2002	2003	2001	2002	2003
Total quantity	12,883	11,904	14,816	2,980	4,522	3,906	3,218	4,672	2,125
Mean (g/RBC)	55.5	55.6	56.3	50.5	50.3	50.8	53.1	51.8	52.6
Standard deviation	7.1	6.9	6.9	5.9	5.8	5.7	7.6	6.8	6.2

Of course, red blood cell collection by apheresis, which allows veritable programming of the quality of collected samples, reduces this variation. However, this technique should not reduce current mean values, as the majority of apheresis techniques in fact do in the preparation of two red blood cell concentrates from a single blood donation.

Better standardization will facilitate the search for an equivalence between the quantity of cellular "active principle" (red blood cells or platelets) considered necessary for patient therapy, and the quantity actually present in the products delivered. It should also be remembered that adapting the dosage leads to better control of the use of labile blood products [36,37]. In France today, this equivalence has been achieved for apheresis platelet concentrates whose platelet content is systematically measured and marked on each product; equivalence is not as easy to achieve for red blood cell concentrates; in the case of the latter, the only guaranteed parameter is a hemoglobin content of at least 40 grams.

Finally, we must point out the great difficulties encountered in practice when attempting to identify the origin of the improvements observed in transfusion safety. On the one hand, over a given period, our activities involve a number of successive developments in different fields, each of which could have a direct or indirect effect on labile blood product quality and safety; on the other hand, each new development is, generally, implemented completely in a very gradual manner. To illustrate, while hemovigilance data showed reduction by half of grade 1 and 3 bacterial contamination incidents between 1998 and 2000 (39 incidents for a million platelet concentrates) and between 2002 and 2004 (20 incidents for a million platelet concentrates), numerous changes that occurred in that period could have contributed to this reduction; among them: gradual installation of the derivation of the first thirty millimeters on apheresis devices, generalization of leukodepletion (in 1998, a few platelet concentrates were not leukodepleted), and implementation of stricter procedures of phlebotomy site decontamination. Consequently, it is hard to establish the role of each of these measures on the progress accomplished. Therefore, it is essential to assess every new technique of labile blood product collection and preparation very rigorously, within the framework of specific prospective studies, before it can be put into effect.

References

1. Mollison PL, Young IM. In vivo survival in the human subject of transfused erythrocytes in various preservative solutions. *Quart J Exp Physiol* 1942 31 : 359.
2. Piertersz RN, de Korte D, Reesink HW, et al. Preparation of leukocyte-poor platelet concentrates from buffy-coats. III. Effect of leukocyte contamination on storage conditions. *Vox Sanguinis* 1988; 55 : 14-20.
3. Price TH, Northway MM, Moore RC. Further results with the COBE Spectra system. Platelet collection using the COBE Spectra. *Infusionstherapie* 1989 ; Suppl. 2 : 44.
4. Andreu G, Masse M, Royer SD, Tardivel R. Leukodepleted blood components: definition of a standard. *Transfus Sci* 1999, 19 : 381-3.
5. Schoendorfer DW, Hansen LE, Kenney DM. The surge technique: a method to increase purity of platelet concentrates obtained by centrifugal apheresis. *Transfusion* 1983; 23 : 182-9.
6. Chabanel A, Andreu G, Carrat F, Hervé P. Quality control of leucoreduced cellular blood components in France. *Vox Sanguinis* 2002 ; 82 : 67-71.
7. Chabanel A, Sensebe L, Masse M, Maurel JP, Plante J, Hivet D, Kannengiesser, Naegelen C, Joussemet M, Marchesseau, Rasongles P, Proust F, David C, Montembalut AM, Bergeat P., Quality assessment of seven types of fresh-frozen plasma leucoreduced by specific plasma filtration. *Vox Sanguinis* 2003 ; 84 : 308-17.
8. *Guide pour la préparation, l'utilisation et l'assurance qualité des composants sanguins.* Editions du Conseil de l'Europe, 2005.
9. Bruneau C, Perez P, Chassaigne M, Allouch P, Audurier A, Gulian C, Janus G, Boulard G, De Micco P, Salmi LR, Noel L. Efficacy of a new collection procedure for preventing bacterial contamination of whole-blood donations. *Transfusion* 2001 ; 41 : 74-81.
10. Pietersz RN, Reesink HW, de Korte D, Dekker WJ, van den Ende A, Loos JA. Storage of leukocyte-poor red cell concentrates: filtration in a closed system using a sterile connection device. *Vox Sanguinis.* 1989 ; 57 : 29-36.
11. Valbonesi M, Frisoni R, Florio G, Ruzzenenti MR, Capra C, Merlo M, Parenti. Single-donor platelet concentrates produced along with packed red blood cells with the Haemonetics MCS 3p: preliminary results. *J Clin Apheresis* 1994 ; 9 : 195-9.
12. Snyder EL, Elfath MD, Taylor H, Rugg N, Greenwalt TJ, Baril L, Whitley P, Brantigan B, Story K. Collection of two units of leukoreduced RBCs from a single donation with a portable multiple-component collection. *Transfusion* 2003 ; 43 : 1695-705.
13. Radtke H, Mayer B, Röcker L, Salama A, Kiesewetter H. Iron supplementation and 2-unit red blood cell apheresis : a randomised, double-blind, placebo-controlled study. *Transfusion* 2004; 44 : 1463-7.
14. Moog R, Bartsch R, Muller N. Concurrent collection of in-line filtered platelets and red blood cells by apheresis. *Ann Hematol* 2002 ; 81 : 322-5.
15. Bertolini F, Rebulla T, Poretti L, Murphy S. Platelet quality after 15-day storage of platelet concentrate prepared from buffy coats and stored in a glucose-free crystalloid medium. *Transfusion* 1992 ; 32 : 9-16.
16. Fijnheer R, Veldman HA, van den Eertwegh AJ, Gouwerok CWN, Homburg CHE, Boogaard MD, de Korte D, Roos D. In vitro evaluation of buffy-coat-derived platelet concentrates stored in a synthetic medium. *Vox Sanguinis* 1991; 60 : 16-22.
17. Janetzko K, Klüter H, van Waeg G, Eichler H. Fully automated processing of buffy-coat-derived pooled platelet concentrated. *Transfusion* 2004; vol. 44 : 1052-8.
18. de Wildt-Eggen, Gullikson H. In vivo and in vitro comparison of platelets stored in either synthetic media or plasma. *Vox Sanguinis* 2003; 84 : 256-64.

19. Oksanen K, Ebeling F, Kekomäti R, Elonen E, Sahlstedt L, Volin L, Myllylä G. Adverse reactions to platelet transfusions are reduced by use of platelet concentrates derived from buffy coat. *Vox Sanguinis* 1994 ; 96 : 356-61.
20. de Wildt-Eggen, Nauta S, Schrijver JG, van Marwikk Kooy M, Bins M, van Prooijen HC. Reactions and platelets increments after transfusion of platelets concentrates in plasma or an additive solution : a prospective, randomized stud. *Transfusion* 2000; 40 : 398-403.
21. Rebibo D, Hauser L, Slimani A, Hervé P, Andreu G. The French Haemovigilance System: organization and results for 2003. *Transf Apheresis Sci* 2004 ; 1 : 145-53.
22. Lin L, Cook DN, Wiesenhahn GP, et al. Photochemical inactivation of viruses and bacteria in platelet concentrates by use of a novel psoralen and long-wavelength ultraviolet light. *Transfusion* 1997; 37 : 423-35.
23. van Rhenen DJ, Gulliksson H, Cazenave JP, Pamphilon D, Davis K, Flament J, Corash L. Therapeutic efficacy of pooled buffy-coat platelet components prepared and stored with a platelet additive solution. *Transfus Med* 2004 ; 44 : 289.
24. Gulliksson H, AuBuchon JP, Cardigan R, van der Meer PF, Murphy S, Prowse C, Richter E, Ringwald J, Smacchia C, Slichter S, de Wildt-Eggen J (for the ISBT). Storage of platelets in additive solutions : a multicentre study of the in vitro effects of potassium and magnesium. *Vox Sanguinis* 2003; 85 : 199-205.
25. Berger G, Hartwell DW, Wagner DD. P-selectin and platelet clearance. *Blood* 1998 ; 92 : 4446-52.
26. Hoffmeister KM, Felbinger TW, Falet H. The clearance mechanism of chilled blood platelets. *Cell* 2003; 112 : 87-97.
27. Hoffmeister K, Josefsson E, Isaac N, Clausen H, Hartwig J, Stossel T. Glycosylation restores survival of chilled blood platelets. *Science* 2003; 301 : 1531-4.
28. Badlou BA, Ijseldijk MJW, Smid WM, Akkerman JWN. Prolonged platelet preservation by transient metabolic suppression. *Transfusion* 2005; 45 : 214-22.
29. Andreu G, Morel P, Forestier F, Debeir J, Rebibo D, Janvier G, Hervé P. Haemovigilance network in France : organization and analysis of immediate transfusion incident reports from 1994 to 1998. *Transfusion* 2002 ; 42 : 1356-64.
30. Horowitz B, Lazo A, Grossberg H, Page G, Lippin A, Swan G. Virus inactivation by solvent/detergent treatment and the manufacture of SD-plasma. *Vox Sanguinis* 1998; 74 : 203-6.
31. Williamson L, Cardigan R, Prowse C. Methylene blue-treated fresh plasma : what is its contribution to blood safety ? *Transfusion* 2003; 43 : 1322-9.
32. McCullough J, Vesole D, Benjamin RJ, et al. Pathogen inactivated platelets using Helinx™ technology are hemostatically effective in thrombocytopenic patients : the SPRINT trial. *Blood* 2001; 98 : 405a.
33. van Rhenen D, Gulliksson H, Cazenave JP, et al. Transfusion of pooled buffy coat platelet components prepared with photochemical pathogen inactivation treatment. The Euro-SPRITE trial. *Blood* 2003 ; 101 : 2426-33.
34. Rhuane PH, Edrich R, Gampp D, Keil SD, Leonard RL, Goodrich RP. Photochemical inactivation of selected viruses and bacteria in platelet concentrated using riboflavin and light. *Transfusion* 2004 ; 44 : 855-77.
35. Giarratana MC, Kobari L, Lapillonne H, Chalmers, Kiger L, Cynober, Marden M, Wajcman H, Douay L. Ex-vivo generation of fully mature human red blood cells from hematopoietic stem cells. *Nature Biotechnology* 2004, on line : 1-5.
36. Arslan O, Toprak S, Arat M, Kayalak Y. Hb content-based transfusion policy successfully reduces the number of RBC units transfused. *Transfusion* 2004 ; 44 : 445-8.
37. Davenport R. Blood components should be labelled for content. *Transfusion* 2005; 45 : 3.

Blood Substitutes:
Challenge or Marginality?*

Patrick Menu, Marie Toussaint-Hacquard, Jean-François Stoltz

Research on the creation of different artificial or biological substitutes for blood functions has been at the center of numerous projects in the 20th century. Although plasma substitutes have been used for a long time in clinical practice (dextran, amidon…), the same is not true for oxygen carriers or platelet function substitutes.

In terms of "oxygen and CO_2 transport", the earliest experiments go back as far as 1925, when Backer and Dodds [1] administered hemoglobin by intravenous injection to rabbits and observed the occurrence of renal problems which they attributed to precipitation of the molecule in the tubules as a consequence of acidosis and increase of saline concentration. In 1940, de Nevasquez [2] showed that these two factors were not responsible for the problems that were observed. Other authors, de Gowin [3, 4] and Bing [5], studied the question but did not arrive at satisfactory answers. In 1948, Hamilton et al. [6], who made a more specific study of the effects of hemoglobin solutions on the kidney, recommended that they should not be used. Later, Rabiner et al. [7] again conducted studies on hemoglobin solutions; they prepared solutions without stroma that they injected to monkeys, and obtained encouraging results: the solution was, for all practical purposes, no longer toxic, and carried oxygen.

In addition, according to Peskin et al., its osmotic properties were close to those of dextran [8].

Despite this unique oxygen-carrying advantage not provided by other substitutes, the use of hemoglobin solutions remained experimental for a long time, given the difficulties of preparation and storage, and poorly controlled adverse effects.

At the same time, interest in artificial oxygen carriers was sparked by the work of Clark and Gollan [9], who showed that a mouse immersed in a fluorocarbon emulsion can survive several hours, although the lungs are filled with liquid. From then on, much research was conducted on the subject, especially in the United States [10] and Japan, including a few clinical trials [11, 12]. It was not until the arrival of the second generation of emulsions that these compounds were subjected to further development [13, 14]; the most advanced compounds should be ready for use in humans in the near future.

---

* Work conducted within the "Euro Blood Substitutes" project of the European Committee, with the support of the Lorraine Region.

Research on the stabilization or substitution of platelet functions (thrombosomes) is much more recent and has given rise to fewer, albeit interesting, studies.

This chapter will review the research and clinical trials related to hemoglobin solutions and to synthesized oxygen carriers, as well as the research on platelet function substitutes. We have not included the recent work on leukocytes and exosomes in antitumoral immunotherapy [15].

Oxygen Carriers: Myth or Reality?

Although blood saving techniques, associated with decreased recourse to transfusion, have made it possible to limit the number of homologous transfusions during surgery, the difficulty of obtaining emergency blood product supplies is still a limitation with respect to their use.

A red blood cell substitute that is universally compatible and can restore blood volume and ensure respiratory gas transport remains of clinical interest, although it can never have all the properties of blood.

Oxygen carriers currently being developed, also called "oxygen therapeutics", must satisfy a variety of requirements that become more and more precise as the solutions in development evolve. Above all, these carriers must have volume expanding capacities (like traditional plasma substitutes) and be able to carry and deliver gases to tissues. They must not provoke major adverse effects, be free of infectious agents and residual toxicity, and demonstrate adequate vascular remanence, at an acceptable cost. Potential indications for such substitutes are many: hemorrhagic shock, ischemia, myocardial infarction, angioplasty, organ and tissue conservation, pre-operative hemodilution, extracorporeal circulation and use in patients who refuse blood transfusion. Thus, this research presents considerable clinical and economic interest. This is why for over forty years many research teams, in cooperation with industry, have been attempting to develop oxygen carriers presenting specific characteristics that could reduce, or even eliminate, the factors limiting their use.

At present, three research perspectives are being explored. The first is based on chemical changes in human or animal hemoglobin; the second, more closely related to transfusion, focuses on producing modifications in the environment of administered hemoglobin and erythrocytes, or in liposomes; and the third studies the potential of fluorocarbon emulsions.

At the same time, the Food and Drug Administration has just published guidelines listing the main criteria for the evaluation of "oxygen therapeutics" efficacy, in anticipation of clinical trials [16].

The various stages of progress and potentials of different substitutes now in development are described below.

Hemoglobin Based Oxygen carriers (HBOC)

Hemoglobin does not have the antigenic properties of erythrocytes, but retains their oxygen-carrying capacity [17].

As we have said above, the first oxygen carriers tested were simple hemoglobin solutions [18, 19]. But they were rapidly shown to be toxic and ineffective. Their harmful effects were attributed to the presence of lipids and proteins originating in erythrocyte membrane debris [20]. Although hemoglobin solutions prepared later were purified by chromatography (producing "stroma-free hemoglobin", SFH) [21], a certain nephrotoxicity remains, mainly due to renal excretion of SFH. Moreover, clearance is rapid and plasma half life is short (2 to 5 hours), due to dissociation of tetramer α2β2 hemoglobin into αβ diamers [17, 20, 21]. Thus, during infusion of stroma-free hemoglobin, the quantities of free hemoglobin in the circulation become excessive, overwhelming physiological regulatory systems and producing renal failure and cytotoxicity inherent to oxydation of free hemoglobin to methemoglobin, with release of free radicals [22].

In addition, due to the current optimization of blood cell concentrate management, unused erythrocyte stocks are limited [20, 23], leading to interest in finding other sources of more easily accessible hemoproteins.

Hemoglobin Sources

- **Human hemoglobin** is only available in limited quantities, it is extracted by lysis from erythrocytes, and can be prepared from outdated blood units. This hemoglobin is purified by ultrafiltration and by chromatography, and then undergoes viral inactivation by heating, filtration and/or solvent-detergent [24]. This inactivates any viral agents potentially present in the red blood cells. Efficacy of these procedures has been validated for many viruses, including HIV, the cytomegalovirus and hepatitis B. In addition, other operations implemented during the manufacturing process, such as ultrafiltration or chromatography, are intended to partly eliminate viruses potentially present, increasing the safety of these solutions [25]. Nevertheless, all risks cannot be formally excluded.

Free hemoglobin prepared in this manner has oxygen affinity that is too high, due to loss of its allosteric effector, 2,3-diphosphoglycerate, responsible for adequate rerelease of oxygen to tissues [13, 17]. Moreover, its possible presence inside endothelial cells [26], and its extravasation and/or excretion require tetrameric stabilization and the addition of an allosteric effector.

- **Bovine hemoglobin,** contrary to human hemoglobin, does not have an allosteric effector; its intrinsic oxygen affinity is low [17]. Therefore, bovine hemoglobin appeared as an interesting alternative to human hemoglobin, particularly since it is available in abundance and at low cost [13]. However, potential risks limit its use (transmission of bovine spongiform encephalitis or possible immune response with production of antibodies after injection of bovine proteins).

- **Recombinant hemoglobins** were obtained, by genetic engineering, in bacteria, yeasts and plant cells [27, 28]. The most common human recombinant hemoglobin is produced by the *Escherichia Coli* bacterium, whose globin coding molecules are integrated in the genome.

The hemoglobin obtained in this manner is superior in terms of tissue oxygen liberation and vascular persistence, due to integration of a glycene link between the two α chains [29].

At present, use of this hemoglobin is limited by the high cost of its production [23]. Somatogen, a firm in the Baxter group, has produced a crosslinked α1-α2 phemoglobin (Optro^{TM}, US) that was polymerized (rHb 2.0, US), but whose development seems to have been halted [29, 30]. A new form of recombinant hemoglobin called *Euroblood Substitute* is currently under study by several collaborating teams including ours, within the framework of the 6th PCRD (2004-2007) [31].

Modified Hemoglobin Solutions and their Limitations

Modified Hemoglobin Solutions

In order to compensate for the disadvantages of native hemoglobin, chemical modifications have been used to stabilize this hemoprotein. Thus, in order to reduce oxygen affinity, coupling with allosteric modulators (such as pyridoxal phosphate) is used, and in order to prolongue half-life, subunits are stabilized by fusion. In order to reduce oncotic pressure, molecular mass is increased by binding to macromolecules (polyethylene, dextran…), by polymerization (glutaraldehyde), or by encapsulating hemoglobin in synthetic microvesicles (liposomes, niosomes). The major physical and chemical characteristics of the developed products are presented at *Table I*.

Table I. Physical and chemical characteristics of the main chemically modified forms of hemoglobin.

Name	Origin	Molecular mass (kDa)	Hb (g/dL)	Viscosity (cPoise)	Oncotic pressure (mmHg)	P50 (mmHg)	Clinical stage
rHb 2.0	Human	Unknown	10	2.3	62	34	In development or halted?
DCLHb	Human	64	10	10	42	32	Halted
Polyheme	Human	64 to 400	15	~ 2.1	~ 23	~ 20	Phase III
o-raffinose--polyHb	Human	64 to 600	10	1.15	~ 24	34	Halted?
Hemopure	Bovine	64 to 500	13	1.3	25	~ 37	Awaited
PHP	Human	187	8	2.9	57	24	Phase III
MP4	Human	95	4.2	2.5	55	6	Phase I
OxyVita	Human, bovine	20 Mda	6	~ 2.5	10	4	Preclinical
HbV/HSA	Human	281 nm diameter	8.6	3	40	33	Preclinical

- **Intramolecular reticulation** between subunits α and β or β and β stabilizes the chains and reduces renal elimination. This technique, developed by the American Army and Baxter HealthCare under the name *Diasprin cross-linked* Hb (DCL Hb), and later *HemAssist*, produced *cross-linked* Hb through chemical modifications α1-lys99, α2-lys99 (bis 3.5 dibromosalicyl fumarate). After trials in trauma, surgery and ischemic settings, development of this product was also halted [17, 20].
- **Hemoglobin polymerization** increases vascular remanence while slowing oxidation. The principle consists of binding several hemoglobin molecules together using agents like glutaraldehyde [13, 20]. Polymerization increases solution viscosity, which appears to be an advantage. Several polymerized hemoglobins have been synthetized from human hemoglobin, particularly:

– PolyHeme[TM] (Northfield Laboratories, US), [β1β2 (pyridoxal 5'phophate) bound and polymerized by glutaraldehyde] now at phase III clinical trial stage (traumatology) [32];

– Hemolink (Hemosol Inc, CN), [β1β2 (bound by o-raffinose chains) and polymerized]; phase II clinical trials [33];

– Hemopure[TM] from bovine hemoglobin (HBOC-201, Biopure Corporation, US), [Hb polymerized by glutaraldehyde], now in preclinical studies before approval by the FDA for orthopaedic surgery, and approved in South Africa as transfusion replacement [34].

- **Conjugated hemoglobin** is obtained by binding the hemoprotein to biocompatible macromolecules such as dextran 40 (Hb-Dex-BTC, Fr) [35, 36] or polyethylene glycol (PEG-Hb; Enzon, US). Development of these products also seems to have been halted.

However, other macromolecules are being evaluated for possible use; among them:

– PHP (PLP-Hb-PEG) produced by Cyracyte Inc. (formerly Apex Bioscience, USA), [β1-β2 bound by pyridoxal phosphate and conjugated with polyethylene glycol], at phase III clinical trial stage [37];

– MP4 (Mal-PEG 4 maleimide-PEG-Hb) produced by Hemospan, Sangart Inc, USA) [38, 39];

– OxyVita (ZL-Hb, fusion $\alpha 1\beta 1$-$\alpha 2\beta 2$ Zero-length and Hb polymerization) produced by IPBL Pharmaceutical (University of Maryland, USA) [40], in preclinical trial phase.

• **Hemoglobin encapsulation** offers an alternative to chemical modification. This method increases intravascular life and allows co-encapsulation of certain molecules, particularly 2.3 DPG and hemoglobin, leading to more rapid fixation and oxygen liberation kinetics for encapsulated hemoglobin than for erythrocytes [20]. Hemoglobin encapsulation can be achieved using liposome-type vectors [41], sometimes coated with polyethylene glycol for better sealing (HbV-PEG) [42], or with Hb PLP in suspension in the presence of human serum albumin (HbV/HAS) developed in Japan [43]. Other approaches, based on the use of biodegradable polymer nanocapsules (polyethylene-glycol-polylactide) containing a small quantity of smaller size hemoglobin, are currently being developed [44].

Finally, in France, a recent study is evaluating hemoglobin loaded on beads (100 to 300 nanometers) of alkylcyanoacrylate and sugar monomers [45].

Limitations of Modified Hemoglobin Solutions

Alayash [46] raises the question of whether modified hemoglobins can really be "tamed", since they almost always cause a change in vascular tonus, attributed to the interaction between hemoglobin and nitric oxide. These vasomotor variations have been detected *in vitro* in isolated artery models, as well as *in vivo*, by blood pressure and local blood volume measurements. Nitric oxide is a powerful vasodilator, produced and liberated by the vascular endothelium, whose action relaxes vascular tonus. One of the probable causes of vasoconstriction observed at injection of hemoglobin solutions could be entrapped nitric oxide [24], with reduction of its bioavailability and consequent elevation of blood pressure. This entrapment by the hemoglobin solution probably takes place in the vascular system during extravasation [46]. Sakai *et al.* have shown that vasoconstriction intensity is correlated with size of hemoproteins [47].

The smallest molecules (crosslinked $\alpha\alpha$ hemoglobin, for example) cross the endothelial barrier easily, while large molecules (HbV-PEG) are far less affected by this phenomenon.

However, Hb-NO interaction is perhaps only the top of the iceberg, indicating many other possible vascular Hb interactions.

It is also clear that the vasoconstriction in question is multifactorial; other mechanisms that could be involved include:

– stimulation of endothelin production (powerful vasoconstrictor) [48];

– potentialization of catecholamine response of $\alpha 1$ and $\alpha 2$ adrenergic receptors [47];

– during hemoglobin auto-oxidation, production of superoxide free radicals which, by reacting with nitric oxide, behave like powerful vasoconstrictors;

– reflex vasoconstriction following excessive oxygenation of peripheral tissues, or following excessively reduced solute viscosity, reducing shear stress applied to internal vessel walls [49].

In a patient in a state of shock, while limited increase of systemic vascular resistances could be beneficial by improving vital organ perfusion (volemic shock, for example), a rise in pulmonary and coronary vascular resistances could produce major adverse effects. This is why numerous studies are attempting to better understand and control these vasomotor phenomena.

Tomorrow's Modified Hemoglobins

New generations of modified hemoglobin will have to show absence of vasopressor effects and/or be "equiped" with enzymes to limit major adverse effects (vasoconstriction or oxidation to methemoglobin), particularly by reducing nitric oxide affinity, or by incorporating antioxidant enzymes. To this end, Chang's team has developed a substitute with antioxidant properties (polyhemoglobin-superoxide-dismutase-catalase or poly-Hb-SOD-CAT) [50]. Tsai et al. use *Escherichia coli*, a recombinant hemoglobin with low oxygen affinity, to produce rHb (beta N108Q), which is relatively stable against oxidation [51]. Tsuchida et al. have developed an original substitute without hypertensive effects: a synthetic heme is "incorporated" in human recombinant albumin [52]. Winslow et al. recommend high molecular weight, high oxygen affinity and considerable intrinsic viscosity favoring better vaso-relaxation [53], which are likely to reduce adverse hemodynamic effects at administration [38]. Based on this principle, other researchers developed hemoglobins with original chemical modifications likely to facilitate vascular remanence. Two French substitutes currently under development can be mentioned in this context: an octomeric hemoglobin produced in *E.coli* from an abnormal hemoglobin gene (rHb beta G83C, INSERM, U473) [54], and a hemoglobin (Roscoff and CNRS and P.&M.Curie University) produced from a sea worm (*Arenicola marina* naturally polymerized extracellular hemoglobin) [55].

Allosteric Hemoglobin or Therapeutic Agent Effectors Encapsulated in Erythrocytes

This technique was developed in the 1980s in France by Ropars et al. [56]; the procedure is used to insert therapeutic agents within erythrocytes by lysis/resealing, without modifying cell viability. The procedure is simple: in response to a controlled osmotic shock, erythrocytes swell and thereby create pores in the membrane, making it possible to insert molecules or therapeutic agents in the cell. When erythrocytes are replaced in an isotonic milieu, the membrane is resealed. Several preliminary studies have validated the therapeutic agent encapsulation principle (thrombotics, iron chelators, allosteric agents, immunosuppressors...) [57, 58]. In transfusion settings, displacement of the oxygen-Hb dissociation curve by 2,3-DPG elevation is important. The technique proposed by Ropars et al., consisting of introducing an allosteric hemoglobin effector (inositol hexaphosphate) by reversible hemolysis, is attractive for P50 modification. Animal studies have shown the method to be feasible, but unfortunately no clinical trials in an ischemic pathology setting have been conducted to date [59]. In addition, the method could be useful for medication vectoring by controlled autotransfusion as an alternative to nanoparticles or liposomes [58].

Fluorocarbon or Perfluorocarbon Emulsions

Perfluorocarbons, inert synthetic hydrocarbons, linear or cyclic in shape, in which all or part of the hydrogen atoms have been replaced by fluor or by bromine, can be used as blood substitutes. This principle dates back to 1966, to the work of Clark and Gollan, who showed that a rat immersed in an oxygenated perfluorocarbon can survive [9].

Fluorocarbon can transport and liberate oxygen and carbon anhydride due to the physical solubility of gases, which is directly proportional to the partial pressure applied [17, 20].

Therefore, in order to increase the quantity of oxygen delivered to the tissues, it is essential to increase oxygen concentration of the air inhaled by the patient ($FiO_2 = 1$), rather than the dose of fluorocarbon. When this is done, the concentration of gas delivered is similar to that of blood. However, fluorocarbons must be administered in the form of a dispersion of fine, stabilized particles, by tensioactive agents. Currently used emulgents (egg yoke lecithin) are relatively well tolerated and provide stable emulsions at ambient temperature [17, 20]. Thus, the quantity of oxygen carried by flyorocarbons is double that of blood (due to absence of binding) and oxygen extraction is increased because of the large fluorocarbon surface exposed by the small size of emulsion particles (2 for 8 µm) [60], making this an interesting substitute for reducing tissue ischemia.

Finally, fluorocarbon emulsions must be diluted in a colloid or HES plasma substitute, in order to have adequate oncotic pressure and viscosity.

Different Generations of Fluorocarbons

The most developed of the first generation emulsions is Fluosol-DA® (Green Cross Corporation, Osaka, Japan). This emulsion is a mixture of 70% perfluorodecalin and 30% perfluorotriproplylamin emulsified by Pluronic F-68. The emulsion has limited efficacy, given its low fluorocarbon content, low intravascular persistance and highly inadequate stability. To be administered, Fluosol-DA® must be thawed (the emulsion is not stable at room temperature), homogenized and oxygenated; this two-hour preparation time is incompatible with emergency use. However, Fluosol-DA® was approved by the Food and Drug Administration for use in percutaneous transluminal coronary angioplasty [61]. But Green Cross Corporation stopped manufacturing the emulsion in 1994 due to limited commercial success [62].

Second generation fluorocarbon emulsions, represented by Oxygent® (perfluorooctyle bromide or perflubron; Alliance Pharmaceutical Co, US) [63], Oxyfluor® (perfluorodichloroctane emulsion; HemaGen, US) and Perftoran (emulsion with 3% per volume perfluoromethylcyclohexylpiperidin and 7% per volume perfluorodecalin, Russia) [64, 65], present three major advantages: increased efficacy due to fluorocarbon concentration four to five times higher than that of first generation emulsions, a better tolerated tensioactive emulgent (egg yoke lecithin), and greater stability (emulsions that are heat-resistant at sterilization can be stored for one year at 5 to 8 °C and are ready for use). However, when used in a human clinical setting, they can produce a dose-dependent flu-like syndrome appearing four to six hours after the injection. The syndrome includes fever, hypotension, tachicardia, hyperleukocytosis and thrombocytopenia; it disappears within 24 hours. At present, it seems that after treatment of 1,400 cases, Alliance has temporarily suspended clinical trials [14].

Potential Clinical Applications of Fluorocarbons

Fluorocarbons could be used to delay transfusions and reduce their volume. Their use, in association with immediate normovolemic hemodilution, increases oxygen transport despite hematocrit levels inferior to the normally tolerated threshold, without compromising tissue oxygenation, and making it possible to delay administration of autologous blood. More severe hemodilution could be tolerated by the patient, in cases of scheduled intervention before which blood collected from the patient is compensated by fluorocarbons, and is reinjected during and after surgery. Recourse to homologous transfusion would be reduced. Clinical phase II and III trials on Perflubron and Perftoran are now in progress to assess this application [66-68].

The small size of the particles and their oxygen-carrying capacity make it reasonable to think that these emulsions could find applications in hypoxic microcirculatory settings (stroke, coronary angioplasty, myocardial infarction...) [17].

In oncology, fluorocarbons would increase cancer cell sensitivity to radiotherapy and chemotherapy [69]. They can also be used for organ storage in view of transplantation. Finally, they are used in pure form for semi-liquid ventilation in pathologies like acute adult respiratory distress syndrome or hyalin membrane disease in newborns [17, 70]. In these settings, fluorocarbons facilitate gas exchange and alveolar recruitment.

The main advantage of perfluorocarbons is that they are entirely synthetic. They have medical and biotechnological applications, most specifically in surgery, as temporary fluids able to oxygenate tissues. As such, they constitute an interesting area for future development.

Can we Create Platelet Substitutes?

Development of platelet substitutes is essentially connected with recurring supply problems (insufficient donors for existing needs) and with storage conditions (maximum 5 days, at 22 °C, with risk of bacterial reproduction). This has made it necessary to consider substitute products. Lee and Blajchman [71] have submitted specifications for a typical platelet substitute. According to these criteria, the product must have haemostatic efficacy without thrombogen effects, must remain active for an adequate duration, must present no immunogenicity and cause no immunodeficiency, must be sterile, must survive a long time in simple storage conditions, and must be easy to administer.

The platelet substitutes proposed are of two types: products derived from platelets and true substitutes not of cellular derivation.

Platelet-derived products

One of the major problems in transfusion today concerns platelet storage at ambient temperature. Many research teams have worked on storing platelets in the cold. These studies revealed hemostatic function changes and reduced survival *in vivo* [72, 73]. In fact, exposure of platelets to cold modulates membrane glycoprotein expression, possibly facilitating elimination of these glycoproteins by hepatic macrophages. Various strategies have been tested to preserve platelet morphology and function during storage at +4 °C, using cytoskeletal assembly inhibitors (cytochalasin B in combination with a calcium chelate) of molecules such as trehalose or "antifreeze" fish glycoproteins, or agents producing platelet enzyme galactosylation, which limits their recognition and, as a result, their elimination by hepatic macrophages [74]. Other teams attempted to freeze their platelets using a cryoprotector like 6% dimethylsulfoxide [75], now a recognized method, which allows platelet storage up to ten years at –80 °C. These platelets present morphological and functional modifications, but preserve their hemostatic properties *in vivo*. However, this method is costly and preparation is delicate. This is why the procedure is used essentially to store autologous platelets for transfusion of allo-immunized patients, in an acute leukemia setting, for example [76]. Recent studies have made it possible to improve the procedure by adding a conservation solution composed of amiloride, adenosine and sodium nitroprusside (ThromboSol™, LifeCell, USA) to the milieu, to obtain inhibition of cell activation and reduce dimethylsulfoxide concentration to 2% [77]. This facilitates subsequent use of the platelets by eliminating the wash stage.

Other researchers are investigating lyophilized platelet preparation. The idea is not new; the first experiments date back to the 1950s [78, 79], but it was only recently that a research team has devised a method of human platelet preparation in paraformaldehyde, frozen in 5% albumin, then lyophilized [80]. *In vitro* evaluation of this preparation showed preservation of platelet morphology and reduced, but residual, expression of most platelet glycoproteins on rehydrated membrane surfaces. Despite absence of aggregation after ADP and collagen stimulation, these platelets seem able to participate in aggregation in the presence of "fresh" platelets, and show procoagulant activity. *In vivo*, the hemostatic properties of these rehydrated platelets were demonstrated in studies on thrombopenic animals (rabbits and dogs); however, activity duration was short, lasting only 4 to 6 hours [81].

Another method uses platelet microvesicles with procoagulant properties that facilitate cellular adhesion. This principle was applied by an American company (Cypress Bioscience), which developed a human platelet microvesicle preparation (In fusible Platelet Membranes, Cyplex®) by means of successive freezing-unfreezing of outdated platelet concentrates [82].

A succession of stages, starting with viral inactivation by heating, followed by formulation in a mixture of saccharose and albumin, and then in a lyophilization mixture, makes this preparation stable for two years at 4 °C. Hemostatic efficacy of this product was demonstrated *in vivo* in a thrombopenic rabbit model, where shortened bleeding time over a period of six hours was observed [82]. No toxicity was detected. Clinical phase I and II trials in humans have been conducted. A phase II trial in thrombopenic patients with refractory hemorrhage showed the product to have a certain hemostatic efficacy, making it possible to stop hemorrhage in some of these patients [76]. However, manufacturing of this product seems to have been halted for the present.

Non-Platelet-Derived Substitutes

In order to solve storage problems and counter insufficient supply, some research teams are working on developing substitute products, in the true sense of the term. All products in this category are still at the preclinical evaluation stage.

One method involves preparing bead or nanoparticle erythrocytes on which a fibrinogen or RGD peptidic sequence is grafted, allowing fibrinogen binding to GPIIbIIIa. However, despite the proaggregating platelet properties they demonstrated *in vitro*, these substitutes showed no hemostatic efficacy *in vivo* [76].

Another method consists of using microcapsules or microspheres coated with fibrinogen. Two preparations of this type have been studied, but this research seems discontinued:

– human albumin microcapsules with a 3.5 to 45 µm diameter, obtained by automation, on which human fibrinogen molecules are immobilized by ionic interaction (Synthocytes™, Andrias, UK). Preclinical trials in thrombopenic animal models have shown that this substitute can shorten bleeding time over a period of 3 hours [83];

– albumin microspheres coated with fibrinogen using a different process (1 to 2 µm diameter particles, Thrombospheres™, Hemosphere, USA) also present hemostatic properties *in vivo* in thrombopenic rabbits. Their effect is surprising: very long duration of action (up to 72 hours after a single bolus, and after the microspheres can no longer be detected in the circulation [84].

Finally, other teams have developed liposomal agents, using various approaches: "plateletsome" liposomes carrying platelet membrane glycoproteins [85], liposomes carrying GPIb von Willebrand factor-binding domain [86], or procoagulant liposomes administered with activated X factor [76]. Each of these compounds shows *in vivo* hemostatic efficacy in thrombopenic animal models. We note, however, that factor Xa-associated liposomes presented significant toxicity in dogs [76].

Future Outlook for Platelet Substitutes

As is the case for all substitution products, platelet substitutes cannot replace all cellular functions. Therefore, each substitute has a limited field of application, and several types of substitutes could be needed. The research conducted so far seems promising, but most products are only at the preclinical stage of development. Moreover, *in vivo* evaluation of the efficacy of these products is very difficult, particularly in a thrombopenia setting, where serious hemorrhage rarely occurs. At the same time, today, other approaches can increase platelet activity (desmopressin acetate), or elevate platelet count (recombinant erythropoietin, thrombopoietin and interleukin-11). Other compounds (antifibrinolytics, recombinant VIIa factor, biological surgical glues) reduce hemorrhage during surgery, limiting transfusion needs [73].

Conclusion

Experimental studies on blood function substitution have been very diversified but, despite half a century of research, they have produced no consistent applications. Oxygen transport remains an important issue, but in the context of blood transfusion it is difficult to know which method is most suitable. Although hemoglobin solutions with or without encapsulation are interesting, sources, preparations and properties related to microbiological safety remain to be defined. Modified erythrocytes and erythrocytes encapsulating allosteric effectors or even therapeutic products are very enticing but, after twenty years, they have not yet been validated in simple clinical models. Finally, perfluorocarbons, which first underwent clinical trials over forty years ago, are still not used in human clinical practice. Platelet function substitution is still at the evaluation stage, and the numerous research projects in progress are essentially attempting to improve storage conditions. In both these fields it is reasonable to expect that reliable, non toxic substitutes with specific applications will be developed for use in specific settings.

References

1. Backer S L, Dodds EC. Obstruction of the renal tubules during the excretion of haemoglobin. *Br J Exp Physiol* 1925 ; 6 : 247-60.
2. de Nevasquez S. The excretion of haemoglobin with special references to the transfusion kidney. *J Path Bact* 1940 ; 51: 413-25.
3. de Gowin EL, Osterhagen MF, Andersch M. Renal insufficiency from blood transfusion. I. Relation to urinary acidity. *Arch Intern Med* 1937 ; 59 : 432-44.
4. de Gowin EL, Wagner ED, Randall WL. Renal insufficiency from blood transfusion. II. Anatomic changes in man compared with those in dogs with experimental hemoglobinuria. *Arch Intern Med* 1938 ; 71: 609-30.
5. Bing RJ. The effect of haemoglobin and related pigments on renal functions of the normal and acidotic dogs. *Johns Hopk Bull* 1944 ; 74 : 161-76.
6. Hamilton PB, Hiller A, Van Slyke DD. Renal effects of haemoglobin infusions in dogs in hemorrhagic shock. *J Exp Med* 1948 ; 87 : 477-87.
7. Rabiner SF, Helbert JR, Lopas H, Friedman LH. Evaluation of a stroma-free hemoglobin solution for use as a plasma expander. *J Exp Med* 1967 ; 126 : 1127-42.
8. Peskin GW, O'Brien K, Rabiner SF. Stroma-free hemoglobin solution: the "ideal" blood substitute? *Surgery* 1969 ; 66 : 185-93.

9. Clark LC Jr, Gollan F. Survival of mammals breathing organic liquids equilibrated with oxygen at atmospheric pressure. *Science* 1966 ; 152 : 5-56.
10. Geyer RP. A fluorocarbon –polyol mixture for essentially total replacement of blood in vivo. Proc. 12 Congr int Soc Blood Transfusion Moscou, 1969. In : *Bibl Haematol*. Basel : Karger, 1971 ; 38 : 802-12
11. Fujita T, Sumaya T, Yokohama K. Fluorocarbon emulsions as a candidate for artificial blood. *Eur Surg Res* 1971 ; 31 : 436-53.
12. Sehgal LR, Sehgal HL, Rosen SA, Gould SA, De Woskin R, Moss GS. Characteristics of polymerized pyridoxylated hemoglobin. *Biomat Artif Cells Artif Organs* 1988 ; 16 : 173-83.
13. Riess JG. Perspectives d'utilisation de transporteurs d'oxygène comme substituts des érythrocytes en chirurgie. *Ann Fr Anesth* 1995 ; 14 : 107-17.
14. Krafft MP, Chittofrati A, Riess JG. Emulsions and microemulsions with a fluorocarbon phase. *Curr Opin Colloid In* 2003 ; 8 : 251-8.
15. Chaput N, André F, Schartz J, Flament C, Angevin F, Escudier B, Zitvogel L. Exosomes et immunothérapie antitumorale. *Bull Cancer* 2003 ; 90 : 695-8.
16. Guidance for industry; criteria for safety and efficacy. Evaluation of oxygen therapeutics as red blood cell substitutes. Draft Guidance. US Department of Health and Human Services, Food and Drug Administration Center for Biologics Evaluation and Research. Octobre 2004, 17 p.
17. Remy B, Deby-Dupont G, D'Ans V, Ernest P, Lamy M. Substituts des globules rouges : émulsions de fluorocarbures et solutions d'hémoglobine. *Ann Fr Anesth* 1999 ; 18 : 211-24.
18. Labrude P, Gaillard S, Vigneron C, Stoltz JF, Benichoux R, Streiff F. Les solutions d'hémoglobine. Etude bibliographique et intérêt. *Bull Assoc Dipl Microbiol Nancy* 1971 ; 124 : 43-9.
19. Standl T, Freitag M, Burmeister MA, *et al.* Hemoglobin based oxygen carrier HBOC-201 provides higher and faster increase in oxygen tension in skeletal muscle of anemic dogs than do stored red blood cells. *J Vasc Surg* 2003 ; 37 : 859-65.
20. Riess JG. Oxygen carriers "blood substitutes" – Raison d'être, chemistry and some physiology. *Chem Rev* 2001 ; 101 : 2797-919.
21. Goodnough L, Scott M, Monk T. Oxygen carriers as blood substitutes : past, present and future. *Clin Orthops Relat R* 1998 ; 357 : 89-100.
22. Ketcham E, Cairns C. Hemoglobin-based oxygen carriers: development and clinical potential. *Ann Emerg Med* 1999; 33 : 326-37.
23. Cohn S. Blood substitutes in surgery. *Surgery* 2000; 127 : 599-602.
24. Buehler P W, Alayash A I. Toxicities of hemoglobin solutions: in search of in-vitro and in-vivo model systems. *Transfusion* 2004 ; 44 : 1516-30.
25. Sharma AC, Gulati A. Yohimbine modulates diaspirin crosslinked hemoglobin-induced systemic hemodynamics and regional circulatory effects. *Crit Care Med* 1995 ; 23 : 874-84.
26. Faivre-Fiorina B, Caron A, Fassot C, Fries I, Menu P, Labrude P, Vigneron C. Presence of hemoglobin inside aortic endothelial cells after cell-free hemoglobin administration in guinea pigs. *Am J Physiol* 1999 ; 176 : H 766-70.
27. Dieryck W, Gruber V, Baudino S, Lenee P, Pagnier J, Merot B, Poyart C. Expression d'hémoglobine humaine recombinante dans les plantes. *Transfus Clin Biol* 1995 ; 6 : 441-7.
28. Hervé P, Lapierre V, Morel P, Tiberghien P. Quelles sont aujourd'hui les nouvelles stratégies susceptibles de faire progresser la sécurité transfusionnelle en France? *Ann Med Interne* 1999 ; 150 : 623-30.
29. Brucker EA. Genetically crosslinked hemoglobin: a structural study. *Acta Crystallogr D* 2000 ; 56 : 812-6.
30. Burhop KE, Doyle MP. The development and preclinical testing of a second-generation recombinant hemoglobin solution, rHb2.0 for injection. In : Messmer K, Burhop KE, Hutter J, eds. *Microcirculatory effects of hemoglobin solutions*. Prog Appl Microcirc. Basel : Karger, 2004, vol. 25 : 48-64.

31. www.eurobloodsubstitutes.com
32. Greenburg AG, Kim HW. Hemoglobin-based oxygen carriers. *Crit Care* 2004 ; 8 : S 61-4.
33. Hsia JC, Song DL, Er SS, *et al*. Pharmacokinetic studies in the rat on a o-raffinose polymerized human hemoglobin. *Biomat Art Cells Immob Biotech* 1992 ; 20 : 587-95.
34 Levy JH, Goodnough LT, Greilich PE, Parr GV, Stewart RW, Gratz I, Wahr J, Williams J, Comunale ME, Doblar D, Silvay G, Cohen M, Jahr JS, Vlahakes GJ. Polymerized bovine hemoglobin solution as a replacement for allogeneic red blood cell transfusion after cardiac surgery: results of a randomized, double-blind trial. *J Thorac Cardiovasc Surg* 2002 ; 12 : 35-42.
35. Quellec P, Leonard M, Grandgeorge M, Dellacherie E. Human hemoglobin conjugated to carboxylate dextran as a potential red blood cell substitute. I. Further physico-chemical characterization. *Artif Cells Blood Substit Immobil Biotechnol* 1994 ; 22 : 669-76.
36. Jia Y, Wood F, Menu P, Faivre B, Caron A, Alayash AI. Oxygen binding and oxidation reactions of human haemoglobin conjugated to carboxylate dextran. *Biochem Biophys Acta* 2004 ; 1672 : 164-73.
37. Talarico TL, Guise KJ, Stacey CJ. Chemical characterization of pyridoxylated hemoglobin polyoxyethylene conjugate. *Biochem Biophys Acta* 2000 ; 476 : 53-65.
38. Vandegriff KD, Malavalli A, Wooldridge J, Lohman J, Winslow RM. MP4, a new nonvasoactive PEG-Hb conjugate. *Transfusion* 2003 ; 43 : 509-16.
39. Winslow RM. MP4, a new nonvasoactive polyethylene glycol-hemoglobin conjugate. *Artif Organs* 2004 ; 28 : 800-6.
40. Matheson B, Kwansa HE, Bucci E, Rebel A, Koehler RC. Vascular response to infusions of a nonextravasating hemoglobin polymer. *J Appl Physiol* 2002 ; 93 : 1479-86.
41. Cedrati N, Bonneaux F, Labrude P, Maincent P. Structure and stability of human hemoglobin microparticles prepared with a double emulsion technique. *Artif Cells Blood Substit Immobil Biotechnol* 1997 ; 25 : 457-62.
42. Sakai H, Takeoka S, Park S, Kose T, Nishide H, Izumi Y, Yoshizu A, Kobayashi K, Tsuchida E. Surface modification of hemoglobin vesicles with poly(ethyleneglycol) and effects on aggregation, viscosity, and blood flow during 90% exchange transfusion in anesthetized rats. *Bioconjugate Chem* 1997 ; 8 : 23-30.
43. Sakai H, Takeoka S, Wettstein R, Tsai AG, Intaglietta M, Tsuchida E. Systemic and microvascular response to hemorrhagic shock and resuscitation with Hb vesicles. *Am J Physiol* 2002 ; 283 : H1191-9.
44. Chang TM, Powanda D, Yu WP. Analysis of polyethylene-glycol-polylactide nano-dimension artificial red blood cells in maintaining systemic hemoglobin levels and prevention of methemoglobin formation. *Artif Cells Blood Substit Immobil Biotechnol* 2003 ; 31 : 231-47.
45. Chauvierre C, Marden MC, Vauthier C, Labarre D, Couvreur P, Leclerc L. Heparin coated poly(alkylcyanoacrylate) nanoparticles coupled to hemoglobin: a new oxygen carrier. *Biomaterials* 2004 ; 25 : 3081-6.
46. Alayash AI. Oxygen therapeutics: can we tame haemoglobin? *Nature Rev Drug Discovery* 2004 ; 3 : 152-9.
47. Sakai H, Hara H, Yuasa M, Tsai A, Takeoka S, Tsuchida E, Intaglietta M. Molecular dimensions of Hb-based O2 carriers determine constriction of resistance arteries and hypertension. *Am J Physiol* 2000 ; 279 : H908-15.
48. Gulati A, Sen AP, Sharma AC, Singh G. Role of ET and NO in resuscitative effect of diaspirin cross-linked hemoglobin after hemorrhage in rat. *Am J Physiol* 1997 ; 273 : H827-36.
49. Menu P, Bleeker W, Longrois D, Caron A, Faivre-Fiorina B, Labrude P, Stoltz JF. In vivo effects of hemoglobin solutions on blood viscosity and rheological behaviour of red blood cells. Comparison with clinically-used volume expanders. *Transfusion* 2000 ; 40 : 1095-103.
50. d'Agnillo F, Chang TM. Polyhemoglobin-superoxide dismutase-catalase as a blood substitute with antioydant properties. *Nature Biotechnol* 1998 ; 16 : 667-71.

51. Tsai CH, Fang TY, Ho NT, Ho C. Novel recombinant hemoglobin, rHb (betaN108Q), with low oxygen affinity, high cooperativity, and stability against autoxidation. *Biochemistry* 2000 ; 39 : 13719-29
52. Tsuchida E, Komatsu T, Matsukawa Y, Nakagawa A, Sakai H, Kobayashi K, Suematsu M. Human serum albumin incorporating synthetic heme : red blood cell substitutes without hypertension by nitric oxide scavenging. *J Biomed Mater Res* 2003 ; 64 : 257-61.
53. Winslow RM. Current status of blood substitute research: towards a new paradigm. *J Intern Med* 2003 ; 253 : 508-17.
54. Fablet C, Marden MC, Green BN, Ho C, Pagnier J, Baudin-Creuza V. Stable octameric structure of recombinant haemoglobin alpha(2)beta(2)83 Gly-->Cys. *Protein Sci* 2003 ; 12 : 690-5
55. Zal F, Green BN, Martineu P, Lallier FH, Toulmond A, Vinogradov SN, Childress JJ. Polypeptide chain composition diversity of hexagonal-bilayer haemoglobins within a single family of annelids, the alvinellidae. *Eur J Biochem* 2000 ; 267 : 5227-36.
56. Ropars C, Tesseire B, Nicolau C, Chassaigne M, Vallez MO. Encapsulation dans les érythrocytes d'un effecteur allostérique de l'hémoglobine. *Médecine Armée* 1984 ; 12 : 77-80.
57. Bailleul C, Borrelly-Villereal M C, Chassaigne M, Ropars C. Modification of partial pressure of oxygen (P50) in mammalian red blood cells by incorporation of an allosteric effector of hemoglobin. *Biotechnol Appl Biochem* 1989 ; 11 : 31-40.
58. Ropars C, Teiseire B, Avenard G, Chassaigne M, Hurel C, Girot R, Nicolau C. Improved oxygen delivery to tissues and iron chelator transport through the use of lysed and resealed red blood cells: a new perspective on Cooley's anemia therapy. *Ann N Y Acad Sci* 1985 ; 445 : 304-15.
59. Boucher L, Chassaigne M, Ropars C. Internalisation and distribution of inositol hexaphosphate in red blood cells. *Biotechnol Appl Biochem* 1996 ; 24 : 73-8.
60. Lowe K. Engineering blood: synthetic substitutes from fluorinated compounds. *Tissue Eng* 2003 ; 9 : 389-99.
61. Kerins DM. Role of the perfluorocarbon fluosol-DA in coronary angioplasty. *Am J Med Sci* 1994 ; 307 : 218-21.
62. Noyé S. Des dérivés d'hydrocarbones bientôt dans nos veines ? *Rev Prat Med Gen* 2001 ; 15 : 1378-81.
63. www.allp.com/Oxygent/OX.HTM
64. Sofronov GA, Selivanov EA Vestn R. New blood substitutes of polyfunctional action. *Akad Med Nauk* 2003 ; 10 : 48-51.
65. www.perftoran.ru/Eng/modules.php?name=News&file=article&sid=20
66. Spahn DR, Van Brempt R, Theilmeier G, Reibold JP, Welte M, Heinzerling H, Birck KM, Keipert PE, Messmer K. Perflubron emulsion delays blood transfusions in orthopedic surgery. European Perflubron Emulsion Study Group. *Anesthesiology* 1999 ; 91 : 1195-208.
67. Hill S, Leone B, Faithfull S, Flaim K, Keipert P, Newman M. Perflubron emulsion (AF0144) augments harvesting of autologous blood : a phase II study in cardiac surgery. *J Cardiothoracic Vasc Anesth* 2002 ; 16 : 555-60.
68. Spahn DR, Waschke KF, Standl T, Motsch J, Van Huynegem L, Welte M, Gombotz H, Coriat P, Verkh L, Faithfull S, Keipert P, The European Perflubron Emulsion in Non-Cardiac Surgery Study Group. Use of perflubron emulsion to decrease allogeneic blood transfusion in high-blood-loss non-cardiac surgery : results of a European phase 3 study. *Anesthesiology* 2002 ; 97 : 1333-4.
69. Sirieix D, Nicolas-Robin A, Baron JF Transporteurs de l'oxygène : solutions d'hémoglobine et fluorocarbones. *Med Thér* 1997 ; 3 : 851-7.
70. Dickson E, Heard S, Tarara T, Weers J, Brueggemann A, Doern G. Liquid ventilation with perflubron in the treatment of rats with pneumococcal pneumonia. *Crit Care Med* 2002 ; 30 : 393-5.

71. Lee D, Blajchman M. Novel treatment modalities : new platelet preparations and substitutes. *Br J Haematol* 2001 ; 114 : 496-505.
72. Vostal J, Reid T, Mondoro T. Liquid cold storage of platelets : a revitalized possible alternative for limiting bacterial contamination of platelet products. *Transf Med Rev* 1997 ; 11 : 286-95.
73. Reid T, Rentas F, Ketchum L. Platelet substitutes in the management of thrombocytopenia. *Curr Hematol Rep* 2003 ; 2 :165-70.
74. Hoffmeister K, Josefsson E, Isaac N, Clausen H, Hartwig J, Stossel T. Glycosylation restores survival of chilled blood platelets. *Science* 2003 ; 301 : 1531-4.
75. Melaragno A, Carciero R, Feingold H, Talarico L, Weitraub L, Valeri C. Cryopreservation of human platelets using 6% dimethyl sulfoxide and storage at –80°C. *Vox Sang* 1985 ; 49 : 245-58.
76. Blachjman M. Substitutes and alternatives to platelet transfusions in thrombocytopenic patients. *J Thromb Haemost* 2003 ; 1 : 1637-41.
77. Currie L, Lichtiger B, Livesey S, Tansey W, Yang D, Connor J. Enhanced circulatory parameters of human platelets cryopreserved with second-messenger effectors : an in vivo study of 16 volunteer platelet donors. *Br J Haematol* 1999 ; 105 : 826-31
78. Klein E, Farber S, Djerassi I, Toch R, Freeman G, Arnold P. The preparation and clinical administration of lyophilized platelet material to children with acute leukemia and aplastic anemia. *J Pediatr* 1956 ; 49 : 517-22.
79. Maupin B. Blood platelets in 1974. Collection, preservation, transfusion. *Rev Fr Transfus Immunohematol* 1975 ; 18 : 155-75.
80. Read M, Reddick R, Bode A, Bellinger D, Nichols T, Taylor K, Smith S, McMahon D, Griggs T, Bringhous K. Preservation of hemostatic and structural properties of rehydrated lyophilised platelets : potential for long term storage of dried platelets for transfusion. *Proc Natl Acad Sci USA* 1995 ; 92 : 397-401.
81. Bode A, Read M. Lyophilized platelets: continued development. *Transfus Sci* 2000 ; 22 : 99-105.
82. Chao F, Kim B, Houranieh A, Liang F, Konrad M, Swisher S, Tullis J. Infusible platelet membrane microvesicles: a potential transfusion substitute for platelets. *Transfusion* 1996 ; 36 : 536-42.
83. Levi M, Friederich PW, Middleton S, de Groot PG, Wu YP, Harris R, Biemond BJ, Heijnen HF, Levin J, Ten Cate JW. Fibrinogen-coated albumin microcapsules reduce bleeding in severely thrombocytopenic rabbits. *Nat Med* 1999 ; 5 : 107-11.
84. Yen R, Ho T, Blachjman M. A new haemostatic agent : thrombospheres shorten the bleeding time in thrombocytopenic rabbits. *Thromb Haemost* 1995 ; 73 : 986.
85. Rybak M, Renzulli L. A liposome based platelet substitute, the plateletsome with haemostatic efficacy. *Art Cells Immob Biotech* 1993 ; 21 : 101-18.
86. Kitaguchi T, Murata M, Iijima K, Kamide K, Imagawa T, Ikeda Y. Characterization of liposomes carrying von Willebrand factor-binding domain of platelet glycoprotein Ibalpha: a potential substitute for platelet transfusion. *Biochem Biophys Res Commun* 1999 ; 261 : 784-9.

The Cell: a Legally Distinct Entity

Jean-René Binet

In a now famous article published in 1989, Mr. Bernard Edelman presented the readers of *Recueil Dalloz* with a new entity to consider in matters of legal doctrine concerning biomedical issues: the human cell [1]. The case at the heart of Mr. Edelman's important contribution to the study of laws governing living matter was being heard before the Supreme Court of California. For many legal practitioners, the case still represents the most extreme deconstruction of the human person. Here are the facts. The plaintiff, John Moore, suffered from leukemia and was admitted to the University of California Medical Center in 1974 for treatment of this terrible illness. Medical investigations revealed that Mr. Moore's blood produced marvellous, unique substances, potentially able to offer hope in treating certain types of cancer, and maybe even AIDS! The doctors who made this discovery decided to examine these precious cells more closely and, for a dozen years, Mr. Moore was subjected – in the interest of his care and treatment, as he was told – to blood tests, biopsies and punctures to obtain skin, serum or bone marrow. These systematic extractions took an even more dramatic turn in October 1976, when the doctors decided to remove his spleen and share it among themselves. Like thieves suspecting each-other of wanting to deprive the others of their share of the spoils, the doctors kept watch at the operating room door, waiting for the surgery to end so they could pounce on the organ, which they divided up as soon as the deed was done.

Thanks to this bit of tissue, a cell line was created and patented on March 20, 1984. Mr. Moore, who learned the truth, brought a law suit. But if the reader assumes that we are speaking of penal action, he will be disappointed to learn that the suit was brought under the terms of industrial property law: Mr. Moore was claiming his part of the commercial gains realized, as it were, from his body but against his will; he was claiming property rights over his cells. We will let the reader peruse on his own the details of the case, brilliantly analysed by Mr. Edelman. For the purposes of the present study, we will only retain certain pertinent elements of the case.

Of course, the Moore case is exceptional, but it illustrates the need for a legal framework where practices involving the human person are concerned. In fact, the human person is, from all possible perspectives, the ultimate reason for the existence of the law, whose obligation it is to protect this person from prejudice to his integrity and dignity. Medical science, which pursues the improvement of the human condition, can only develop within the limited framework assigned to it by the law. This might seem obvious, but when we read certain invectives made by doctors and scientists against the right of the Law to intervene in their professional practices, we feel impelled to point out why the Law has a role to play in these matters [2].

Above all, the Moore case reveals the interests involved in legal reflection on the human cell. Inasmuch as the cell can have therapeutic uses, either for the benefit of the person from whom it was collected or for the benefit of someone else, these uses, that are solely in the sphere of medical science, must be defined, made possible and rendered safe. Recourse to the law is needed to bring this about.

Thirty years after the Moore case, biomedical fields are just as interested in the cell, if not more. Once again, as in many other instances, this medical object has become a legal concern. In fact, the human cell has acquired legal status and been recognized as a legal "entity" (to refer to the theme I was asked to develop). Analysis of the definitions that ensued reveals that human cells now have a plurality of legal statuses. If we look at the Code of Public Health drafted after the issuing of the August 6, 2004 law on bioethics [3] and the August 9, 2004 law on public health policy [4], we find a considerable number of clauses dealing with cells[1]. On closer examination, although most of these clauses deal with the conditions of donation and the use of components and products of the human body, certain clauses concern embryology and procreation.

Cells as Components and Products of the Human Body

Legislative and regulatory stipulations relating to human cells defined as components and products of the human body constitute the largest category. The legislative aim was to decide what type of law would govern activities involving cells. Once these provisions were formulated, the administrative tribunal attempted to include embryonic stem cells in this category.

Legal Framework of Activities Involving Cells as Components and Products of the Human Body

The stated objective of the bill relating to bioethics, supported by government representatives who see this field as "an immense construction site" [5], was to institute, for the cell, a single legal status instead of the multiple statuses previously in effect [6]. The reason for the complexity was that depending on whether or not cells were intended for genetic or cell therapies, the rules governing their procurement, storage and distribution were different.

Therefore, a single legal status was instated, regardless of the intended use of the cells collected[2]. However, because stipulations regarding hematopoietic stem cells from bone marrow, previously in the organ transplant category, are now included in the tissue and cell category, two legal statuses still apply: a status specific to these cells, and a general status[3].

---

[1] 110 articles contain the word "cell" in the sense of human cell, and 49 articles contain the word "cellular". Many clauses of the Penal Code also concern them. On the other hand, the word is not used in article 16 and in subsequent articles of the Civil Code, that concern larger categories in which cells are included.

[2] Subsection VI of book II of the first part of the Code of Public Health is now entitled: "Clauses pertaining to related medicinal products". The first two chapters of the book are annulled: L.2004-800, art.14, 1. Specific stipulations validate, under the new rules, the authorizations previously granted: L.no.2004-800, art.35, I and II.

[3] Collection of tissues, cells and products of the human body *post mortem* is, as before, governed by articles L.1232-1 and subsequent articles of the Code of Public Health: C.sant.publ., art.L.1241-6, L.2004-800, art.12, II, 4. A decree issued by the Conseil d'Etat is expected to specify the legal provision authorizing this: L.1241-7, 3; L.2004-800, art.12, II, 4.

This distinction is only made in relation to procurement of "tissues, cells isolated from the human body, and their by-products" [4]. We will review these modes of procurement before examining the rules regarding accreditation of establishments performing collection, and the rules governing preparation, storage and use of tissues, cells and their by-products.

Procurement of Tissues and Cells

Tissue and cell collection for donation purposes is a medical activity [7] governed by different rules depending on whether or not the collection involves hematopoietic cells. We will present a brief review of the general status laws applying to cells, before looking at stipulations specific to hematopoietic cells.

General Legal Status of Cells

Before the law of August 6, 2004 entered into force, collection of tissues and cells could be practiced for research or therapeutic purposes. The new law upholds this decision, but authorizes an additional intention for these collections. Now, they can be practiced for purposes of manufacturing or evaluating medical devices, for diagnostic purposes or for quality assurance [8], making their authorized uses identical to those of blood and blood components [9]. The text of the law also provides that, excluding tissues collected as part of the procedures of a biomedical research project, the only tissues that can be procured for therapeutic donation purposes are those listed in the decree of the Conseil d'Etat [10].

When this condition is fulfilled, harvesting can only take place if the donor gives written consent after being informed of the purpose, consequences and risks of the donation. This consent can be rescinded without warning at any time[5]. Moreover, the conditions for obtaining consent are those that apply to organ collection from living donors, when the nature of the procurement and its consequences for the donor justify it [11]. In addition, the prohibition of collection from a minor or adult living subject protected by article L.1241-2 is maintained [12].

However, lawmakers have created a new donor category: the presumed living donor. This allows tissues, cells and products of the human body collected during surgery performed for the benefit of the person undergoing the surgery, as well as the placenta, to be used for therapeutic or scientific purposes, unless the said person is opposed to such use after being informed of it [13]. The text of the law specifies that in case of a minor or an adult under guardianship, subsequent use of the elements or products procured in this manner shall be subordinated to absence of objection expressed by any means by parental authorities or guardians duly informed of the intended uses of these materials. Refusal by the minor or adult subject shall prevent these uses. Similar stipulations exist regarding organ procurement [14] and a new paragraph 2 of article L.1211-2 included in the "General Principles" sets out a principle in accordance with these rules.

Stipulations Governing Hematopoietic Cells from Bone Marrow

Previously included in the category of organ procurement, hematopoietic cells from bone marrow could only be harvested in the same conditions of consent as those required for organ procurement from living donors. As we have said, lawmakers have now included these cells in the category of tissues, cells and products of human origin. However, the

---

[4] This is the new wording of subsection IV of book II of the first part of the Code of Public Health, L.2004-800, art.12, I.

[5] These conditions are sanctioned by penal law : Penal Code, art. 511-5, par.1; L.no.2004-800, art.15, 2.

intent was to maintain the previous level of protection for this type of harvesting, given the seriousness of the procedure for the donor. Therefore, these stipulations only apply to hematopoietic cells from bone marrow, and are not intended to regulate the procurement of such cells from peripheral blood.

Regarding procurement of hematopoietic cells from bone marrow, paragraph 3 of article L.1241-1 of the Code of Public Health provides for consent procedures requiring intervention of the president of the "Tribunal de Grande Instance", or of the Public Prosecutor, in cases where human life is in danger [15]. In addition, the principle prohibiting procurement from incompetent subjects, laid down in article L.1241-2, applies equally to hematopoietic cells from bone marrow. However, derogations have been provided for cases where no therapeutic solutions exist. In these conditions, procurement from a minor is authorized, when it is practiced for the benefit of his brother or sister [16], or even for the benefit of a first cousin, an uncle, an aunt, a nephew or a niece, when no other solution exists. This type of procurement requires consent – revocable at any time – from duly informed parental authority holders, obtained in the same conditions as those applicable to competent subjects [17]. Refusal by the minor able to express his wishes shall prevent this procurement [18]. Finally, a committee of experts created by the law to replace previous expert committees regulating bone marrow harvesting, is responsible for authorizing these procurements [19]. A decree issued on May 10, 2005 sets out the conditions of these procurements [20]. The said conditions are presented in articles R.1241-3 and subsequent articles of the Code of Public Health. All these conditions are sanctioned by the Penal Code [21].

Accreditation of Cell and Tissue Establishments

Harvesting of tissues and cells of human origin can only be performed in health establishments accredited by the public Authority [22] with the consent of the Biomedical Agency[6]. However, harvesting for autologous application of certain cells[7] shall be possible in all health establishments, and can also be performed by doctors and dentists practicing outside these establishments [23].

Preparation, Storage and Use of Tissues, Cells and their By-Products

Lawmakers have established very clear terminological and procedural distinctions within the legal framework applying to the preparation, storage and use of tissues, cells and their by-products.

Definitions

First, the heading of chapter III of subsection IV, in book II of the first part of the Code of Public Health was modified to read "Preparation, storage and use of tissues, cells and their by-products" [24]. Article L.1243-1, the first clause of the chapter, defines cellular products with therapeutic uses, excepting labile blood products, as being "human cells used for medicinal autologous or allogeneic purposes, whatever their degree of transformation, and including their by-products" [25].

---

[6] Constituted by the present law; see articles L.1418-1 to L.1418-7 of the Code of Public Health. Regarding the status, functions and organization of the Biomedical Agency, see Binet J-R, *Le nouveau droit de la bioéthique*, op.cit., spec.no.17 to 30.

[7] A list of these cells is to be issued by the Ministry of Health.

They can then be given one of two statuses.

• **The first status** defines them as therapeutic products for human use [26]. In essence, lawmakers wished to avoid submitting them to the monopoly of pharmaceutical companies[8].

For this reason, subsection II of book I of the fifth part, dealing with medicinal products for human use, has now added two definitions to article L.5121-1: preparation of gene therapies and preparation of xenogeneic cell therapies. These preparations are thus expressly exempted from the requirement that manufacturing, importing, exporting and wholesale distribution of therapeutic products for human use be performed exclusively by pharmaceutical companies [27]. However, these activities have to be approved by the AFSSAPS [28]. For the same reason, book II of the fourth part, dealing with the pharmaceutical professions, now contains new derogations from the monopoly of the pharmaceutical industry [29]; these derogations concern preparation, storage, distribution, licensing, importing and exporting of gene therapy and xenogeneic cell therapy products. These activities can be carried out by establishments and institutions authorized by the AFSSAPS, after consent from the Biomedical Agency.

Finally, a new chapter entirely dedicated to gene therapy and xenogeneic cell therapy products has been added to the penal clauses in book IV of the fifth part of the Code of Public Health [30].

• **The second status** conferred by lawmakers is that of cell therapy products. Under this designation, only the stipulations of this chapter apply to these products.

Finally, another definition provided by legislators is that of "human biological sample collection", which designates the assembling, in view of scientific research, of biological samples taken from a group of persons identified and selected according to clinical and biological characteristics in one or several members of the group, and any by-product of such samples [31]. This constitutes, in practice, a DNA bank or biobank[9].

Authorization and Declaration Procedures

The law of August 6, 2004 has instituted procedures of authorization or declaration for practices related to the preparation, storage and use of tissues and of cell therapy products.

Authorization relating to the preparation, storage, distribution and licensing, for therapeutic autologous or allogeneic purposes, of tissues and their by-products, and of cell therapy preparations is granted to establishments and institutions that apply for it through the AFSSAPS, after consent from the Biomedical Agency. Authorization is granted for five years, and is renewable. In case of modification of elements specified in the initial authorization, a new application for authorization must be submitted [32]. The AFSSAPS must also authorize the use of tissues, by-products and cell therapy products [33].

The constitution of a collection of human biological samples must make the object of a prior declaration by the institution undertaking it for the purposes of its own research programs.

The declaration is submitted to the Minister in charge of Research, as well as to the Director of the Regional Hospitalization Agency (RHA), the local competent authority, if the organization is a health institution. Consent from the Committee for the Protection of

---

[8] Stipulations introduced by amendment at first reading in the Senate, JO Sénat CR, January 29, 2003.

[9] It will be remembered that such a collection of genetic data on the Icelandic population has been compiled since 1998 and is starting to produce spectacular results, *Le Figaro*, Nov. 2, 2004.

the Person[10] is also required. The Minister and, if the situation warrants it, the Director of the RHA, can oppose the implementation of the proposed activities, or prohibit them if they no longer satisfy established criteria, either in terms of safety, in terms of information and consent of subjects, or in terms of ethical and research relevance of the project [34].

When storage and preparation of tissues and cells of human origin are carried out in view of their licensing for a scientific purpose, either as part of a commercial project or on a no profit basis, the institution conducting these activities must obtain an authorization granted by the Minister in charge of Research. A supplementary authorization from the local competent authority, the RHA Director, is also required if the organization is a health institution [35].

Moreover, in principle, tissue transplants and administration of cell therapy products can only be performed in health establishments which are required to obtain special authorization when the cost of these activities is high, or when they require special stipulations[11]. Exceptionally, tissues and cell therapy products appearing on a list issued by the Minister of Health can be used by doctors and dentists outside health establishments [36].

Finally, hematopoietic cell allografts can be performed by health establishments pursuing teaching and research activities, and by affiliated establishments, with public health authorization granted after AFSSAPS consent.

"Components and Products of the Human Body" Status not Applicable to Embryonic Cells

The administrative tribunal attempted to include embryonic cells in the category of components and products of human origin. Subsequently, the legislative body rejected this opinion and confirmed the obvious status of embryonic cells as falling under the stipulations applying to procreation and embryology[12]. But the initial attempt is of interest because it allows understanding of the factors that prevailed against it.

The Case before the Administrative Tribunal

On June 20, 2001, the bill "relative to bioethics" was brought before the National Assembly by Elisabeth Guigou, Minister of Employment and Solidarity, on behalf of Prime Minister Lionel Jospin [37]. This bill prposed that a section under the heading "Research on the embryo and embryonic cells" be included in the Code of Public Health, to stipulate the conditions required for research on embryos and their cells. The bill, which was adopted after first reading by the National Assembly on January 22, 2002 [38], resulted in the drafting of article L.2151-3 stipulating: "Authorization is granted for research on human embryos and embryonic cells, conducted for medical purposes, provided that such research cannot be conducted by another method with comparable effectiveness given the present state of scientific knowledge". In addition, a new Public Health Code article, L.2151-3-1, provides that: "importing of embryonic or fetal tissues and cells requires prior authorization from the Minister in charge of Research."

---

[10] After the August 9, 2004 law came into effect, the Committee for the Protection of the Person replaced the Committee for the Protection of Persons in Biomedical Research (CPPBR), created by the Huriet law of December 20, 1988. See Code of Public Health, art.L.1123-1 and subsequent articles.

[11] A decree issued by the Conseil d'Etat must define these activities : Code of Public Health, art.L.1243-9, 1; L.2004-800, art.12, IV.

[12] See above.

Encouraged by the adoption of the bill after first reading, and anticipating to some extent on the ensuing legal process, Roger-Gérard Schwartzenberg, then Minister of Research, issued two decrees on April 30, 2002[13]. The first authorized a National Scientific Research Center laboratory to import two human embryonic stem cell lines from Australia. The second authorized conducting research on these cells. When an association called for summary proceedings, objecting that these two decrees were illegal, the Paris administrative tribunal refused to suspend their enforcement [39]. The petitioning association submitted an appeal to the Conseil d'Etat.

On November 13, 2002, a ruling of the Palais-Royal, made in chambers, overturned the decision of the administrative tribunal, citing the stipulations of article L.2141-8 of the Code of Public Health, as it was then in effect [40]. The Conseil d'Etat declared specifically that "the Minister of Research, who could not legally base his decision on the stipulations of the bill on bioethics, under study in Parliament when he made his ruling, disregarded the aforementioned parliamentary stipulations, which were the only ones in force on the date of the authorization granted". This threw serious doubt on the legality of the appealed decision, justifying suspension of the ministerial decree contested for a period of four months starting on the date of the decision. This interval was intended to allow the Paris administrative tribunal the time to investigate and make a decision regarding a request for suspension of the previous decision.

Thus, the administrative tribunal had to make a new decision, this time involving a fundamental issue: the legality of the decrees of April 30, 2002 [41]. Its decision rejected the appeal, enforcing a very restrictive interpretation of the prohibition principle in article L.2141-8 of the Code of Public Health, and a questionable qualification of embryonic cells as falling under the stipulations governing tissues, cells and products of human origin.

In fact, to save the legality of the ministerial decree authorizing importing of embryonic cells, the Paris administrative tribunal upheld the application of the stipulations of article L.1245-4 of the Code of Public Health, based on the text then in effect. This text stated that only institutions authorized by the AFSSAPS, with supplementary authorization from the Minister in charge of Research when importing is undertaken in view of scientific research, could import tissues and cells of human origin onto the national territory. In the opinion of the administrative tribunal, "embryonic stem cells constitute cells of human origin", so that "their importing requires prior authorization delivered by the Minister of Research". In practice, as we have seen, this authorization was not going to be denied.

Obstacles to the Qualification Determined by the Administrative Tribunal

At first sight, the qualification determined by the administrative tribunal seems attractive. But careful examination of the category in question leads to contesting the validity of the inclusion.

---

[13] He declared before the National Assembly his desire to issue such decrees if the article authorizing research on embryos was adopted : "If your assembly enacts this text authorizing research on supranumerary embryonic cells, it is perhaps time to respond favorably to the request submitted by four Nobel Prize winners who wish to import existing stem cell lines, providing they do not originate from nuclear transfer. The signatories of this request, very high-level scientists as we all agree, emphasize that the duration of parliamentary procedure will prevent the law from taking effect before 2003, delaying the progress of French research, while researchers are already at work in this field in the United States, Great Britain, Australia and elsewhere. Therefore, I feel more justified in authorizing the importing of these cells than I did until now." JOAN CR, third session, January 17, 2002.

THE CELL: A LEGALLY DISTINCT ENTITY

The first part of the Code of Public Health, dedicated to the "General protection of health", comprises a book II entitled "Donation and use of products and elements of human origin". Section I of this book sets out its "General Principles". The latter specify that licensing and use of components and products of human origin are governed by the stipulations of articles 16 to 16-9 of the Civil Code, as well as by the stipulations of Book II of the Code of Public Health[14].

Examination of these stipulations reveals that they comprise four sub-categories: human blood [42], organs [43], tissues, cells and products [44], and finally, gene and cell therapy products and related products [45]. The January 21, 2003 tribunal decision includes embryonic cells in the third sub-category.

The "General Principles" in subsection I of book II [46] and subsection IV of this book [47] apply to this sub-category, as do the penal stipulations outlined in the seventh subsection of the same book [48].

What do these stipulations say? Article L.1241-1 presents the general legal framework for collection of tissues and cells, which can only be performed "on a living person", according to this text, "for research or therapeutic purposes". The following article specifies that collection "cannot be performed on a living person who is a minor or on a living person who is an adult under legal guardianship". As for collection "on a deceased person", article L.1241-3 provides that the conditions outlined in article L.1232-1 and subsequent articles must be respected; that is, the stipulations initially formulated by the Caillavet law are in effect. Therefore, collection is always performed on a person, living or dead. This interpretation is confirmed by the "General Principles", which state that "collection of components of the human body and collection of its products cannot be performed without prior consent of the donor" (art.L.1211-2), that "no payment […] can be made for allowing the taking of elements of one's body" (art.L.1211-4), and that "the donor cannot have knowledge of the identity of the recipient". Even with a great effort of imagination, it is difficult to see how these stipulations could apply to embryonic cells, unless we consider the embryo a person. But even then, collection would be prohibited. If the embryo was in fact considered a living person, it would necessarily be a minor. And we have seen that collection on a living person who is a minor is prohibited. If the embryo was considered a deceased person, things would not be simpler, because it is hard to see how doctors could establish decease in accordance with article R.1232-1 and subsequent articles of the Code of Public Health.

Can we deny that the general principles in articles L.1211-1 to L.1211-9 do not apply to embryonic cells pursuant to article L.1211-8 of the Code of Public Health, which stipulates that "the present subsection does not apply to products of the human body which are normally exempted from all of the principles established in articles L.1211-2 to L.1211-6"? Clearly, we cannot, because when we consult the list of these products [49], we see that they have nothing to do with embryonic cells, since they consist of hair, nails, body hair and teeth.

In effect, if we have trouble seeing how embryonic cells can be governed by the stipulations applying to the collection of tissues, cells and products of the human body, it is because these stipulations never concerned embryonic cells. Some uncertainty is possible regarding cells and tissues from dead embryos or foetuses, collected after spontaneous or elective abortion.

These cells, which were not directly addressed by the July 29, 1994 law, are sometimes considered part of the "tissues, cells and products of human origin collected during a medical pro-

---

[14] Since this judgement, the Public Health Code stipulations referred to above have been modified to conform to the previously mentioned Decree 2004-800 issued on August 6, 2004 relating to bioethics. Unless otherwise indicated, the text referred to herein is that in force at the time of the administrative tribunal decision, given that its arguments are founded solely on this version.

cedure" category [50]. However, aside from the fact that application of this text to embryonic and fetal cells – relegated to the status of surgical waste – raises certain problems[15], making this qualification unacceptable for some[16], it goes without saying that this principle cannot be extended, in any circumstances, to the *in vitro* human embryo and its cells[17].

For these components – if we want to give them a distinct status – another qualification is legally appropriate: the one rejected by the Paris administrative tribunal because of its restrictive interpretation of article L.2141-8 of the Code of Public Health which, in the text in force at the time, stipulated the prohibition of research on *in vitro* human embryos. Consequently, the question is settled, since the legislature expressly considers that embryonic stem cells should be governed by stipulations applying to embryology and procreation.

Cells Governed by Stipulations Applying to Embryology and Procreation

Stipulations applying to embryology and procreation provide legal definitions for two types of cells: fetal cells and embryonic cells.

Concerning fetal cells, the August 6, 2004 law defines the legal framework for diagnostic, therapeutic[18] or research use of embryonic or fetal tissues originating from abortions [51].

These uses are only possible with the consent of the mother, given in writing after she decides to end the pregnancy and after she has received appropriate information. Moreover, the Biomedical Agency is responsible for monitoring scientific uses.

But, more importantly, the bioethics law defines a legal framework for *in vitro* research on human embryos and their cells [52] by reaffirming the prohibition principle, while providing possibilities for derogation in conducting research, as well as a transitional legal framework.

Reaffirmation of the Prohibition Principle Applying to Research on Embryonic Cells

The study of parliamentary proceedings held between June 2001 and August 2004 shows that the question of embryonic research had not lost the importance that had been accorded to it in 1994 [53] [19].

---

[15] This is why the bill relative to bioethics contained, from its earliest version, stipulations aimed "at filling the legal void in matters of procurement, storage and use of these cells", to quote Madame Guigou : AN (2001-2002), no.3166, Summary of motives, P.57.

[16] See "*Dict.perm.bioétich, biotech.*": "Tissues, cells and products of human origin", spec.no.26 : "It seems therefore hazardous, in view of biological reality, of the respect due to the human embryo and fetus [...] to interpret, within the closed sphere of the law, a text that regulates the disposal of surgical waste, as also applying to, and deciding by a stroke of the pen, the very delicate and controversial question of use of human embryos and foetuses deceased as a result of a medical procedure".

[17] Since Law 2004-800 entered into force on August 6, 2004, the legislature established a specific legal framework for the procurement and use of embryonic or fetal cells in a setting of elective abortion : Code of Public Health, art.L.1241-5, see above.

[18] Use of fetal cells has recently made it possible for a woman with retinitis pigmentosa to recover her sight. See *Le Figaro*, Oct.30, 2004.

[19] This question was presented as "the most important aspect of this bill" by Madame Guigou when the bill was filed : JOAN CR, January 15, 2002 session. Addendum, Claeys A : "Extension of embryonic

Like in 1994, lawmakers excluded the question of a legal status for the embryo, and only considered scientific reality: an embryo is the start of a human life [54]. Therefore, once again, parliamentarians had to consider the consequences of this reality in deciding whether to uphold or to bring into question the prohibition principle applying to embryonic research. The study of the debate on this very important question reveals the existence of two seemingly irreconcilable positions.

According to some, the prohibition principle had to be reversed, that is, a principle authorizing research on the embryo had to be established. It was for this reason that the bill was proposing a change in the law, to make it possible "to conduct research on *in vitro* embryos no longer part of a parental project […]". This request for extended authorization was "motivated by the concern with not impeding progress in the area of treatment of as yet incurable diseases, which could result from research involving embryonic stem cells" [55].

This was the perspective that prevailed when the bill was adopted after first reading in the National Assembly.

But other parliamentarians wished to maintain the prohibition principle, essentially for two complementary reasons: one ontological and the other pragmatic. Mr. Mattei, then Member of Parliament, explained that the need expressed by researchers to work with embryonic cells was sporadic and did not justify disregarding a principle as old and fundamental ad the protection of human life at its beginnings. He added that "it would be to our country's honour to implement all modes of research on adult stem cells in order to become a leader in the field, rather than trailing behind in embryonic research" [56].

In the end, an intermediary opinion prevailed quite rapidly during the debate. In effect, the report presented by Senator Giraud on behalf of the Commission of Social Affairs recommended reaffirming the prohibition principle in embryonic research [57]. However, in order not to risk impeding French research, the Commission considered that it was essential to make an assessment of the potential of embryonic cells compared to that of adult stem cells.

In order to allow this comparative assessment, request for a derogatory transitional legal provision was submitted to the Senate. This provision would only authorize research on embryos and their cells for this express purpose and in strictly defined conditions.

---

research constitutes the major innovation compared to the choices made in 1994", *ibid*. On this subject in general, see Feuillet-Le-Mintier B (ed.), *L'embryon humain : approche multidisciplinaire*, Rennes conference, Nov. 9-10, 1995, Economica 1996; Labrusse-Riou C, Mathieu B, Mazen N-J (ed.), *La recherche sur l'embryon : qualifications et enjeux*, RGDM spec.no., 2000; *Ethique. La vie en question*, "L'embryon", no.3 et 4, Société française de réflexion bioéthique, 1992; Binet J-R. *La recherche sur l'embryon humain in vitro. Variations sur le thème de l'interdit*, RGDM 2004, no.14 : 225-45 ; Byk C. *La recherche sur l'embryon humain*, JCP G 1996, I, 3949 ; *L'embryon jurisprudentiel*, Gaz.Pal. 1997, 2, doctr : 1391 ; Herzog-Evans M. *Homme, homme juridique et humanité de l'embryon*. RTD civ.2000 : 165 ; Le Dourian N, Puigelier C. *L'expérimentation à partir de cellules souches embryonnaires humaines*. JCP G 2002, I, 127 ; Martin R. *Les premiers jours de l'embryon. A propos du projet de loi relatif à la bioéthique*. JCP G 2002, I, 115 ; Mathieu B. *Génome humain et droits fondamentaux*. Economica/PUAM, 2000, spec.p.48 and following ; *La recherche sur l'embryon au regard des droits fondamentaux constitutionnels*. D 1999, chron p.451 ; *De la difficulté d'appréhender l'emploi des embryons humains en termes de droits fondamentaux*, RTDH, spec.no.54/2003 *Progrès scientifiques ou techniques et droits de l'homme*, April 2003 : 387-401 ; Mémeteau G. *L'embryon législatif*, D 1994, chron : 355 ; Neirinck C. *L'embryon humain ou la question en apparence sans réponse de la bioéthique*. Petites affiches, March 9, 1998 ; *L'embryon humain : une catégorie juridique à dimension variable*, D.2003, chron : 841 ; Pédrot P. *La recherche sur l'embryon : un consensus impossible ?* in Feuillet-Le-Mintier B.(ed.). *Les lois « bioéthique » à l'épreuve des faits. Réalités et perspectives*, Paris : PUF, 1999 :243-60 ; Seuvic J-F. *Variations sur l'être humain comme valeur pénalement protégée*. In : « mélange Christian Bolze », Economica, 1999 :339.

The Commission was proposing a modified text defining the principle as: prohibition of embryonic research; maintaining the exception regarding research that preserves the integrity of the embryo; a derogation: the transitional possibility of conducting research to evaluate the therapeutic potential of embryonic cells. This proposition is at the origin of article L.2151-5 of the Code of Public Health.

Derogatory Transitional Provision for Certain Research on Embryos and Embryonic Cells

As Mr. Mattei explained, the new legal framework for research on embryos and their cells is a three-tier system: "the basic prohibition, research studies, and derogation for research on embryonic stem cells" [58]. Therefore, application of the new provision requires strict respect of the conditions[20] outlined by legislators careful to be clearly understood by those whom the law concerns. In fact, during the debate, amendments were frequently filed to ask the Government or the Commission for laws specifying their intentions regarding the conditions of derogation in embryonic research. For instance, during the first discussion after initial reading in the Senate, Mr. Vasselle stated that it was "necessary that *Le Journal officiel* report the spirit in which we adopt these stipulations; and that when the research protocols will be examined, Members of Parliament will "keep an eye out" and remind researchers, if need be, of the reasons for adopting these stipulations, in order to prevent them from going beyond the limits of the derogation outlined in the text, after reaffirmation of the prohibition of embryonic research [59]".

Thus, derogation from the prohibition principle applying to research on embryos involves several conditions related to the embryos in question, to the aim of the proposed research and to the procedure of authorization.

Embryos Involved in the Derogation Procedure

The law only authorizes research on embryos no longer part of a parental project: that is, supernumerary embryos conceived within a project of medically assisted procreation, and initially stored by freezing in view of ulterior re-implantation into the womb, and the cells of these embryos [60]. Therefore, on the one hand, naturally conceived embryos that developed *in utero* are excluded, even if they were expulsed from the maternal womb during development[21]. On the other hand, as legislators stated very clearly, *in vitro* creation of embryos or constitution by cloning of human embryos for research purposes [61], as well as for industrial or commercial purposes [62], or for therapeutic purposes [63], is prohibited and sanctioned by penal law[22]. Therefore, in case of infringement of this prohibition, the very existence of embryos created in this manner would exclude the possibility of their use for research purposes. It should be stressed that embryos used for research purposes in conformity with the provisions of the law cannot be re-implanted subsequently [64]. Finally, in addition to *in vitro* embryos available on the national territory, it will be possible to conduct research on embryonic tissues and cells imported with consent from the Biomedical Agency [65], provided they were obtained in accordance with the fundamental principles set out in articles 16 to 16-8 of the Civil Code [66].

---

[20] Exceptions, in law, are always given a strict interpretation.

[21] These embryos are governed by stipulations of the new article L.1241-5 of the Code of Public Health; see above.

[22] Seven-year prison sentence and 100,000 euro fine; Penal Code, art. 511-17, 511-18, 511-18-1; Code of Public Health, art. L.2163-3, L.2163-4 and L.2163-5.

Objectives of the Research Considered

The legislature intended to make possible research on *in vitro* human embryos in order to investigate the potential of therapeutic applications related to human embryonic cells.

Specifically, given that research on adult stem cells had already demonstrated its efficacy[23] and that this field is given preference by the Government[24], it seemed that the possibility that embryonic cells could give better results should not be excluded, and that comparing the results of the two types of research was reasonable[25]. Therefore, starting from the date of publication in the Conseil d'Etat of the decree specifying the conditions of application of article L.2151-5 of the Code of Public Health, for a period of five years this type of research will be possible on two conditions: absence of an alternative method affording similar efficacy, and likelihood of contributing to major therapeutic progress [67]. Parliamentarians have been very clear regarding these conditions: "Not only is prior animal research required, particularly on large primates, but this research must have produced results that are significant enough to justify going on to human research." [68]. Therefore, before starting research on human embryonic research, animal research will have to produce convincing results. Moreover, as the reporter in the National Assembly emphasized: "This research is only conceivable if it becomes clear that expected advances can only be achieved by working with the human embryo and nothing else" [69]. That is, if major therapeutic progress can be made simultaneously through embryonic cells or through adult stem cells, only the latter path, which poses no ethical problem, should be pursued.

In order to better serve the comparison objective, a structure of assessment has been created. Article 26 of the bioethics law stipulates that six months before the end of the five-year period, the Biomedical Agency and the Parliamentary Office of Scientific and Technological development must prepare a report evaluating the respective results of embryonic cell Research, so that the Parliament can re-evaluate the stipulations concerning them. Lawmakers foresee *ab initio* putting an end to the temporary provisions in case of absence of proof of the usefulness of *in vitro* embryonic research, considering that "in five years embryonic stem cells will perhaps no longer be necessary" [70].

However, article L.2151-5 provides that research projects whose protocols could not be completed within the authorized five-year period can be continued under the conditions set forth by the law.

Procedural Conditions

In vitro research on human embryos no longer part of a parental project can only be conducted if the prospective parents gave prior consent to this type of research, and if the Biomedical Agency has given its approval.

First, the research cannot take place without prior written consent obtained from the couple donating the cells [71]. In cases where the parental project is abandoned following the death of one partner, consent given by the surviving partner is sufficient. In all cases,

---

[23] See results published by the Washington Times, Dec. 30, 2003, in reference to Parkinson's disease, diabetes, heart disease and ophthalmology.

[24] J.-F. Mattei, *JO Sénat CR*, Jan. 30, 2000 session : "We will develop research on adult stem cells, for which the Ministry of Research and INSERM, the National Institute of Health and Medical Research, are now preparing a call for tenders. This is the research area we in fact intend to encourage."

[25] J.-F. Mattei, *ibid.*: "We have to accept as unavoidable that, by derogation, research on embryonic stem cells will be legalized for five years. This will make it possible to compare them to adult stem cells, and to orient the future of medicine, without making a definitive and irreversible decision."

the persons whose authorization is requested must be informed of the possibility that another couple could receive the embryos, or that their conservation could be ended. Such consent, which in principle must be confirmed after a three-month legal reflection period, can be rescinded at any time and without motive.

In addition, this type of research can only be undertaken if its protocol has been authorized by the Biomedical Agency. Article L.2151-5, paragraph 5, of Code of Public Health specifies that this decision is made based on the scientific relevance of the research project, on the ethical considerations involved in its implementation, and on its contribution to public health. The project proposal is submitted to the Minister of Health and the Minister of Research who can deny authorization or prevent implementation if they consider that scientific relevance is not established and that ethical principles are not safeguarded. On the other hand, when the Biomedical Agency refuses the protocol, the Ministers can request, in the interest of public health or scientific research, that the project be re-examined within thirty days [72].

Finally, in addition to these conditions, legal procedure is expected to be elucidated by an awaited Conseil d'Etat decree specifying requirements for the authorization and implementation of this type of research [73].

Introduction of Transitional Legislation Authorizing Embryonic Cell Research

In order to allow researchers to rapidly submit applications for approval of research on embryonic stem cells, legislators introduced a transitional system [74] which was expected to be clarified by a Conseil d'Etat decree, published in the "Journal officiel" on September 30, 2004 [75].

This jurisprudence was to remain in force until the issuing of two decrees: the Conseil d'Etat decree requested at article L.2151-8 of the Code of Public Health, expected to specify the conditions in which rules relating to embryonic research apply, and a decree issued by the Director of the Biomedical Agency.

Given that the May 9, 2005 decree issued by the Director of the Biomedical Agency has been published [76], only the other decree is still pending before the transitional legislation loses effect. In any case, since the jurisprudence in question will be of short duration, we will limit our description to its essential elements.

The legislative rule instituted by the September 28, 2004 decree subjects authorization of research to the same conditions as those outlined in article L.2151-5, paragraph 3.

But the said conditions only apply to embryonic stem cells imported with authorization from the Ministers of Research and of Health [77], obtained through a process set down in the September 28, 2004 decree as well. The text imposes respect of the fundamental principles outlined in articles 16 to 16-8 of the Civil Code. The text also specifies that these cells must originate from embryos conceived *in vitro* within a medically assisted fertility project, and which are no longer part of a parental project. Finally, the couple from whom the embryos originate must have given prior consent to the use of these embryos for research purposes [78].

Pursuant to this transitional jurisprudence, the Ministries of Health and of Research [79] have issued three series of joint decisions authorizing the importing and storage of embryonic stem cells, as well as research protocols using them [80]. In conformity with article 10 of the September 28, 2004 decree, research and storage authorizations granted in these conditions will lose effect after the expiration of a five-year period [81] starting on the date of issuing of the decree that governs them.

References

1. Edelman B. *L'homme aux cellules d'or*, 1989 : 225. V. aussi : Edelman B. *La Personne en danger*. Paris : PUF, 1999 : 289-304.
2. Langaney A. *La Philosophie… biologique*. Paris : Belin, 1999 : 117-8. (L'auteur y dénie toute compétence aux « foules de juristes… » qui ont « envahi[…] » « les récents colloques sur l'éthique biologique et médicale », se présentant « comme experts de questions auxquelles ils n'avaient rien compris ».)
3. Loi n° 2004-800, 6 août 2004, relative à la bioéthique : JO, 7 août, p. 14040. V. Binet JR. *Le Nouveau Droit de la bioéthique*, Litec, 2005.
4. L. n° 2004-806, 9 août 2004, relative à la politique de santé publique. JO, 11 août 2004, p. 14277.
5. Claeys A. JOAN CR, 2ème séance, 17 janv. 2002.
6. *Doc. AN (2000-2001)*, n° 3166, pp. 25-35.
7. Code de la santé publique, art. L. 1245-3, L. 2004-800, art. 12, VI.
8. Code de la santé publique, art. L. 1241-1, al. 1er, L. 2004-800, art. 12, II, 1°.
9. Code de la santé publique, art. L. 1221-8, al. 1, L. 2004-800, art. 8, 3°.
10. Code de la santé publique, art. L. 1241-7, 1°, L. 2004-800, art. 12, II, 4°.
11. Code de la santé publique, art. L. 1241-1, al. 2, L. 2004-800, art. 12, II, 1°. (Un décret en Conseil d'État devra déterminer les conditions d'application de ces dispositions : Code de la santé publique, art. L. 1241-7, 2°, L. 2004-800, art. 12, II, 4°.)
12. Sous la sanction de l'article 511-3 al. 2 du Code pénal, L. n° 2004-800, art. 15, 1°.
13. Code de la santé publique, art. L. 1245-2, L. 2004-800, art. 12, VI.
14. Code de la santé publique, art. L. 1235-2, L. n° 2004-800, art. 9, VI, 2°.
15. Code de la santé publique, art. L. 1241-1, al. 3, L. 2004-800, art. 12, II, 1°. Comp. Code de la santé publique, art. L. 1231-1, al. 3, L. n° 2004-800, art. 9, II, 1°, v. *supra*.
16. Code de la santé publique, art. L. 1241-3, al. 1er, L. 2004-800, art. 12, II, 3°. (Des dispositions similaires sont prévues pour les majeurs protégés, avec une différence de protection selon que la personne est, d'une part, sous tutelle ou, d'autre part, sous curatelle ou sauvegarde de justice : Code de la santé publique, art. L. 1241-4, L. 2004-800, art. 12, II, 3°.)
17. Code de la santé publique, art. L. 1241-3, al. 3, L. 2004-800, art. 12, II, 3°.
18. Code de la santé publique, art. L. 1241-3, al. 3 *in fine*, L. 2004-800, art. 12, II, 3°.
19. Code de la santé publique, art. L. 1241-3, al. 4, L. 2004-800, art. 12, II, 3°. (Jusqu'à l'installation de ces comités, les mandats des membres des comités d'experts chargés d'autoriser les prélèvements de moelle osseuse sur une personne mineure en application des dispositions législatives et réglementaires applicables avant la date d'entrée en vigueur de la loi du 6 août 2004 sont prorogés : L. n° 2004-800, art. 33. Le nouveau comité est également compétent pour autoriser le prélèvement de cellules hématopoïétiques issues de la moelle osseuse sur majeur protégé (art. L 1241-4). Il doit, en outre, autoriser le prélèvement d'organes sur toutes les personnes visées par l'article L. 1231-1, alinéa 2.)
20. D. n° 2005-443 du 10 mai 2005 relatif aux prélèvements d'organes et de cellules hématopoïétiques issues de la moelle osseuse et modifiant le Code de la santé publique (partie réglementaire). *JO* 11 mai 2005 : 8155.
21. Code pénal, art. 511-5, al. 2, L. n° 2004-800, art. 15, 2°.
22. Code de la santé publique, art. L. 1242-1, al. 1er, L. 2004-800, art. 12, III, 1°. (Les autorisations antérieurement accordées pour les prélèvements de moelle osseuse sont prorogées pendant un an à compter de la date de publication de la loi (7 août 2004) : L. n° 2004-800, art. 34, I. En cas d'insuffisance régionale, les directeurs des ARH peuvent autoriser les établissements à prélever des cellules hématopoïétiques issues de la moelle osseuse : L. n° 2004-800, art. 34, II.)
23. Code de la santé publique, art. L. 1242-1, al. 3, L. 2004-800, art. 12, III, 1°.

24. L. 2004-800, art. 12, IV.
25. Code de la santé publique, art. L. 1243-1, al. 1er, L. 2004-800, art. 12, IV.
26. Code de la santé publique, art. L. 5121-1 et s.
27. Code de la santé publique, art. L. 5124-1, L. n° 2004-800, art. 19, III, B, 1°.
28. Code de la santé publique, art. L. 5124-13, L. n° 2004-800, art. 19, III, B, 2°.
29. Code de la santé publique, art. L. 4211-8 et s., L. n° 2004-800, art. 19, I et II.
30. Code de la santé publique, art. L. 5426-1, L. n° 2004-800, art. 20, I.
31. Code de la santé publique, art. L. 1243-3, al. 2, L. 2004-800, art. 12, IV.
32. Code de la santé publique, art. L. 1243-2, L. 2004-800, art. 12, IV.
33. Code de la santé publique, art. L. 1243-5, L. 2004-800, art. 12, IV.
34. Code de la santé publique, art. L. 1243-3, L. 2004-800, art. 12, IV. (La procédure concerne, plus largement, la conservation et la préparation à des fins scientifiques de tissus et de cellules issus du corps humain ainsi que la préparation et la conservation des organes, du sang, de ses composants et de ses produits dérivés. Pour les activités exercées avant l'entrée en vigueur de la loi du 6 août 2004, une obligation de déclaration dans un délai de deux ans est instituée : L. n° 2004-800, art. 36, I.)
35. Code de la santé publique, art. L. 1243-4, L. 2004-800, art. 12, IV. Pour les activités exercées avant l'entrée en vigueur de la loi du 6 août 2004, la demande d'autorisation doit être présentée dans un délai de deux ans est instituée : L. n° 2004-800, art. 36, II.
36. Code de la santé publique, art. L. 1243-6, L. 2004-800, art. 12, IV.
37. AN (2001-2002), n° 3166, Projet de loi relatif à la bioéthique.
38. AN (2001-2002), n° 763.
39. Ordonnance du 18 juin 2002.
40. CE, 13 novembre 2002, *Petites affiches*, 3 avril 2003 (n° 67), pp. 8-13, note B. Pauvert.
41. Trib. adm. Paris, 21 janvier 2003, *Petites affiches*, 1er octobre 2003, n° 196, pp. 7-10 note B. Pauvert.
42. Code de la santé publique, art. L. 1221-1 à L. 1224-4.
43. Code de la santé publique, art. L. 1231-1 à L. 1235-4.
44. Code de la santé publique, art. L. 1241-1 à L. 1245-6.
45. Code de la santé publique, art. L. 1261-1 à L. 1263-4.
46. Code de la santé publique, art. L. 1211-1 à L. 1211-9 et, par renvoi, C. civ., art. 16 à 16-9.
47. Code de la santé publique, art. L. 1241-1 à L. 1245-6.
48. Code de la santé publique, art. L. 1272-1 à L. 1272-8 ; Code pénal, art. 511-2 à 511-8-2.
49. Code de la santé publique, art. R. 1211-49 auquel renvoie l'article L. 1211-9, 4°.
50. Code de la santé publique, art. L. 1245-2.
51. Code de la santé publique, art. L. 1241-5, L. n° 2004-800, art. 27. Les art. 28, 8° et 32 B de la loi prévoient des dispositions pénales sanctionnant le respect de ces conditions.
52. Code de la santé publique, art L. 1241-5, L. n° 2004-800, art. 27. Les art. 28, 8° et 32 B de la loi prévoient des dispositions pénales sanctionnant le respect de ces conditions.
53. V. Binet JR. *Droit et progrès scientifique. Science du droit, valeurs et biomédecine*. Paris : PUF, 2002, préf. Labrusse-Riou C, postface Beignier B. spéc. chapitre « L'abandon sollicité : l'embryon humain » : 59-92.
54. Chérioux M, *JO Sénat CR*, séance du 30 janv. 2003 : « Dans son ensemble, le monde scientifique [...] admet que l'embryon humain ne peut être considéré comme une chose, que, à l'évidence, un embryon est le début d'une vie d'homme et que, à ce titre, il mérite le respect. Pour ces raisons, il n'est pas utile de définir un statut juridique de l'embryon. Il suffit simplement de reconnaître la réalité. »
55. *AN (2001-2002)*, n° 3166, exposé des motifs, p. 55. Adde, Mme Guigou, *JOAN CR*, Séance du 15 janv. 2002 : « Les perspectives de traitement des maladies dégénératives incurables de nos jours, comme la maladie d'Alzheimer, la maladie de Parkinson ou l'insuffisance hépatique, nous commandent de nous pencher sur cette question, tout comme l'espoir d'une meilleure connais-

sance des bases de la différenciation cellulaire, qui pourrait apporter des informations essentielles à la compréhension de la formation des cancers, ou encore celui d'une amélioration des techniques d'assistance médicale à la procréation. »

56. JOAN CR, 3ème séance du 15 janv. 2002.
57. Sénat (2002-2003), n° 128 : 47.
58. Mattei JF, JO Sénat CR, séance du 30 janv. 2003.
59. Vasselle A, *ibid* Ayant suscité un « D'accord » de M. Giraud, rapporteur à l'origine du régime en question, *ibid*.
60. Code de la santé publique, art. L. 2151-5, al. 4
61. Code de la santé publique, art. L. 2151-2.
62. Code de la santé publique, art. L. 2151-3.
63. Code de la santé publique, art. L. 2151-4.
64. Code de la santé publique, art. L. 2151-5, al. 7.
65. Créée par cette loi : Code de la santé publique, art. L. 1418-1
66. Code de la santé publique, art. L. 2151-6, al. 1er.
67. Code de la santé publique, art. L. 2151-5, al. 3.
68. F. Giraud, JO Sénat CR, séance du 30 janv. 2003
69. AN (2002-2003), n° 761, p. 161.
70. Mattei JF, JO Sénat CR, séance du 30 janv. 2003.
71. Code de la santé publique, art. L. 2151-5, al. 4
72. Code de la santé publique, art. L. 2151-5, al. 6
73. Code de la santé publique, art. L. 2151-8
74. L. n° 2004-800, art. 37-II.
75. D. n° 2004-1024, JO 30 sept., p. 16802. V. Binet JR. Le régime transitoire d'autorisation des recherches sur les cellules souches embryonnaires. JCP 2004, act. 540.
76. JO 10 mai 2005 : 8106.
77. L. n° 2004-800, art. 37, II, al. 1er, 1°.
78. L. n° 2004-800, art. 37, II, al. 1, 2°.
79. D. n° 2004-1024, art. 8.
80. Arr. 16 fév. 2005, JO 3 mars ; arr. 21 mars 2005, JO 1er avril ; arr. 22 mars 2005, JO 8 avril.
81. D. n° 2004-1024, art. 10.

Cellular Engineering and Transfusion: a Continuum?

Pierre Tiberghien

Cell or tissue therapy can be defined as the use, for therapeutic purposes, of isolated cells or clusters of cells (tissue) of autologous, allogeneic or xenogeneic origin [1, 2]. Cell and tissue engineering comprises all the stages necessary for the preparation of these cell or tissue therapies. These stages are very diverse and include collection, qualification, storing, distribution and delivery, as well as all the associated aspects such as quality assurance, traceability and biovigilance.

The Scope of Cell and Tissue Engineering

The scope of this type of engineering has widened considerably in recent years. After the use of "whole blood" and the advent of erythrocyte or platelet concentrates, development of cell apheresis techniques has made it possible to obtain purified cell populations such as platelet units from a single donor, granulocyte concentrates and mononuclear cells that can contain hematopoietic stem cells and/or immunocompetent cells (T-lymphocytes, natural killer cells, monocytes).

Possible sources of hematopoietic stem cells have also become much more diversified, once it was shown that these cells could be harvested from peripheral blood after mobilization by hematopoietic growth factors [3], or obtained from placental blood [4]. *Ex vivo* cellular engineering techniques have gradually developed thanks to semi-automated methods and closed-system methods that allow collection and cryopreservation of cell and tissue therapy products, *ex vivo* selection of cell populations, or expansion of hematopoietic progenitors [5].

At the same time, these methods, originally developed in the field of transfusion medicine, have been applied successfully to non hematopoietic cells and tissues such as the cornea, vessels, bone and skin, as well as, in a more experimental fashion, to Langerhans islets, hepatocytes or fetal origin neuroblasts [6-8]. Finally, the recent demonstration that "adult" stem cells can be isolated, or that it is possible to count on a certain degree of cellular plasticity by cellular "transdifferentiation" or fusion [9, 10] has made an important contribution to the potential field of cell therapy, a field whose future development could perhaps be ensured by the use of embryonic stem cells [11].

Are Cell and Tissue Therapy Products Medicinal?

Whether or not cell and tissue therapy products should have the status of "medicinal products" is subject to intense debate. This debate has already brought to light a number of specific characteristics of cell and tissue therapy products that clearly differentiate them from medicinal products in the classic sense of the term. A cell or tissue therapy product is often "patient-specific" or "donor and recipient-specific". This specificity makes it necessary to adapt quality control and lot approval criteria, which must take into account factors such as donor availability, possibility of collection and preparation of the cell therapy product and, of course, clinical state and indication for the patient. Thus, a hematopoietic stem cell graft from a single donor for a child with a malignant hemopathy will not necessarily be refused because it contains a germ whose antibiogram shows it to be reactive to available antibiotics. These specificities also make close cooperation necessary between cell and tissue engineering teams and clinical teams, so that "production" can be adapted on a daily basis to patient needs.

The use of biological material as "starting material" makes it indispensable that every effort should be made to ensure safety and enforce vigilance [12]. The tragedy of the HIV contaminated blood and, more recently, health alerts related to severe acute respiratory syndrome (SARS) [13], to avian influenza [14], to Creutzfeldt-Jakob variant [15] or to West Nile virus [16] make it mandatory to provide optimal response in the form of perfect biovigilance and traceability. Development of therapeutic innovations using cell therapy products does not follow the classic path where the pharmaceutical industry plays a key role and brings all its know-how into play. This relative absence of major industrial partners is also a financial handicap, making it difficult to conduct and organize clinical trials in the field of cell and tissue therapy.

Regulations Governing Cellular Biotherapies

In order to ensure patient safety, the French Health Regulatory Agency (AFSSAPS) has created a regulatory system comprising specific stipulations regarding:

– establishments which prepare these products;

– cell and tissue therapy products and procedures;

– implementation of clinical trials involving cell and tissue therapy;

– ethics and public health measures applicable to donations and to the use of components of the human body;

– importing and exporting of cells and cell and tissue therapy products [17].

This set of regulations is intended to guarantee the patient optimal collection, transformation and administration conditions involving products of human origin. Hepatitis B virus contamination of hematopoietic grafts cryopreserved in liquid nitrogen [18], serious *Clostridium* infections associated with an osteo-tendinous graft [19], and the development of encephalitis following West Nile virus contamination in four recipients of organs from the same donor, himself contaminated after a transfusion of red blood cells from an infected donor [20], point out the importance of establishing and maintaining principles of good practice in cell and tissue engineering, in transfusion and in transplantation.

Cellular Biotherapies

Such quality assurance practices are equally important in a related field, but not one truly connected, at present, with the other actors in cell and tissue engineering: assisted reproductive technology. In fact, in many ways, activities like sperm or oocyte collection, cryopreservation of gametes, *in vitro* fertilization, injection of spermatozoons in oocyte cytoplasm, cryopreservation of gametes and embryos, encounter problems very similar to those associated with transfusion and with cell and tissue engineering: monitoring, biological qualification, white rooms, traceability [21, 22]. Therefore, it seems essential to encourage close interaction between somatic cell producers and germinal and embryonic cell producers in order to establish joint means of ensuring optimal safety.

The probable future use of embryonic cells differentiated *ex vivo* [23] should facilitate this cooperation.

Advances in Transfusion

Rapid advances in cell and tissue therapy have been made possible in large part by the progress already achieved in transfusion medicine. Thus, collection and cell separation techniques using apheresis, automation and closed systems were applied directly to hematopoietic stem cell collection. The same is true for cryobiology, which benefited from developments in cryopreservation procedures, rapidly applied to hematopoietic grafts and tissue grafts such as vessels. Similarly, progress in risk reduction related to infectious agent transmission through labile blood products was directly applied to the preparation of cell and tissue engineering products. This field has implemented very effective qualification systems which are used at present for serologic and genomic diagnosis [24] and could be applied in the future to new methodologies derived from proteomics [25]. Considerable innovations made today in the area of bacterial risk reduction associated with labile blood products, the major cause of transfusion-related mortality [26], will also benefit the field of cell and tissue therapy [27, 28]. Adopting permanent rules of sample collection based on knowledge of health risks (temporary contraindications, emergency implementation of new screening techniques such as those recently used in a specific high-risk region in France to detect the West Nile virus [29], ...) has become standard procedure in transfusion medicine, and this know-how can certainly contribute to increased safety in the field of cell and tissue therapy. Motivated by the "contaminated blood tragedy", by the continued existence of infectious risk, minimal but real, and by the notion of possible "emerging" risks, transfusion medicine has created a system of traceability and monitoring of recipients (and donors) that can claim to be optimal and can be applied directly to the other cell and tissue biotherapies. In day-to-day practice, transfusion centers have established close relations, beneficial to all concerned, with blood donors and their associations. Medical and scientific expertise in transfusion medicine can also benefit the field of cell therapy. In addition, we must keep in mind that wherever donors are involved, the use of allogeneic tissues or cells is associated with immunologic risks such as alloimmune hemolysis [30], graft rejection or graft-*versus*-host disease [31]. Many of these alloimmune risks are well known and controlled in transfusion medicine.

This know-how can be extremely beneficial in the administration of other cell and tissue therapy products.

Finally, the most important aspect of the experience acquired in transfusion, and likely to benefit cell and tissue therapy, is that related to the large number of donors and recipients.

Frequently, cell therapy is limited to phase 1 and 2 trials involving a small number of patients. In these settings, organizational concerns, circuit safety, trans-contamination risk or labelling error risk... are not the greatest concern. When the numbers increase, the situation changes. For example, in 2004, the Bourgogne/Franche-Comté regional blood bank counted 273 collected grafts and 140 recipients; the placental blood bank counted 1,100 collected grafts, 208 cryopreserved, and 30 recipients; the cornea bank counted 1,608 corneas received and 803 recipients; for labile blood products, there were 81,000 donors, 26,400 products and 19,000 recipients. Quality assurance expectations and problems related to the management of such large numbers of donors, therapeutic products and recipients are both considerable and highly specific. The know-how and experience acquired in transfusion are already contributing to the development of cell and tissue therapy.

Transfusion and Cellular Biotherapy: Legitimacy and Added Benefits

The French National Blood Service (Etablissement Français du Sang: EFS) started to develop cell and tissue engineering activities over twenty years ago, when it created a network of cell and tissue engineering platforms located all across the country. In 2003, 40% to 50% of hematopoietic blood or marrow stem cell grafts were prepared in one of the cell therapy units of the EFS for about 2000 patients. The EFS has contributed greatly to the creation of the French network of placental blood. Founded in 2003, this network is comprised of three banks (Besançon, Bordeaux and Annemasse), each one within the EFS and producing about 500 placental blood grafts per year. These grafts are cryopreserved and made available to transplant teams. This important contribution of the EFS is reproduced in the field of tissue engineering, specifically in corneal tissue preparation, with over 60% of preparation units organized in a blood transfusion center. In 2003, 59% of corneal grafts made available for patients in France were prepared in one of the cell and tissue engineering Units of the EFS. One third of the bone grafts distributed in France comes from a Unit of the EFS. The EFS is also very active in the field of vessels, valves, skin and amniotic membranes for therapeutic purposes.

Finally, the EFS has demonstrated its ability to develop and control the production process of innovative cell therapy products such as hematopoietic progenitors expanded *ex vivo* [32], genetically modified T-lymphocytes [33, 34], and more recently, cytotoxic lymphocytes directed against viruses like the Epstein-Barr virus, as well as dendritic cells for immunomodulation purposes.

Thus, transfusion medicine can and must play an essential role in cell and tissue engineering.

It draws its legitimacy from the combined know-how of transfusion fields, its expertise in most stages of the production chain, functioning based on directly transferable quality, a national network under a single authority, and optimized safeguards in research and development activities in the important fields of biological qualification of donations, production processes and transfusion medicine.

The added value of this strategic role for a transfusion medicine actor such as the EFS consists in the possibility of developing, with a view to the long term, its know-how and the various transfusion fields by relying on existing collection, engineering, qualification and distribution structures. This development can also contribute to attract and to keep top level medical and scientific minds, while ensuring the sharing of knowledge and experience between cell and tissue therapy – whose therapeutic benefits have been established (for example: transfusion, hematopoietic graft, corneal transplant), and more innovative and experimental cellular biotherapy approaches.

Management of cell and tissue engineering development by transfusion medicine also constitutes an important added benefit for society, as development costs of these biotherapy approaches can be very high. Integration of these developments in the technical systems designed for collection, engineering and quality control, which already exist and function at "top speed" in transfusion medicine, can result in considerable savings. The "precautionary principle" has led transfusion medicine to make huge investments in order to accomplish what could seem like minimal safety gains [35]. It would be regrettable for cell and tissue therapy to have to acquire the necessary equipment and know-how "from scratch". In the same way, sharing of monitoring and vigilance structures by the fields of transfusion and cell and tissue biotherapy should make it possible to guarantee improved quality and better responsiveness in the face of known, poorly controlled or emerging risks.

A Successful Continuum

In order to successfully integrate therapeutic cell and tissue engineering into the activities of transfusion medicine, additional reflection and a specific action plan are needed in several areas:

– affirming the intent of "being able to produce any cell or tissue product for any patient in France or in Europe", and to formulate a development strategy allowing the implementation of this intention;

– ensuring harmonious, homogenous and complementary development of technical systems across the country, in order to create an efficient network;

– offering "cell and tissue engineering" services to public and private partners: this offer can cover the whole process from research to distribution and monitoring, or can be limited to a variable number of "modules": "design-development-collection-production/qualification-storage-distribution-traceability";

– developing research and development capabilities in cooperation with public scientific and technical establishments such as INSERM or the CNRS, universities and industry, in order to benefit from optimal synergy, but also to allow actors in transfusion to effectively anticipate and keep pace with scientific progress. *In vitro* production of red blood cells for therapeutic use [36], or the contribution of micro-nanotechnologies or of proteomics [25] for biological qualification of biotherapy products, are examples of important potential developments in which transfusion medicine can play a major role. A particularly good illustration of this is the use, at the start of the 1980s, of the CD4/CD8 ratio at Stanford (United States) to screen for blood donors contaminated by a virus (HIV) for which no screening test existed at the time [37];

– creating strong partnerships in "sensitive" or "critical" fields for the development of cell and tissue engineering activities. At present, the difficulty of obtaining clinical quality cytokines is still a major obstacle, particularly in the field of hematopoietic progenitor expansion. Moreover, most *ex vivo* cell separation methods require monoclonal antibodies that must be of therapeutic quality. In addition, several biotherapy approaches that combine a therapeutic cellular product with *in vivo* administration of monoclonal antibodies are being developed. Finally, the possibility of producing cells that express, in a stable manner, a transgene of therapeutic interest depends on availability of transcomplementary cells of therapeutic quality for the production of viral vectors;

– contributing to the establishment of standards of excellence in clinical investigations and biological monitoring in the field of biotherapies;

– working toward coherence and unification of authorization and follow-up procedures of cell and tissue engineering activities, applied by different administrative agencies within the European Union;

– finally, facilitating cooperation and joint activities with the other cell and tissue biotherapy sectors: organ transplant and assisted reproductive technology.

Conclusion

Cell and tissue engineering represents great potential in terms of the treatments transfusion medicine can offer. Actors in transfusion medicine are knowledgeable in all the areas involved and possess the necessary skills for the production of cell and tissue therapy products. Development difficulties are not related to the specific techniques required to obtain cell and tissue therapy products, but rather to the creation of a context of good manufacturing practices, safeguards and optimal responsiveness to donors, recipients, therapeutic indications and possible biological risks. Thus, the aim of transfusion medicine is not to specialize in one or several areas of cell and tissue engineering, but to carry out its intention of being able to prepare any cell and tissue therapy product for any patient. The transfusion medicine network and its expertise can guarantee efficient scientific and economic development of these new therapeutic approaches that hold great promise for patients. At the same time, implementation of such joint activities guarantees long-term continuity for transfusion activities and skills, and reinforces the central role of transfusion medicine in medical progress.

References

1. Gage FH. Cell therapy. *Nature* 1998 ; 392(Suppl.) : 18-24.
2. Maeno A, Naor J, Hung Ming L, Hunter W, Rootman D. Three decades of corneal transplantation: indications and patient characteristics. *Cornea* 2000 ; 19 : 7-11.
3. Kessinger A, Armitage JO, Landmark JD, Smith DM, Weisenburger DD. Autologous peripheral hematopoietic stem cell transplantation restores hematopoietic function following marrow ablative therapy. *Blood* 1988 ; 71 : 723-7.
4. Rocha V, Labopin M, Sanz G, Arcese W, Schwerdtfeger R, Bosi A, Jacobsen N, Ruutu T, de Lima M, Finke J, Frassoni F, Gluckman E; Acute Leukemia Working Party of European Blood and Marrow Transplant Group; Eurocord-Netcord Registry. Transplants of umbilical-cord blood or bone marrow from unrelated donors in adults with acute leukemia. *N Engl J Med* 2004 ; 351 : 2276-85.
5. Reiffers J, Cailliot C, Dazey B, Attal M, Caraux J, Boiron JM. Abrogation of post-myeloablative chemotherapy neutropenia by ex-vivo expanded autologous CD34-positive cells. *Lancet* 1999 ; 354 : 1092-3.
6. Robertson RP. Islet transplantation as a treatment for diabetes – a work in progress. *N Engl J Med* 2004 ; 350 : 694-705.
7. Borderie VM, Touzeau O, Allouch C, Scheer S, Carvajal-Gonzalez S, Laroche L. The results of successful penetrating keratoplasty using donor organ-cultured corneal tissue. *Transplantation* 1999 ; 67 : 1433-8.
8. Bachoud-Levi AC, Remy P, Nguyen JP, Brugieres P, Lefaucheur JP, Bourdet C, Baudic S, Gaura V, Maison P, Haddad B, Boisse MF, Grandmougin T, Jeny R, Bartolomeo P, Dalla Barba G, Degos JD, Lisovoski F, Ergis AM, Pailhous E, Cesaro P, Hantraye P, Peschanski M. Motor and cognitive improvements in patients with Huntington's disease after neural transplantation. *Lancet* 2000 ; 356 : 1975-9.

9. Rafii S, Lyden D. Therapeutic stem and progenitor cell transplantation for organ vascularization and regeneration. *Nat Med* 2003 ; 9 : 702-12.
10. Coulombel L. Cellules souches adultes: seing is not being. *Médecine /Science* 2003 ; 19 : 683-94.
11. Rosenthal N. Prometheus's vulture and the stem-cell promise. *N Engl J Med* 2003 ; 349 : 267-74.
12. Zou S, Dodd RY, Stramer SL, Strong DM; Tissue Safety Study Group. Probability of viremia with HBV, HCV, HIV, and HTLV among tissue donors in the United States. *N Engl J Med* 2004 ; 351 : 751-9.
13. Weinstein RA. Planning for epidemics-the lessons of SARS. *N Engl J Med* 2004 ; 350 : 2332-4.
14. Hien TT, de Jong M, Farrar J. Avian influenza-a challenge to global health care structures. *N Engl J Med* 2004 ; 351 : 2363-5.
15. Wilson K, Ricketts MN. Transfusion transmission of vCJD: a crisis avoided ? *Lancet* 2004 ; 364 : 477-9.
16. Pealer LN, Marfin AA, Petersen LR, Lanciotti RS, Page PL, Stramer SL, Stobierski MG, Signs K, Newman B, Kapoor H, Goodman JL, Chamberland ME; West Nile Virus Transmission Investigation Team. Transmission of West Nile virus through blood transfusion in the United States in 2002. *N Engl J Med* 2003 ; 349 : 1236-45.
17. Moussaoui S, Lucas S, Zorzi P, Le Saulnier C, Trouvin JH. Le cadre réglementaire des produits de thérapie cellulaire. *Bull Cancer* 2003 ; 8-9 : 779-88.
18. Tedder RS, Zuckerman MA, Goldstone AH, Hawkins AE, Fielding A, Briggs EM, Irwin D, Blair S, Gorman AM, Patterson KG, et al. Hepatitis B transmission from contaminated cryopreservation tank. *Lancet* 995 ; 346 : 137-40.
19. Kainer MA, Linden JV, Whaley DN, Holmes HT, Jarvis WR, Jernigan DB, Archibald LK. *Clostridium* infections associated with musculoskeletal-tissue allografts. *N Engl J Med* 2004 ; 350 : 2564-71. Erratum in: *N Engl J Med* 2004 ; 351 : 397-8.
20. Dwamoto M, Jernigan DB, Guasch A, Trepka MJ, Blackmore CG, Hellinger WC, Pham SM, Zaki S, Lanciotti RS, Lance-Parker SE, DiazGranados CA, Winquist AG, Perlino CA, Wiersma S, Hillyer KL, Goodman JL, Marfin AA, Chamberland ME, Petersen LR; West Nile Virus in Transplant Recipients Investigation Team. Transmission of West Nile virus from an organ donor to four transplant recipients. *N Engl J Med* 2003 ; 348 : 2196-203.
21. Maertens A, Bourlet T, Plotton N, Pozzetto B, Levy R. Validation of safety procedures for the cryopreservation of semen contaminated with hepatitis C virus in assisted reproductive technology. *Hum Reprod* 2004 ; 19 : 1554-7.
22. Practice Committee of the American Society for Reproductive Medicine. American Society for Reproductive Medicine/Society for Assisted Reproductive Technology position statement on West Nile Virus. *Fertil Steril* 2005 ; 83 : 527-8.
23. Hochedlinger K, Jaenisch R.Nuclear transplantation, embryonic stem cells, and the potential for cell therapy. *N Engl J Med* 2003 ; 349 : 275-86.
24. Stramer SL, Glynn SA, Kleinman SH, Strong DM, Sally C, Wright DJ, Dodd RY, Busch MP; National Heart, Lung, and Blood Institute Nucleic Acid Test Study Group. Detection of HIV-1 and HCV infections among antibody-negative blood donors by nucleic acid-amplification testing. *N Engl J Med* 2004 ; 351 : 760-8.
25. Papadopoulos MC, Abel PM, Agranoff D, Stich A, Tarelli E, Bell BA, Planche T, Loosemore A, Saadoun S, Wilkins P, Krishna S. A novel and accurate diagnostic test for human African trypanosomiasis. *Lancet* 2004 ; 363 : 1358-63.
26. Morel P, Deschaseaux M, Bertrand X, Naegelen C, Talon D. Transfusion-transmitted bacterial infection: residual risk and perspectives of prevention. *Transfus Clin Biol* 2003 ; 10 : 192-200.
27. Larsen CP, Ezligini F, Hermansen NO, Kjeldseri-Kragh J. Six years' experience of using the BacT/ALERT system to screen all platelet concentrates, and additional testing of outdated platelet concentrates to estimate the frequency of false-negative results. *Vox Sang* 2005 ; 88 : 93-7.

28. Morel P, Roubi N, Bertrand X, Lapierre V, Tiberghien P, Talon D, Herve P, Delbosc B. Bacterial contamination of a cornea tissue bank: implications for the safety of graft engineering. *Cornea* 2003 ; 22 : 221-5.
29. Gallian P, De Lamballerie X, De Micco P, Andreu G. Virus West Nile : généralités et implications en transfusion sanguine. *Transfus Clin Biol* 2005 ; 12 : 11-7.
30. Lapierre V, Kuentz M, Tiberghien P. Allogeneic peripheral blood hematopoietic stem cell transplantation: guidelines for red blood cell immuno-hematological assessment and transfusion practice. Société Francaise de Greffe de Moelle. *Bone Marrow Transplant* 2000 ; 25 : 507-12.
31. Devetten MP, Vose JM. Graft-versus host disease: how to translate new insights into new therapeutic strategies. *Blood Marrow Transplant* 2004 ; 10 : 815-25.
32. Reiffers J, Cailliot C, Dazey B, Attal M, Caraux J, Boiron JM. Abrogation of post-myeloablative chemotherapy neutropenia by ex-vivo expanded autologous CD34-positive cells. *Lancet* 1999 ; 354 : 1092-3.
33. Robinet E, Certoux JM, Ferrand C, Maples P, Hardwick A, Cahn JY, Reynolds CW, Jacob W, Hervé P, Tiberghien P. A closed culture system for the ex vivo transduction and expansion of human T lymphocytes. *J Hematother* 1998 ; 7 : 205-15.
34. Tiberghien P, Ferrand C, Lioure B, Milpied N, Angonin R, Deconinck E, Certoux JM, Robinet E, Saas P, Petracca B, Juttner C, Reynolds CW, Longo DL, Hervé P, Cahn JY. Administration of Herpes simplex-thymidine kinase-expressing donor T cells with a T-cell-depleted allogeneic marrow graft. *Blood* 2001 ; 97 : 63-72.
35. McClelland B, Contreras M. Appropriateness and safety of blood transfusion. *Br Med J* 2005 ; 330 : 104-5.
36. Giarratana MC, Kobari L, Lapillonne H, Chalmers D, Kiger L, Cynober T, Marden MC, Wajcman H, Douay L. Ex vivo generation of fully mature human red blood cells from hematopoietic stem cells. *Nat Biotechnol* 2005 ; 23 : 69-74.
37. Galel SA, Lifson JD, Engleman EG. Prevention of AIDS transmission through screening of the blood supply. *Annu Rev Immunol* 1995 ; 13 : 201-27.

Stem Cells and their Therapeutic Promise for Tomorrow's Regenerative Medicine

Ali Turhan, Anne-Lise Bennaceur Griscelli

In the recent years, very few fields have developed as rapidly as the domain of stem cell and cell therapy, both at the theoretical and the applied level, making it possible to foresee therapeutic uses that were unimaginable only fifteen years ago. After the "genomic" revolution, stem cells seem to offer new prospects that could revolutionize 21st century medicine.

At the theoretical level, in a very short time, certain established principles were revised. For example, the presence of tissue-specific adult stem cells had only been associated with certain organ systems, like bone marrow [1]. Their presence was demonstrated in medullary cells by the ability of the latter to produce long-term hematopoiesis reconstitution after myeloablative treatments. For other organs like the brain and the liver, presence of stem cells in adults was a more recent discovery [2, 3]. Recently, it has been suggested that the adult heart has c-kit+ cells able to regenerate cardiac cells after induced ischemia [4]. The most surprising revelations were, on the one hand, the discovery that adult stem cells can produce cells of another embryologic layer, a phenomenon called "plasticity" [5]; and on the other hand, the discovery of multipotent adult stem cells whose characteristics resemble those of embryonic stem cells [6]. At the same time, developments in embryonic stem cell research have shown that these cells can repair certain adult tissues in several systems. The challenge for their future use in regenerative medicine will be to understand the underlying mechanisms explaining their potential for specialized differentiation. At the applied level, and in a manner unrelated to direct knowledge transfer, certain observations have already been applied to the treatment of human diseases, and other applications can be foreseen in the next few decades. As in all scientific fields, progress will be slow, understanding of mechanisms will be incomplete, but cellular "regenerative" medicine is likely to become clinical reality.

"Therapeutic" Cells

Cell Therapy: Changes in Basic Assumptions

Therapeutic use of stem cells, known as cell therapy in the wide sense of the term, has, in fact, been part of medical practice ever since it became possible to perform autologous and allogeneic grafts. In hemato-oncology, these practices are standard therapy for treating several types of leukemia and lymphoma, as well as certain cancers where intensified chemotherapy makes it possible to produce therapeutic effects on the tumor. In these cases, "therapeutic" cells are essentially hematopoietic cells, autologous or allogeneic. When allogeneic cells are used, real immunologic cell therapy takes place, thanks to the anti-leukemia effect produced by graft-*versus*-host disease [7]. As far as autologous grafts are concerned, *ex vivo* manipulation of progenitors using growth factors resulted in the development of expansion techniques serving to abrogate post-transplantation aplasia [8]. In areas other than hemato-oncology, cell therapies by functional cell replacement are used to treat insulin-dependent diabetes by Langerhans islet transplantation, which has already proven effective at least in the middle term [9]. However, use of autologous cells from other tissues, to replace a deficient function, was inconceivable before the characterization and implementation of mesenchymal cell culture techniques [10]. In effect, mesenchymal stem cells were used, for instance, to generate bone cells needed in traumatism or congenital bone disease settings [11]. In the field of cardiac cell therapy, use of autologous striated muscle cells amplified *ex vivo* and transplanted into the cardiac parenchyma to repair myocardial ischemia foci was an important therapeutic innovation that showed myocardial performance improvement in a pilot study [12]. A clinical randomized trial now in progress, where patients receive a placebo or autologous myoblasts cultivated *ex vivo*, will determine cell therapy efficacy in heart failure.

In all of these cell therapy approaches, the tissues used were embryologically related to those that had to be repaired, because accepted principles posited a strict relation between embryologic origin of a given tissue and its potential in adult life; for example, hematopoietic cells can only be used to generate hematopoietic cells and, based on another assumption, in adults, stem cells only exist in certain organs capable of constant cell renewal, like bone marrow and the epidermis, which maintains homeostasis by renewal of cells with a short half-life.

At the end of the 1990s, a series of studies revealed that in mice having received a marrow transplant it was possible to detect donor muscle cells [13, 14]. This result could be obtained by transplanting whole bone marrow or stem cells enriched with a side population (SP) able to efflux Hoechst; in a murine muscular dystrophy model, this method made it possible to generate muscular fibers able to synthesize dystrophin [14]. Surprisingly, it was also possible to reconstitute hematopoiesis in lethally irradiated mice after transplantation of muscle-derived SP cells [15].

In addition, it has been shown that neuronal cell transplantation can generate lympho-myeloid hematopoietic cells [16] and that donor neuronal cells are present after marrow transplant [17, 18]. Function generation by transplanted cells has been demonstrated in the myocardial, hepatic and neural systems. In fact, experiments involving marrow transplant in a fumarylacetoacetate hydrolase (FAH) deficit model responsible for hereditary murine tyrosinemia has demonstrated the possibility of correcting FAH deficit in FAH-/- mice by transplanting hematopoietic cells from a FAH+/+ mouse [19].

It has also been shown that injecting purified hematopoietic cells into a myocardial infarction site can produce contractile GFP+ cardiac cells [20]. Functional Purkinje cells can also be detected in the cerebellum of mice after marrow transplant [21].

This experimental data involving several types of cells (*Table I*) has created great enthusiasm concerning the potential of cell therapies, although the frequency of phenotype changes was very low in almost all the experiments conducted.

Table I. Multipotent cell populations and their tissues of origin.

Whole bone marrow (BM)	Muscle, neuron, hepatocytes, cardiomyocytes, pancreatic β-cells
Sca1+c-kit+lin-(BM)	Hepatocytes, cardiomyocytes
SP* cells (BM)	Muscle
Whole muscle	Hematopoiesis
SP cells (muscle)	Hematopoiesis
SP/CD45 (muscle)	Hematopoiesis

SP: *side population*

What Mechanisms?

Several types of mechanisms have been invoked to explain cell phenotype changes after transplantation (*Figure 1*). The most common explanation is that the donor tissue possesses a very primitive stem cell able to give rise to different phenotypes following a change of the microenvironment in response to local conditions: this would suggest a "training" mechanism, leaving the primitive character of the cell undetermined. In most experimental conditions, the need for pre-existing tissue injury (toxin injection or irradiation) pointed to the importance of the tissue environment to induce the phenotypic conversion of the "stem" cell that migrated to the injured site. The multipotent character of the stem cell responsible for this effect has been examined in experiments involving single hematopoietic stem cell transplants; these experiments produced evidence of the contribution of these single cells to pulmonary epithelial cells and to hepatocytes [22]. The role of the environment was clearly demonstrated by studies involving co-culture of neural stem cells also able to differentiate into new phenotypes upon contact with muscle tissue [23]. Overall, the potential for conversion was observed mainly in hematopoietic cells (*Table I*).

However, another possible explanation demonstrated experimentally in certain settings is cellular fusion (*Figure 1*). Thus, experiments involving marrow transplants producing regeneration of liver cells, have shown that the original donor liver cells were polyploid, with presence of both donor and recipient markers [24]. However, two-way programming was documented in this context, because the hematopoietic cells from FAH+/+ animals, which fused with hepatic FAH-/- cells, stopped expressing hematopoietic markers (CD45) and, at the same time, triggered FAH synthesis, FAH being a substance that, at the physiological level, is not expressed in hematopoietic cells.

This reactivation of epigenetic-like expression gave rise to the hypothesis of "healing fusion", and could become the source of a new cell therapy theory [24]. At present, it is likely that cells at the origin of this type of fusion are differentiated myelomonocytic cells [24].

Cellular fusion likely explains other phenotype conversions, such as those involving striated muscle [25].

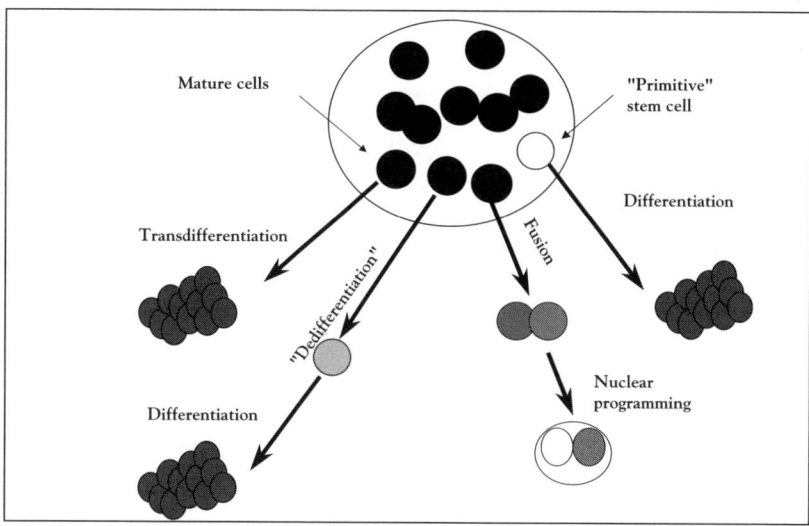

Figure 1. Graphic representation of the hypotheses explaining plasticity. The first hypothesis invokes the "transdifferentiation" of a mature cell already directed toward a specific differentiation, perhaps including an intermediary "dedifferentiation" stage (the two arrows on the left). Another hypothesis postulates the persistence in adult tissues of a primitive "somatic" stem cell able, in certain conditions (but perhaps never *in vivo* at the basal level), to initiate a differentiation pathway leading to structures other than those corresponding to the initial tissue. Finally, it has been shown that cellular fusion could explain phenotypic conversion phenomena (see text).

The controversy concerning the role of fusion is far from over. In fact, recent observations show that phenotypic change without cellular fusion can exist in certain contexts, indicating the possibility of actual transdifferentiation [26, 27]. Recent experiments show, for example, that it is possible to generate in one week, from purified hematopoietic cells, hepatocytic phenotype cells, when the latter are cultivated with hepatic tissue regenerating in a culture system, without any contact [26]. In the same way, the culture of neural stem cells in contact with paraformaldehyde-fixed murine endothelial cells causes human neural cells to change phenotype and become endothelial cells [27]. Nuclear programming with or without fusion appears, therefore, to be a reality, confirming nuclear programming possibilities observed in other experiments, specifically for inducing a T-cell phenotype from monocytic cells [28].

Another possible explanation for plasticity mechanisms observed by researchers is the existence of tissue-specific stem cells found in different locations in the adult, probably due to the existence of "niches" allowing the survival and self-regeneration of these stem cells [29].

The best known example is the striated muscle which, in mice, contains stem cells with hematopoietic potential: recent experiments show that these "extramedullary" cells possess a hematopoietic phenotype and have major reconstitution potential, although we do not know why they are present in striated muscle [30]. The phenotype conversion mechanism is not related, in this case, to cell "plasticity", but rather to the activity of a stem cell at an extramedullary location [31].

Finally, another "plasticity" mechanism resembling two-stage programming could consist of dedifferentiation followed by direction toward another differentiation path.

In fact, in experimental conditions, it is possible to change the phenotype of a mature muscle cell (multinucleate myoblast) to a more primitive phenotype by overexpression of Msx1, a MyoD inhibitor [32]. Cells overexpressing Msx1 can then be directed, in the presence of specific growth factors, toward osteoblastic or chondrocytic differentiation [32].

In the same way, in the neural system, oligodendrocytes can be directed toward a more stem cell-like phenotype, then redirected toward more specific differentiation [33].

In Drosophilia, germinal stem cells can be reconstituted from spermatogonia already engaged in the differentiation process, suggesting dedifferentiation in these cells [34].

"Regenerative" Cells

Cells involved in regeneration are, for the most part, very clearly characterized, as is the case for tissue-specific stem cells like hematopoietic stem cells and mesenchymal cells. These cells offer a distinct contrast with multipotent stem cells that have wider differentiation potential, which also exist in a number of adult tissues. In any case, we know today that bone marrow probably constitutes a real "reservoir" of different types of stem cells.

Tissue-Specific Stem Cells

First in this category are hematopoietic stem cells, which have been used either in whole marrow transplantation, or after purification of specific subpopulations such as Sca 1+, c-kit+, or "side population" phenotype cells (SP) able to efflux Hoeschst 33342 (*Table I*). In addition, the SP phenotype can serve to effect stem cell enrichment in other tissues, such as muscles, which also contain stem cells with hematopoietic potential [15]. Whatever their phenotype, hematopoietic stem cells could become a major tool for regenerative cell therapy in the future, given that isolation, purification and *ex vivo* manipulation techniques involving them have existed for a long time in hemato-oncological applications. Other cellular phenotypes with plasticity potential should be examined to determine the possibility of *ex vivo* manipulation of this potential in culture systems.

Moreover, bone marrow also contains mesenchymal stem cells that have already demonstrated their capacity to generate bone cells, representing one of the first examples of regenerative medicine [11, 35]. Plasticity is an inherent property of these cells, at least for generating osteoblastic, adipocytic and chondrocytic cells [36, 37], but recent studies show that they could have very wide regenerative potential *in vivo*, particularly in the repair of cardiac damage [38], renal damage [39, 40] and respiratory damage [41]. In these models, mesenchymal cells appear to be integrated into the damaged tissue, but it is difficult to determine if this is due to a fusion mechanism, to transdifferentiation or to a throphic effect, particularly in the heart, where the mesenchymal cells induce VEGF secretion and neovascularization. Finally, mesenchymal stem cells have the remarkable capacity of producing immunologic tolerance through a mechanism that remains unknown. This property could be very promising for potential use of these cells in the prevention or modulation of graft-*versus*-host reactions [42]. As far as other tissue-specific cells are concerned, neural stem cells are probably programmable, but clinical applications involving use of these cells are difficult to achieve at present. The bulbar stem cells of the pilose system have epidermic and pilose potentiality, suggesting their possible use in regenerative cellular skin therapies. Stem cells isolated from the dermis could also have wide potentiality, mainly of the neural type [43]. The adipose system, another easily accessible tissue, contains stem cells that could have endothelial and muscular potential [44].

Multipotent Adult Stem Cells

In 2001, Verfaillie's team showed, both in mice and in humans, the existence of a multipotent cell designated as the "Multipotent Adult Stem Cell" (MAPC) [6]. These cells were isolated from human and murine bone marrow, as well as from other tissues such as muscle and brain in rodents, starting with a CD45-population, after a culture period of several weeks in the presence of epidermal growth factor and platelet-derived growth factor, provided these were very low density cultures. These cells have major duplication potential, up to over 120 duplications, while maintaining mesodermic, endodermic and ectodermic differentiation potential [6]. Therefore, these cells could become a major tool in future cell therapy, but isolating them is very difficult because they can only be detected in culture after several weeks, raising the question of their existence *in vivo*, and of their appearance in culture through a mechanism resembling "differentiation" of a committed stem cell.

Since the initial description of multipotent adult stem cells, other multipotent stem cells have been described more recently. For example, a population of very primitive stem cells obtained from cord blood and known as "Unrestricted Somatic Stem Cells" (USSC) [45] can be amplified in the absence of cytokine, and could be relatively easier to isolate and cultivate. These cells are believed to have a proliferation potential identical or superior to that of MAPCs, and the potential to differentiate into the cells of the three embryologic layers, at least *in vivo* in the sheep hematopoiesis model [45].

Finally, other types of multipotent cells have been described in adult tissues, such as the cells called "Miami cells" (Marrow-Inducible Activated Multipotent Cells) [46] or stem cells isolated from adipose tissue, known as hMAD [47].

At present, the most important questions concern the presence of these cells in certain privileged organs, their existence *in vivo* and the techniques that could make it possible to isolate them in a single step. In reality, based on their description, it will be difficult to give MAPC cells clinical applications, given the difficulty of their culture and preservation.

If multipotent adult stem cells do, in fact, exist, they could have major therapeutic potential in the future, provided that their multiple differentiation capacity can be manipulated *ex vivo*.

Plasticity of the Differentiated State

Stem cell "plasticity", for both adult and embryonic cells, is inherent to their function, because their genetic programming is sufficiently primitive to make specialization dependent on external stimuli or on the activation of certain specific genetic programs. Inversely, cloning experiments have clearly shown that a differentiated adult cell can be programmed, confirming genomic plasticity. Plasticity of the "differentiated state" described in the experimental conditions of the heterokaryon study [48] is a concept implying that a differentiated cell can be "reprogrammed" to acquire different fates than the fate of its embryonic origin. Experimental examples involving use of myoblast or oligodendrocyte lines [32, 33] indicate that adequate *in vitro* conditions for programming exist, but *in vivo* extrapolation of this phenomenon seems too minimal to explain plasticity in general. Finally, we must point out that induction of a given phenotypic characteristic does not make it possible to conclude that there is function generation. Although plasticity of the differentiated state is an experimental reality, its clinical use will require, in coming decades, the development of programming techniques, probably through use of external pharmacological or exogenous molecular stimuli.

Regenerative Medicine : Therapeutic Applications

Today

In the last few years, some research-produced findings have been given clinical applications, particularly in cardiology. In fact, following initial description of generation of GFP+ contractile myocardial cells after graft of c-kit+ stem cells in rats, several clinical trials were conducted, to apply a cardiac repair strategy after myocardial ischemias in view of preventing post-infarction heart failure. These trials consisted of intramyocardial injection of autologous hematopoietic cells, followed by investigation of myocardial function. Injected cells were of different types (whole bone marrow, CD34+, AC133+, mobilized blood cells) and, in most cases, produced improvement of myocardial performance tests in the months following local injection. In another randomized trial with sixty participants, intracoronary injection of autologous bone marrow cells produced very significant improvement of left ventricular function after infarction in thirty patients, compared to the control group which did not receive medullary cells [49]. Similarly, stem cell mobilization by G-CSF seems to improve post-infarction myocardial function in certain cases. But it must be noted that, in one randomized clinical trial, intracoronary injection of peripheral stem cells mobilized by G-CSF produced restenosis, resulting in halting of the trial [50]. The mechanism responsible for improvement is still undetermined; it could involve local neovascularization or a trophic effect, rather than transdifferentiation.

The use of stem cells as a regenerative medicine approach can also find applications in the field of angiology, offering the possibility of repairing limb ischemia by hematopoietic cell injection. Certain clinical results have already been obtained [51]. It has been shown that administration of bone marrow cells by local injection at ischemic sites could stimulate ischemic tissue revascularization. Protocols are now being designed in view of improving these strategies by changing the means of administration or by using purified cells from bone marrow or from mobilized peripheral blood. Overall, the mechanisms of this proangiogenic cell therapy are unknown: there could be a trophic effect related to hematopoietic and/or stromal cells grafted onto the ischemic site, or there could be a true angiogenic effect originating in a locally implanted precursor from the bone marrow. Finally, we must point out that long-term results of these repair strategies are not known, and that their usefulness will have to be determined by randomized clinical trials.

In neurology, stem cells from embryos have already been used in the treatment of certain degenerative diseases. Based on results obtained in experimental conditions, we can foresee developing regenerative strategies to treat neurological diseases. But the use of adult hematopoietic stem cells is still experimental, although it has been suggested that it could be possible to produce neuronal regeneration after marrow transplantation [52]. Similarly, hematopoietic stem cells could be used to treat degenerative retinopathies, given that in a murine model of retinal degeneration, local injection of lin-bone marrow stem cells produced retinopathy improvement [53]. Contradictory results were obtained with use of bone marrow stem cells in an attempt to generate pancreatic β cells [54]. While certain studies showed the possibility of generating pancreatic cells [55] from bone marrow cells without evidence of fusion [56], in other studies, specifically a GFP+ marrow cell transplantation model in mice with previously induced pancreatic lesion, it was not possible to identify any donor mouse cells [57]. Conflicting study results could be due to differences in experimental conditions, and only further studies can lead to conclusive results.

Finally, the ability of bone marrow cells (be they stem cells or differentiated cells) to achieve fusion could be used in the treatment of myopathies and hepatocellular insufficiencies. Occurrence of this type of fusion has been demonstrated after allogeneic transplantation in humans, but therapeutic application will require greater frequency of the fusion phenomenon in a setting where the objective is hepatic regeneration. In addition, clinical applications of the fusion strategy require judicial selection of therapeutic models, in order to demonstrate the clinical usefulness of therapeutic fusion. However, the functional consequences of poliploidy induced by this process have to be evaluated in experimental conditions, taking into account the target tissues.

Tomorrow

Programming Adult Cells

In the past few years, despite much controversy, it became clear that the adult cell genome has a potential identical to that of the embryonic cell. In fact, cloning experiments show the "plasticity" of the genome and the capacity of its genes to be reactivated by external or internal stimuli that remain to be defined. The most recent results have revealed three *a priori* programming mechanisms that could prove beneficial in future therapeutic applications:

1. cellular fusion, that is, programming of the donor cell nucleus in receiver cell cytoplasm;

2. programming by means of external stimuli, which, in some cases, could propagate within the receiver cell to be programmed;

3. programming of an adult cell by introducing an intermediate "stem" cell state through a dedifferentiation mechanism, as has been shown in experimental conditions [33, 34] (*Figure 1*).

In this context, certain results make it possible to suppose that the microenvironment could play a major role in programming, particularly through contact with adherent cells, which provide the viable cells in culture with an inert support. To illustrate, it has been shown that it is possible to produce an endothelial phenomenon starting with human neural stem cells when the latter are co-cultivated with adherent, and therefore dead, murine endothelial cells [27].

These observations indicate that "programming" molecules capable of dissemination could be developed in the future to induce certain phenotypes from differentiated cells. We know, for example, that a synthetic molecule known as reversine, a purine analog, can transform muscle cells which can later be directed toward osteoblastic or adipocytic differentiation [58].

Therapeutic Use of Adult Stem Cells

In 2005, experimental results showed that several technical problems must be solved before we can realistically plan to use multipotent adult stem cells in regenerative medicine. Multipotent cells are difficult to obtain in a reproducible manner in humans. Although their multiple potential opens major therapeutic perspectives in regenerative as well as hemato-oncological medicine, it is still too early to imagine therapeutic strategies using multipotent adult stem cells. In addition, experiments will have to examine hierarchical relations between multipotent cells described as unrestricted somatic stem cells obtained from cord blood, whose capacity for multilineage differentiation and for proliferation makes them resemble multipotent adult stem cells, but which are easier to produce in culture [45]. Finally, other types of adult stem cells, isolated from bone marrow or from adipose tissue [46, 47], could have clinical applications earlier than multipotent adult stem cells, in ischemia or myopathy settings.

Human Embryonic Stem Cells

Human embryonic stem cells, whose use gave rise to ethical problems, represent a major therapeutic tool for the regenerative medicine of the future. They were at the center of intense controversy and wide-spread debate, particularly due to the conditions of their procurement and propagation, and fears connected to reproductive cloning [59]. In experimental conditions, these cells have theoretically unlimited proliferation potential, making it possible to obtain large quantities of cells. These cells are also theoretically totipotent, because they contribute to the generation of all the tissues in the body. In mice, and to a certain extent in humans, the conditions of cell differentiation toward many lineages have been established. Despite these advantages, several practical problems will have to be solved before these cells can acquire therapeutic uses in regenerative medicine applied to humans. At present, several human embryonic stem cell lines exist in the world, but their clinical use would hardly be acceptable due to traceability problems regarding their prior handling. In France, the Bioethics Law allows the use of human embryonic stem cells for research purposes, but generation of new cell lines will require the creation of cell therapy structures that will probably form networks and that will be able to generate and characterize these cells in good practice conditions. Experiments involving murine cells show that embryonic stem cells, that are theoretically immortal, do nevertheless lose their differentiation potential with successive passages, making it imperative to ensure rigorous and traceable banking conditions.

Table II. Clinical applications of regenerative cell therapy using "heterologous" tissue.

Cells	Means of administration	Pathology	References
Bone marrow	Local injection	Lower limb arteriopathy	[51]
Bone marrow, CD34+, CSP	Intracoronary local injection	Ischemic cardiopathies	[49, 50]
Myoblasts	Local injection	Ischemic cardiopathies	[12]
Buccal epithelial cells	Local graft	Corneal repair	[61]
Mesenchymal cells	Graft IV	Osteogenesis imperfecta	[11, 35]

From a scientific point of view, one of the major challenges is to establish rigorous differentiation conditions, because human embryonic stem cells need only stromal cells for their growth. Monitoring their differentiation *in vitro* is essential, particularly in order to prevent the persistence of totipotent embryonic cells that could be responsible for oncogenesis. *In vivo* injection of embryonic stem cells, particularly for neural repair after medullary compression or in cardiomyopathy treatment, could be a strategy of choice. We know, for example, that human embryonic stem cells injected in pig heart differentiate into cardiogenic cells with a "pace-maker" function, causing disappearance of experimental auricular/ventricular blockages [60]. Finally, clinically acceptable culture and cryopreservation conditions will have to be developed, just as they will have to be developed for adult cells, in cell therapy centers specifically designed for these activities.

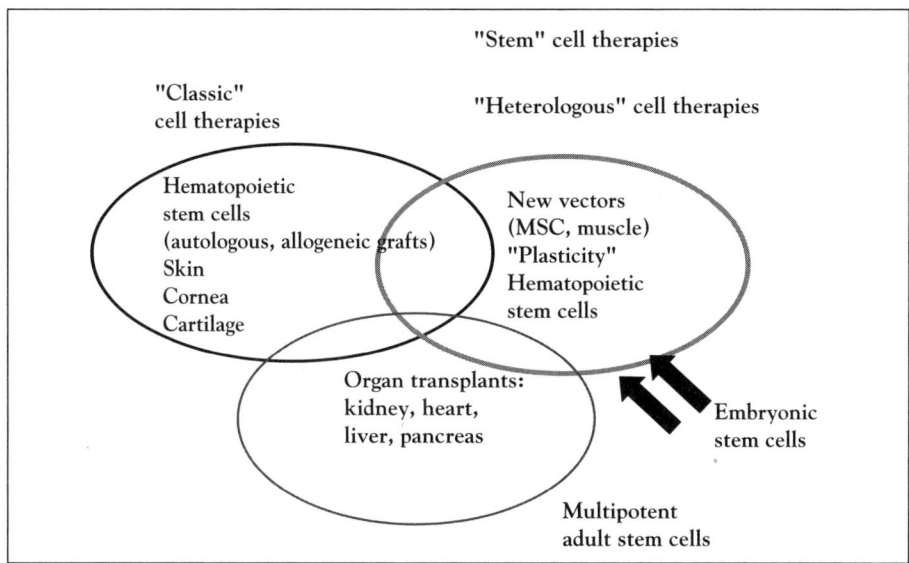

Figure 2. Evolution of cell therapy concepts.

Future Prospects and Conclusion

The major advances made recently in the field of stem cell biology make it reasonable to suppose that regenerative cell therapy will become part of standard practice in several branches of medicine in the 21st century. This therapy will develop thanks to the experience acquired in classic cell therapy (autologous and allogeneic grafts, skin grafts) and the experience acquired in organ transplantation (*Figure 2*). Finally, thanks to the introduction in clinical practice of new cellular vectors such as mesenchimal cells, and the discovery of new types of adult "stem" cells (MAPC, USSC…) or embryonic cells, regenerative medicine could one day become an alternative to transplantation in a number of pathologies.

References

1. Prchal JT, Throckmorton DW, Carroll AJ 3rd, Fuson EW, Gams RA, Prchal JF. A common progenitor for human myeloid and lymphoid cells. *Nature* 1978 ; 274 : 590-1.
2. Gage FH. Mammalian neural stem cells. *Science* 2000 ; 287 : 1433-8.
3. Strain AJ, Crosby HA. Hepatic stem cells. *Gut* 2000 ; 46 : 743-5.
4. Beltrami AP, Barlucchi L, Torella D, Baker M, Limana F, Chimenti S, Kasahara H, Rota M, Musso E, Urbanek K, Leri A, Kajstura J, Nadal-Ginard B, Anversa P. Adult cardiac stem cells are multipotent and support myocardial regeneration. *Cell* 2003 ; 114 : 763-76.
5. Blau HM, Brazelton TR, Weimann JM. The evolving concept of a stem cell: entity or function? *Cell* 2001 ; 105 : 829-41.
6. Jiang Y, Jahagirdar BN, Reinhardt RL, Schwartz RE, Keene CD, Ortiz-Gonzalez XR, Reyes M, Lenvik T, Lund T, Blackstad M, Du J, Aldrich S, Lisberg A, Low WC, Largaespada DA, Verfaillie CM. Pluripotency of mesenchymal stem cells derived from adult marrow. *Nature* 2002 ; 418 : 41-9.
7. Jiang YZ, Kanfer EJ, Macdonald D, Cullis JO, Goldman JM, Barrett AJ. Graft-versus-leukaemia following allogeneic bone marrow transplantation: emergence of cytotoxic T lymphocytes reacting to host leukaemia cells. *Bone Marrow Transplant* 1991 ; 8 : 253-8.

8. Reiffers J, Cailliot C, Dazey B, Attal M, Caraux J, Boiron JM. Abrogation of post-myeloablative chemotherapy neutropenia by ex-vivo expanded autologous CD34-positive cells. *Lancet* 1999 ; 354 : 1092-3.
9. Rother KI, Harlan DM. Challenges facing islet transplantation for the treatment of type 1 diabetes mellitus. *J Clin Invest* 2004 ; 114 : 877-83.
10. Deans RJ, Moseley AB. Mesenchymal stem cells: biology and potential clinical uses. *Exp Hematol* 2000 ; 28 : 875-84.
11. Horwitz EM, Prockop DJ, Fitzpatrick LA, Koo WW, Gordon PL, Neel M, Sussman M, Orchard P, Marx JC, Pyeritz RE, Brenner MK. Transplantability and therapeutic effects of bone marrow-derived mesenchymal cells in children with osteogenesis imperfecta. *Nat Med* 1999 ; 5 : 309-13.
12. Menasche P, Hagege AA, Scorsin M, Pouzet B, Desnos M, Duboc D, Schwartz K, Vilquin JT, Marolleau JP. Myoblast transplantation for heart failure. *Lancet* 2001 ; 357 : 279-80.
13. Ferrari G, Cusella-De Angelis G, Coletta M, et al. Muscle regeneration by bone marrow-derived myogenic progenitors. *Science* 1998 ; 279 : 1528-30.
14. Gussoni E, Soneoka Y, Strickland CD, et al. Dystrophin expression in the mdx mouse restored by stem cell transplantation. *Nature* 1999 ; 401 : 390- 4.
15. Jackson KA, Mi T, Goodell MA. Hematopoietic potential of stem cells isolated from murine skeletal muscle. *Proc Natl Acad Sci USA* 1999 ; 96 : 14482-6.
16. Bjornson CR, Rietze RL, Reynolds BA, Magli MC, Vescovi AL. Turning brain into blood: a hematopoietic fate adopted by adult neural stem cells in vivo. *Science* 1999 ; 283 : 534-7.
17. Brazelton TR, Rossi FM, Keshet GI, Blau HM. From marrow to brain: expression of neuronal phenotypes in adult mice. *Science* 2000 ; 290 : 1775-9.
18. Mezey E, Chandross KJ, Harta G, Maki RA, McKercher SR. Turning blood into brain: cells bearing neuronal antigens generated in vivo from bone marrow. *Science* 2000 ; 290 : 1779-82.
19. Lagasse E, Connors H, Al-Dhalimy M, Reitsma M, Dohse M, Osborne L, Wang X, Finegold M, Weissman IL, Grompe M. Purified hematopoietic stem cells can differentiate into hepatocytes in vivo. *Nat Med* 2000 ; 6 : 1229-34.
20. Orlic D, Kajstura J, Chimenti S, Jakoniuk I, Anderson SM, Li B, Pickel J, McKay R, Nadal-Ginard B, Bodine DM, Leri A, Anversa P. Bone marrow cells regenerate infarcted myocardium. *Nature* 2001 ; 410 : 701-5.
21. Priller J, Persons DA, Klett FF, Kempermann G, Kreutzberg GW, Dirnagl U. Neogenesis of cerebellar Purkinje neurons from gene-marked bone marrow cells in vivo. *J Cell Biol* 2001 ; 155 : 733-8.
22. Krause DS, Theise ND, Collector MI, Henegariu O, Hwang S, Gardner R, Neutzel S, Sharkis SJ. Multi-organ, multi-lineage engraftment by a single bone marrow-derived stem cell. *Cell* 2001 ; 105 : 369-77.
23. Galli R, Borello U, Gritti A, Minasi MG, Bjornson C, Coletta M, Mora M, De Angelis MG, Fiocco R, Cossu G, Vescovi AL. Skeletal myogenic potential of human and mouse neural stem cells. *Nat Neurosci* 2000 ; 3 : 986-91.
24. Wang X, Willenbring H, Akkari Y, Torimaru Y, Foster M, Al-Dhalimy M, Lagasse E, Finegold M, Olson S, Grompe M. Cell fusion is the principal source of bone-marrow-derived hepatocytes. *Nature* 2003 ; 422 : 897-901.
25. Doyonnas R, LaBarge MA, Sacco A, Charlton C, Blau HM. Hematopoietic contribution to skeletal muscle regeneration by myelomonocytic precursors. *Proc Natl Acad Sci USA* 2004 ; 101 : 13507-12.
26. Jang YY, Collector MI, Baylin SB, Diehl AM, Sharkis SJ. Hematopoietic stem cells convert into liver cells within days without fusion. *Nat Cell Biol* 2004 ; 6 : 532-9.
27. Wurmser AE, Nakashima K, Summers RG, Toni N, D'Amour KA, Lie DC, Gage FH. Cell fusion-independent differentiation of neural stem cells to the endothelial lineage. *Nature* 2004 ; 430 : 350-6.

28. Hakelien AM, Landsverk HB, Robl JM, Skalhegg BS, Collas P. Reprogramming fibroblasts to express T-cell functions using cell extracts. *Nat Biotechnol* 2002 ; 20 : 460-6.
29. Watt FM, Hogan BL. Out of Eden: stem cells and their niches. *Science* 2000 ; 287 : 1427-30.
30. Farace F, Prestoz L, Badaoui S, Guillier M, Haond C, Opolon P, Thomas JL, Zalc B, Vainchenker W, Turhan AG. Evaluation of hematopoietic potential generated by transplantation of muscle-derived stem cells in mice. *Stem Cells Dev* 2004 ; 13 : 83-92.
31. McKinney-Freeman SL, Jackson KA, Camargo FD, Ferrari G, Mavilio F, Goodell MA. Muscle-derived hematopoietic stem cells are hematopoietic in origin. *Proc Natl Acad Sci USA* 2002 ; 99 : 1341-6.
32. Odelberg SJ, Kollhoff A, Keating MT. Dedifferentiation of mammalian myotubes induced by msx1. *Cell* 2000 ; 103 : 1099-109.
33. Kondo T, Raff M. Oligodendrocyte precursor cells reprogrammed to become multipotential CNS stem cells. *Science* 2000 ; 289 : 1754-7.
34. Brawley C, Matunis E. Regeneration of male germline stem cells by spermatogonial dedifferentiation in vivo. *Science* 2004 ; 304 : 1331-4.
35. Horwitz EM, Gordon PL, Koo WK, Marx JC, Neel MD, McNall RY, Muul L, Hofmann T. Isolated allogeneic bone marrow-derived mesenchymal cells engraft and stimulate growth in children with osteogenesis imperfecta: implications for cell therapy of bone. *Proc Natl Acad Sci USA* 2002 ; 99 : 8932-7.
36. Prockop DJ, Gregory CA, Spees JL. One strategy for cell and gene therapy: harnessing the power of adult stem cells to repair tissues. *Proc Natl Acad Sci USA* 2003 ; 100 : 11917-23.
37. Liechty KW, MacKenzie TC, Shaaban AF, Radu A, Moseley AM, Deans R, Marshak DR, Flake AW. Human mesenchymal stem cells engraft and demonstrate site-specific differentiation after in utero transplantation in sheep. *Nat Med* 2000 ; 6 : 1282-6.
38. Mangi AA, Noiseux N, Kong D, He H, Rezvani M, Ingwall JS, Dzau VJ. Mesenchymal stem cells modified with Akt prevent remodeling and restore performance of infarcted hearts. *Nat Med* 2003 ; 9 : 1195-201.
39. Herrera MB, Bussolati B, Bruno S, Fonsato V, Romanazzi GM, Camussi G. Mesenchymal stem cells contribute to the renal repair of acute tubular epithelial injury. *Int J Mol Med* 2004 ; 14 : 1035-41.
40. Yokoo T, Ohashi T, Shen JS, Sakurai K, Miyazaki Y, Utsunomiya Y, Takahashi M, Terada Y, Eto Y, Kawamura T, Osumi N, Hosoya T. Human mesenchymal stem cells in rodent whole-embryo culture are reprogrammed to contribute to kidney tissues. *Proc Natl Acad Sci USA* 2005 ; 102 : 3296-300.
41. Wang G, Bunnell BA, Painter RG, Quiniones BC, Tom S, Lanson NA Jr, Spees JL, Bertucci D, Peister A, Weiss DJ, Valentine VG, Prockop DJ, Kolls JK. Adult stem cells from bone marrow stroma differentiate into airway epithelial cells: potential therapy for cystic fibrosis. *Proc Natl Acad Sci USA* 2005 ; 102 : 186-91.
42. Le Blanc K, Rasmusson I, Sundberg B, Gotherstrom C, Hassan M, Uzunel M, Ringden O. Treatment of severe acute graft-versus-host disease with third party haploidentical mesenchymal stem cells. *Lancet* 2004 ; 363 : 1439-41.
43. Fernandes KJ, McKenzie IA, Mill P, Smith KM, Akhavan M, Barnabe-Heider F, Biernaskie J, Junek A, Kobayashi NR, Toma JG, Kaplan DR, Labosky PA, Rafuse V, Hui CC, Miller FD. A dermal niche for multipotent adult skin-derived precursor cells. *Nat Cell Biol* 2004 ; 6 : 1082-93.
44. Planat-Benard V, Silvestre JS, Cousin B, Andre M, Nibbelink M, Tamarat R, Clergue M, Manneville C, Saillan-Barreau C, Duriez M, Tedgui A, Levy B, Penicaud L, Casteilla L. Plasticity of human adipose lineage cells toward endothelial cells: physiological and therapeutic perspectives. *Circulation* 2004 ; 109 : 656-63.
45. Kogler G, Sensken S, Airey JA, Trapp T, Muschen M, Feldhahn N, Liedtke S, Sorg RV, Fischer J, Rosenbaum C, Greschat S, Knipper A, Bender J, Degistirici O, Gao J, Caplan AI,

Colletti EJ, Almeida-Porada G, Muller HW, Zanjani E, Wernet P. A new human somatic stem cell from placental cord blood with intrinsic pluripotent differentiation potential. *J Exp Med* 2004 ; 200 : 123-35.

46. D'Ippolito G, Diabira S, Howard GA, Menei P, Roos BA, Schiller PC. Marrow-isolated adult multilineage inducible (MIAMI) cells, a unique population of postnatal young and old human cells with extensive expansion and differentiation potential. *J Cell Sci* 2004 ; 117 : 2971-81.
47. Rodriguez AM, Elabd C, Delteil F, Astier J, Vernochet C, Saint-Marc P, Guesnet J, Guezennec A, Amri EZ, Dani C, Ailhaud G. Adipocyte differentiation of multipotent cells established from human adipose tissue. *Biochem Biophys Res Commun* 2004 ; 315 : 255-63.
48. Blau HM, Pavlath GK, Hardeman EC, Chiu CP, Silberstein L, Webster SG, Miller SC, Webster C. Plasticity of the differentiated state. *Science* 1985 ; 230 : 758-66.
49. Wollert KC, Meyer GP, Lotz J, Ringes-Lichtenberg S, Lippolt P, Breidenbach C, Fichtner S, Korte T, Hornig B, Messinger D, Arseniev L, Hertenstein B, Ganser A, Drexler H. Intracoronary autologous bone-marrow cell transfer after myocardial infarction: the BOOST randomised controlled clinical trial. *Lancet* 2004 ; 364 : 141-8.
50. Kang HJ, Kim HS, Zhang SY, Park KW, Cho HJ, Koo BK, Kim YJ, Soo Lee D, Sohn DW, Han KS, Oh BH, Lee MM, Park YB. Effects of intracoronary infusion of peripheral blood stem-cells mobilised with granulocyte-colony stimulating factor on left ventricular systolic function and restenosis after coronary stenting in myocardial infarction: the MAGIC cell randomised clinical trial. *Lancet* 2004 ; 363 : 751-6.
51. Shintani S, Murohara T, Ikeda H, Ueno T, Sasaki K, Duan J, Imaizumi T. Therapeutic angiogenesis for patients with limb ischaemia by autologous transplantation of bone-marrow cells: a pilot study and a randomised controlled trial. *Lancet* 2002 ; 360 : 427-35.
52. Cogle CR, Yachnis AT, Laywell ED, Zander DS, Wingard JR, Steindler DA, Scott EW. Bone marrow transdifferentiation in brain after transplantation: a retrospective study. *Lancet* 2004 ; 363 : 1432-7.
53. Otani A, Dorrell MI, Kinder K, Moreno SK, Nusinowitz S, Banin E, Heckenlively J, Friedlander M. Rescue of retinal degeneration by intravitreally injected adult bone marrow-derived lineage-negative hematopoietic stem cells. *J Clin Invest* 2004 ; 114 : 765-74.
54. Hussain MA, Theise ND. Stem-cell therapy for diabetes mellitus. *Lancet* 2004 ; 364 : 203-5.
55. Hess D, Li L, Martin M, Sakano S, Hill D, Strutt B, Thyssen S, Gray DA, Bhatia M. Bone marrow-derived stem cells initiate pancreatic regeneration. *Nat Biotechnol* 2003 ; 21 : 763-70.
56. Ianus A, Holz GG, Theise ND, Hussain MA. In vivo derivation of glucose-competent pancreatic endocrine cells from bone marrow without evidence of cell fusion. *J Clin Invest* 2003 ; 111 : 843-50.
57. Choi JB, Uchino H, Azuma K, Iwashita N, Tanaka Y, Mochizuki H, Migita M, Shimada T, Kawamori R, Watada H. Little evidence of transdifferentiation of bone marrow-derived cells into pancreatic beta cells. *Diabetologia* 2003 ; 46 : 1366-74.
58. Chen S, Zhang Q, Wu X, Schultz PG, Ding S. Dedifferentiation of lineage-committed cells by a small molecule. *J Am Chem Soc* 2004 ; 126 : 410-1.
59. Jaenisch R. Human cloning – the science and ethics of nuclear transplantation. *N Engl J Med* 2004 ; 351 : 2787-91.
60. Kehat I, Khimovich L, Caspi O, Gepstein A, Shofti R, Arbel G, Huber I, Satin J, Itskovitz-Eldor J, Gepstein L. Electromechanical integration of cardiomyocytes derived from human embryonic stem cells. *Nat Biotechnol* 2004 ; 22 : 1282-9.
61. Nishida K, Yamato M, Hayashida Y, Watanabe K, Yamamoto K, Adachi E, Nagai S, Kikuchi A, Maeda N, Watanabe H, Okano T, Tano Y. Corneal reconstruction with tissue-engineered cell sheets composed of autologous oral mucosal epithelium. *N Engl J Med* 2004 ; 351 : 1187-96.

Gene Transfer: from the Laboratory to Clinical Practice

Fabienne Rolling, Michel Weber, Gilles Folléa, Philippe Moullier

What follows attempts to show the link between transfusion and cell and vector production for gene transfer, a link which is still virtual today, but will certainly gain in strength and legitimacy tomorrow.

As knowledge of the human genome advances and the molecular foundations of physiopathology are solidified, tools making it possible to enclose and transport genes become available. The transfer of a therapeutic gene has become a reality. In fact, hundreds of clinical trials are now studying a multitude of applications, from hereditary genetic diseases like hemophilia to acquired diseases like cancer.

The first gene transfer experiments were described over fifty years ago (1944), when researchers "transformed" bacteria by inserting a heterologous gene in them. About twenty years later, in 1968, virus genes were transferred into mammalian cells by using a simple salt precipitate derived from calcium phosphate, to form a gene complex that served as a rudimentary vector facilitating absorption and integration in the target cell. In 1971, the first conference on gene therapy was held in the United States; *in vitro* experiments on gene transfer to treat genetic diseases like hemoglobinopathies were described. Since then, mapping of the human gene has made exciting advances and contributes to "theoretical" opportunities for therapeutic gene transfer both in oncology and in the field of genetic diseases.

But transferring a gene into a living organism is a complicated operation that poses ever more complex problems as the process develops. For example, although fifteen years of research have finally given us effective vectors able to transport and transfer therapeutic genes to mammalians, a whole series of questions has arisen. Some of these questions are very fundamental and would require time consuming reflection… Once they become apparent. For instance, can we presume to introduce a so-called "therapeutic" gene, often by overexpressing protein (because we don't know how to control protein expression), purely on the basis that the genetic progenitors involved are not functional? Is definitive insertion of a gene from the researcher's laboratory into a person's genome really without risk, as some of us were still maintaining not long ago? Other than the evaluation of probable risk associated with insertion mutagenesis, what safety measures can we take when we introduce such material into the "genetic heritage"? What do we know about the consequences of introducing one or several copies of a "therapeutic" gene into endogenous gene expression? Because, in reality, the present state of scientific knowledge cannot accomplish substitution of a defective gene by a normal copy of the same gene, give or take one base pair. However, recent experiments seem to show that "surgical" corrections precise within a nucleotide are possible [1, 2]. Can we imagine that this type of more "physiologic" approach could be developed on a large scale in a large number of target cells?

In other words, are we on the brink of change from "rough" gene therapy with potentially devastating side effects, to a human intervention resembling the "perfect procedure"? Even if we could attain this degree of refinement in the procedure, transcriptome (intermediary gene expression product) analysis might reserve some surprises.

Moreover, does an organism genetically modified by science recognize the transgene product as "self"?

It would be reasonable to expect gene therapy to develop through long and patient research with alternating successes and setbacks, but society's relation to science is not likely to accommodate this cautious progression.

How is a Gene Transferred into a Living Organism?

Although the idea of transferring a DNA fragment into an organism to compensate or correct a failing function is easy to understand, putting it into practice has proven to be very complex. In fact, although DNA treatment has very specific characteristics and the concept of therapeutic DNA defined in 1933 [3] and again, more recently, in 2004 [4] by Axel Kahn, remains truer than ever, we must draw attention to its particularities. Fortunately for us, DNA is a very stable molecule, resistant to many physical and chemical agents, as demonstrated by the fact that today we can use PCR amplification on DNA extracted from Egyptian mummies.

It is the remarkable stability of this molecule that has enabled paleopathology to reveal the viral or zoonotic infections existing in the time of the Pharaohs. This resistance of the DNA to the ravages of time is such an exceptional property, and so legitimately noteworthy given its role in the continuity of our heritage, that British sociobiologist Richard Dawkins used it as his crucial argument for displacing, albeit excessively, Darwinian competition from the scale of the species to the scale of the gene [5]. Be that as it may, the stability of this molecule is a true advantage from the therapeutic point of view, since what could be more disturbing for a therapist than to work with a molecule whose structure changes unpredictably over time?

However, this property becomes very relative once the DNA is introduced "naked" into a living organism. The half-life of a gene injected into the circulation is so short, because of the effect exercised on it by several types of enzymes present in biological fluids, that its integrity is quickly lost and its therapeutic action becomes uncertain. This unfortunate destiny can be partly avoided by attaching the naked DNA to other chemical molecules; but even then, overall effects are still not very significant. Although some of these macromolecular complexes improve therapeutic DNA stability, they also elevate its clearance by various natural phagocytic mechanisms that are often very primitive and unstoppable (Küpffer cells, alveolar macrophages, the reticulo-endothelial system in general...).

Even if a gene were to arrive intact at the point of contact with the target cell, it still has to penetrate the cell. Different forms of endocytosis allow non specific capture and integration of this genetic material, and it has been clearly shown that exogenic DNA can be detected in the cytoplasm... but mainly in the early vesicular compartments, and then in late compartments that enclose lysosomes. In fact, there is no physical or chemical reason for a naked DNA fragment, or even for a fragment attached to "protective" chemical molecules, to escape this endosomal compartment. In 1995, Jean-Paul Behr's Illkirch team discovered that polyethylenimine (PEI) attached to therapeutic DNA enables the latter to escape from the vesicles. Although this important observation contributed to advances in the field [6], its therapeutic application *in situ* and *in vivo* is still uncertain to date.

Finally, let us imagine that part of this therapeutic DNA escapes – by necessity or by chance –lisosomal dissolution; it still has to reach the nucleus, to penetrate, to migrate in a nuclear environment suitable to its transcription – to say nothing of having or not having to be integrated – and finally, in a genetic disease therapy setting, it has to persist (and its transcription as well) in the long term… And all these pitfalls are multiplied by the number of target cells to be treated and, in some pathologies, by the number of organs involved!

These, then, are the most obvious obstacles to overcome in order to produce an effect on the phenotype after gene transfer. But from the point of view of the geneticist, the fact that exogenous DNA has such a small chance of reaching the chromatin and of lodging itself there, even temporarily, is fortunate and absolutely necessary for the survival of the species…

To explain, imagine what would happen if each time we ate cabbage its DNA could reach our chromatin in a functional form: we would really have something to worry about!

Thus, transfer of a functional gene is not a natural event, and any attempt to do this qualifies as "genetic engineering" and brings about a made-to-measure genetically modified organism.

Therefore, the first difficulty encountered by the scientific and medical community was finding an effective and reproducible method of transporting therapeutic DNA from the test tube to the heart of the target cell nucleus. Like in the film scrip written by Richard Fleischer, director of the 1966 movie "Fantastic Voyage", in which Raquel Welsh and Stephen Boyd slip into the *Proteus*, the miniature submarine that will allow the heroes (and the traitor) to travel through the body of a diplomat in a coma, molecular biologists use the virus to transport therapeutic genes. The virus cannot replicate without penetrating the cell by inserting its own genetic material in the nucleus. This parasitism is optimal because behind this relation there are millions of years of evolution and almost as much diversity. This has led to a considerable variety of viral envelopes and capsids which enrich – at least theoretically – the pharmacopeia of the therapist/geneticist. Viruses use the cell's own membrane motifs as receptors with more or less high affinity; they take advantage of cellular internalization mechanisms and, in certain cases, succeed in escaping from vesicular compartments. Viruses have also developed mechanisms that allow polymerisation of intermediary microfilaments of the cytoskeleton to actively and effectively carry their genetic material – naked or protected by the capsid – to the entrances of nuclear pores. Once there, this material is often actively transferred into the nucleus, where, usually, proteic factors of viral origin and/or nucleotidic motifs of the viral genome facilitate its migration into nuclear compartments favourable to its transcription and replication. In short, from a Darwinian point of view, selection imperatives in the viral world have always explained, and still do, that each stage of the process is probably optimal.

Certain viruses, like the adeno-associated virus, are found in the nucleus as quickly as twenty minutes after contact with the cell membrane [7]. This being so, transferring a therapeutic gene by using a viral vector means substituting the wild-type viral genome for the genome we want to see expressed in the patient. This play of substitution depends on the conservation of genetic elements of viral origin that are indispensable for maintaining certain properties, on condition that all the other properties are deleted, particularly the sequences involved in replication, and in the synthesis of the capsid and the envelope. In short, ideally, we must delete the greatest number of wild-type viral genomes possible, to make room for therapeutic

DNA cloning, but also to "inactivate" the wild type virus by depriving it of the functions usually responsible for its pathogenic effect, such as replication. This play of substitution generates recombinant viral vectors, also called "replication defective", because they cannot replicate *in vivo*. In practice, it is essential to "make room" because therapeutic DNA can be long (for example, dystrophine, CFTR...) and requires association of elements essential for its expression (promoters) and for mRNA maturation (polyadenylation signal), the whole structure being known as an "expression cassette". This maximum available capacity concept resembles, once again, the submarine *Proteus* that can only take on its "fantastic voyage" a limited number of heroes... one too many and the hatchway will not close.

In the same way, a few hundred nucleotides too many and the vector virus capsid will remain immature and therefore unable to carry optimal infection.

In the end, the final product consists of a virus whose architecture is identical to that of the wild-type virus, but whose genetic material is a recombinant product unable to support virus replication, but able to deliver a therapeutic expression cassette. This scenario achieves gene transfer after infection of the target cell, but then it fails because the transfer is not followed by replication of the viral particle. This scenario is a modern version of the Greek legend of the Trojan horse, only different in that, although the therapist/geneticist wishes to insert the therapeutic gene by tricking the cell, once inside, he wants it to remain unnoticed. We will see in the sections that follow that solving this problem, considered secondary a few years ago, has now become a "sacred quest".

Once we understand this process of replacement of a wild-type genome by a recombinant genome, it is possible to deduce that production *in vitro* of these vectors requires *trans*-expression of the wild functions initially deleted. These functions, that we do not want to transfer and to be expressed in the organism to be treated, are, nevertheless, necessary at the production stage in order to provide capsid and envelope factors, and possibly other viral factors involved in the assembly of the recombinant vector. Thus, taken to the extreme, isolated expression of these *trans* functions into a cell will lead to the creation of viral or "empty" vector particles, or virus-like particles (VLP) (that is, without encapsidated recombinant genome). If we were to introduce, into the same cells, the genome that we want the viral vector to transport, the latter will be selectively encapsidated in the viral particles if we add the nucleotidic sequence called "encapsidation" sequence of the parental virus. This encapsidation sequence is particular to each virus and is usually made up of about one hundred nucleotides; its natural function is to promote selective encapsidation of the wild-type viral genome, or of any other associated nucleotidic sequence (that is, the therapeutic gene) during virion assembly. But here again, as is often the case in biology, encapsidation is certainly not a binary process. In other words, if the presence of a nucleotidic encapsidation sequence is well cloned by contact with the therapeutic genome, the latter will be preferentially encapsidated in the vector; but what happens to cellular or plasmidic DNA or RNA whose sequences can resemble viral encapsidation signals? This question becomes even more relevant given large scale production methods of these recombinant vectors, that overexert cellular mechanisms for the sake of increased vector assembly production. This problem has only recently become evident.

What are the Rational Stages before Patient Treatment?

As is the case in the development of any pharmaceutical product, assessment in animals is an indispensable stage in the modern scientific process whose objective is to find, as much as possible, substitute methods *in vitro*. This alternative process is supported by the European Community through its research funding policies. Although our scientific community has to reflect on animal experiments even beyond strict "politically correct" requirements, the fact remains that evaluating vector-assisted gene transfer involves phenotypic correction usually in murine models, and then biodistribution and toxicity studies in large animals such as dogs and primates. This is easy to say but complicated to carry out, since it requires the coming together of many types of experts who can work jointly in a coordinated fashion.

In effect, how could we consider injecting a vector in the subretinal space or the putamen of a primate if scientists, engineers and technicians did not ensure the production of therapeutic vectors of exceptional quality? How could we perform the surgical procedure without veterinarians with expertise in anesthesia, postoperative care and pain control? How could we administer the vector to a dog or a primate in a clinically useful way if the procedure was not performed by the ophthalmologist, the neurosurgeon or a surgeon in the specialty involved? How could we carry out valid anatomical screening without the modern means of medical imagery at the disposal f the radiologist? And how could we make reliable analyses of the tissues exposed to the vector, and therefore genetically modified, if these analyses were not carried out by pathologists who can interpret murine, canine or primate tissue, and who are also familiar with recombinant vectors? The culmination of the process is a magic moment when all these actors come together to interpret results, each one bringing his particular vision to the overall process. This is when two things become clear: the importance of the principal investigator who has to create a coherent picture, and the difficulty of advancing methodically toward application in patients. Concretely, the difficulty is related to the fact that results have to be interpreted depending on the purity of the vector, its concentration, the excipient used, the speed of injection of the vector, the volume chosen, the type of needle, local or systemic administration, as well as individual variability, especially in large animals like primates (which is also what makes them valuable). Finally, there are the characteristics of the expression cassette transferred; the nature and level of expression of the therapeutic gene are generally related to the nature of the promoter chosen, as well as to sequences called enhancers which facilitate transduction, like the WPRE sequence [8]. The expression levels of the genes we introduce at present are no doubt surrealistic and certainly much too high in most cases. Frequent use of constitutive promoters of viral origin leads to overexpression (very often unnecessary) of the gene introduced.

Not so long ago (before 1996), when the speciality did not possess effective vectors, it was useful to have recourse to such powerful promoters to "compensate", as it were, the vector's lack of efficiency.

Today, availability of the adeno-associated virus (AAV) or of vectors derived from lentivirus allows long-term expression in a variety of tissues, and makes it possible to effect satisfactory phenotypic corrections in genetic diseases in mice and, more and more often, in large animals.

It has now become possible to consider the importance of expression level of the gene introduced; using the natural promoter of the therapeutic gene is the preferred choice whenever possible, because it facilitates obtaining a more physiologic protein level, as well as its restriction to the cells that normally express it. For example, expressing in the retinal epithelium the gene encoding for the RPE65 protein in Leber's congenital amaurosis (severe degenerative retinopathy) is certainly more satisfactory when the natural promoter RPE65 is chosen, rather than any other promoter, particularly if RPE65 is only slightly expressed naturally. Unfortunately, we are often forced to choose "artificial" strategies with high therapeutic synthesis levels, because vector technology is still imperfect. This is the case in clinical trials investigating hemophilia B or alpha antitrypsine (AAT) deficit, which involve transfer of the factor IX gene and of AAT respectively, into skeletal muscle. Rather than taking surgical risks by transferring the gene into the liver (natural synthesis site of the two proteins) using more complex procedures, the investigator opted for intramuscular injections, relying on the striated muscle to sustain the secretion of these therapeutic proteins. Given that the number of "transduced" (genetically modified) muscle cells remains relatively low in relation to the hepatic mass which ensures this synthesis, partial compensation can be obtained by using a powerful promoter like RSV, CMV or promoters called "chimera", which combine enhancers/promoters of different origins, often very powerful. This approach makes it possible to obtain therapeutic levels of factor IX and AAT in mice, and to treat hemophiliac dogs [9]. Phase I and II trials are now in progress for these two indications at the University of Pennsylvania (factor IX) and the University of Florida (AAT deficit).

These two examples illustrate the frequently used strategy consisting of overexpressing a therapeutic gene from a limited number of genetically modified cells. Recently, quantitative PCR assays have confirmed that *in vivo* gene transfer often produces several dozen vector copies per transduced cell. Now that viral vectors have finally become efficient tools capable of transferring genes into a variety of organs, we are discovering that we are breaking genome homeostasis. We now have to ask, for example, whether a macaque should reasonably possess 400 transgene copies per myotube after a single intramuscular injection of a recombinant AAV (Toromanoff et al. unpublished results), for a number of years. It is only common sense to admit that this imbalance is not desirable, but what practical solution can we offer? Here is where we appreciate the importance of the anatomo-pathologist, who can interpret the phenotypical corrections and the toxicity associated with vector use and with transgene expression. These conclusions have an impact on all the actors in this network, in terms of methodological choices for recombinant vector production and purification, as well as in terms of the nature of the vector chosen, the surgical technique employed, the mode of administration and the preclinical protocol. At the same time, the scientist, the engineer or the technician can suggest an innovation in the method of obtaining the vector, but this method can be judged to be inappropriate by the practitioner, who can consider, for example, that changing the excipient buffer is incompatible with the target tissue. Inversely, the practitioner can propose the use of a more concentrated viral solution, rejected by the scientist because of spontaneous precipitation in the syringe; the pathologist will support this objection, based on his own fear of a toxic effect; the immunologist will agree with them, given innate immune response and the ensuing secretion of cytokines. Finally, clinical trial results provide data that systematically revise notions of the vector and its expression cassette at all stages of the process, including production, administration and dosage. For example, introduction of the vector near an oncogen, and persistence in the vector of a functional promoter belonging to the parental virus, could be one possible reason, among others, for the three cases of leukemia that appeared among about ten children with severe immune deficit treated at the Necker Hospital in Paris. At present, studies are in progress to help us arrive at a better understanding of the conditions that led to this complication; these studies involve the entire network of specialties associated with the two principal investigators, Alain Fischer and Marina Cavazzano-Calvo. The conclusions submitted to the regulatory agencies will make it possible to conduct these trials again with a modified vector and, no doubt, other changes related to the protocol(inclusion criteria, vector concentration to use during gene transfer into hematopoietic stem cells…).

The development of gene transfer for therapeutic purposes is a process of back-and-forth communication among these actors with different but complementary training, whose common objective is to arrive at a "genetically modified patient" who has been treated. Gene therapy is not the only field that develops in this way; the same process applies to cell therapy and, in general, to the development of any therapeutic product. It takes a dozen years for an anti-inflammatory or an anti-cancer drug to reach the phase I trial stage, and biotherapies follow a similar progression, although – in response to market and media pressure – the tendency is to accelerate the process by taking shortcuts [10].

What is the Status Quo Today?

In summary, after twenty years of advances and setbacks, where does gene therapy stand in 2006? To answer this question, it might be useful to review the short history of the field. Those of us who, at the end of the 1980s, were trying to transfer a gene into a cell, had no vectors at our disposal. Chemical molecules forming complexes with DNA in order to protect the latter from the extracellular milieu were, essentially, not very effective *in vitro*, and could not effect gene transfer *in vivo*. These so-called "inert" or "chemical" vectors are still the focus of intense research, but although a certain progress has been made, they have still not shown systematic ability to produce long-term expression of a transgene in large animal models.

In the beginning, only murine retroviruses like the murine leukemia virus (MLV) and recombinant viruses were able to transfer genes *in vitro* and *in vivo*. However, MLV use requires division of the target cell in order for gene transfer to take place. This constraint limited transduction to so-called *ex vivo* protocols involving isolation of the organism from the target cells whose division is provoked *in vitro* when incubation with the MLV vector takes place. In practice, this type of approach only concerns hematopoietic stem cells, and even then there has to be a selective advantage in order to produce a possible therapeutic effect [11].

The adenovirus is effective for gene transfer *in vivo* by direct injection into a large variety of organs because, contrary to the MLV, it can infect the quiescent cell nucleus (G0) and transport the genetic material to this nucleus; this is an advantage, given that the great majority of the cells in our organs are in a quiescent state, the only exceptions being certain compartments of the hematopoietic system and, to a far lesser extent, a fraction of the digestive or respiratory epithelial cells. In addition to allowing transfer *in situ*, the adenovirus has two particularities that could constitute an advantage in oncology applications and a disadvantage in the treatment of genetic diseases. In fact, the replication cycle of most adenovirus serotypes does not depend on integration in the genome of the infected cell, implying that the vector produced cannot support long-term expression of the therapeutic gene. The other particularity of this vector is its toxicity, whose origins are diverse: they are related at once to the nature of the capsid and to the persistent expression of certain reading frames of the parental virus [12]. The result of introducing a recombinant virus into an organ is activation of the innate and adaptative (humoral and cellular) immune system, with a host of ensuing inflammatory, cytokinic and destructive reactions. In practice, these two characteristics produce, *in vivo*, peek expression of the therapeutic gene introduced between two and three weeks after vector administration, and its complete disappearance beyond that interval.

How Has Gene Therapy Evolved Historically?

In summary, after the discovery in the early 1980s that a vector could be derived from a virus [13] and that vectors could be produced in controlled conditions [14], until 1995 the scientific community used mainly the MLV vector, which was not very effective in terms of therapeutic effect, unless we worked with particular models in which very low transgene expression could produce positive visible consequences; when this was the case, transgene expression could be definitive. The archetypical example is that of lysosomal storage diseases, which were among the first to be treated with quite spectacular results in mice [15, 16].

The other vector we had was the one derived from the recombinant adenovirus. Effective but toxic, this vector did not allow long-term expression. Therefore, it was developed essentially for oncologic applications and remains a very dynamic research area for this type of clinical application. Thus, in 1995 the situation was not too promising, and an important report written by a committee presided over by Stuart. H. Orkin, M.D. (Harward Medical School) and Arno G. Motulsky, M.D. (University of Washington) recommended halting clinical trials and focusing on vector performance. This was the equivalent of recommending a return to basic principles. The following is an excerpt of the report: "While the expectations and the promise of gene therapy are great, clinical efficacy has not been definitively demonstrated at this time in any gene therapy protocol, despite anecdotal claims of successful therapy and the initiation of more than 100...approved protocols (...). Significant problems remain in all basic aspects of gene therapy. Major difficulties at the basic level include shortcomings in all current gene transfer vectors and an inadequate understanding of the biological interaction of these vectors with the host."

In 1996 a second technological breakthrough occurred. Two articles described the use of two categories of derived vectors: a non autonomous parvovirus, the AAV and a lentivirus, the HIV. In fact, the recombinant AAV had been described as early as the end of the 1980s [17] by Richard Samulski's team at the University of North Carolina; this team demonstrated in 1989 that a single injection of recombinant AAV in the striated muscle of mice is non toxic and allows expression of the transgene for the entire lifetime of the animal (almost two years) [18]. At the same time, Didier Trono's team at the Salk Institute in San Diego transformed a fearful virus – the HIV – into a vector unable to replicate but able to effectively transduct quiescent cells *in vivo*, such as nervous system cells and particularly neurons [19].

In both cases, these vectors can be injected directly *in situ* in the organ, and produce effective transduction, non toxic and stable over time. These three characteristics fulfilled in large measure the requirements that the therapeutic gene transfer community had defined as its key objectives.

Since 1996, biological data obtained on these two vectors has revealed their main characteristics. The latter seem to be complementary, at least as far as two of them are concerned, since the AAV vector is not integrated (at least not in a manner that can be detected, except in particular experimental settings [20], while the HIV-derived vector is integrated in a stable manner in the genome of the target cell. In both cases, transgene expression is permanent; the best illustration of this has been published recently by Jim Wilson's team at the University of Pennsylvania [21]; the team showed that after a single intramuscular administration of AAV encoding for expression of the erythropoietin gene (Epo) in macaques, the vector expressed the transgene for the entire duration of the follow-up, that is, for six years! Why does the AAV vector, which is not integrated, effect stable expression, while the adenovirus does not? This question is still subject to debate. Examples of long-term expression with HIV vectors have also been observed in different organs, particularly in mice, and even in complex settings like transducted human CD34+ followed for several months after engraftment in NOD/SCID mice [22].

Finally, one last point to underline is the remarkable abundance of ideas since 1996, in an effort to obtain derivatives of these two vectors and to enrich the pharmacopoeia of the genetic therapist. Today, there are about a dozen AAV vectors with different tropisms, that have been derived from the natural serotypes of the AAV. The same is true for HIV vectors, each of which can be engrafted with a variety of envelopes with different tropisms. In this case too, about a dozen of these "pseudotypes" have been studied *in vivo* [23-25].

Thus, the availability of these two categories of vectors has made it possible to obtain very significant therapeutic results. First in mice, either those with spontaneous genetic diseases or those actually man-made through transgenesis ("transgenic mice"). Thus, in less than five years we were able to treat a hemophiliac mouse, a mouse with myopathy, a mouse with lysosomal storage or a mouse with degenerative retinopathy..., simply by injecting, one time only, a few microliters of vector suspension in the liver, a muscle, the retina or the brain. These are tangible results, involving several genetic disorders (but far from all), and they confirm that the gene transfer principle can produce long-term therapeutic effects in an organism as complex as a mouse.

Since the beginning of the current decade, there have been more and more attempts to transfer these results to larger animals. Before 1996, it would have been unimaginable to systematically conduct such experiments, and even less for them to be successful [26].

Today, genetic diseases in dogs are treated, some with spectacular phenotypic correction. This is the case for hemophilia B [9, 27, 28], for Leber's congenital amaurosis, retinal dystrophy [29, 30], affections of the hematopoietic system [31-33] and glucose-6-phosphatase deficit [34]. Primates are used in biodistribution and viral preparation toxicity studies [35-41], but also in the evaluation of gene transfer in induced models, most often for central nervous system diseases. Here too, AAV vectors and lentiviruses produce significant results that are obtained more and more often [42-45].

This overview illustrates how the "center of gravity" of gene therapy has shifted from vector design (1985-1996), to treatment of genetic murine models (1996-2000), to the first tangible results in large animals (since 2000). This progress is now accompanied by a few very encouraging examples in patients such as those suffering from x-linked severe combined inmmune deficit [46] or from chronic septic granulomatosis, another x-linked disorder (Manuel Grez, Francfort, clinical trial in progress, unpublished), although there are adverse effects which raise the problem of risk/benefit assessment. In this context, it is reasonable to foresee that this recent availability of effective gene transfer vectors compatible with clinical use will start to impose this assessment more and more. In addition to the question of vector integration – whether the vector is of MLV or HIV origin, a question only recently examined in a relevant manner [47], at least two other questions remain important now that we can really transfer therapeutic genes *in vivo* effectively:

– What are the consequences of expression of a "new" gene on the physiology of the organ?

– Is a therapeutic protein newly expressed in an individual recognized as non self?

Having to ask these questions points out the need for the speciality to continue its development and progress through the search for the physiological mechanisms involved, beyond the simple transfer of an expression cassette. This demonstrates once again the continuous exchange between the scientist who produces the vector and the "carried" material, and the practitioner responsible for the clinical trial. But since the short history of gene therapy clearly shows that legitimately the path we are following leads to clinical trials, it seems reasonable and strategically justified to foresee technological procedures able to provide the medical hospital milieu with vectors for clinical use. Paving the way to such procedures will take time because the regulations governing the production of a recombinant viral vector for clinical use are complex, with few precedents, and extremely demanding when they concern a product intended for administration to patients. This brings the regulatory agencies into the back-and-forth exchange mentioned above, not as partners but as independent observers and regulators. To illustrate, on January 24, 2005, the regulatory agency reacted to a third case of T-lymphocyte proliferation in the DICS X children's trial by issuing a press release whose conclusion stated: "Studies are now under way to type this lymphoproliferation. Based on this information, the decision to halt the trial again has been made by the investigators and the sponsor, in agreement with the regulatory agencies, while awaiting the results of investigations in progress."

But what Does Gene Therapy Have to Do with the Future of Transfusion Medicine? Where is the Common Ground?

Production of recombinant viral vectors uses the cell as its starting material. The cell is, in fact, the essential ingredient, since it is at the origin of vector assembly. Depending on the source virus, encapsidation of the therapeutic gene and maturation of the vector capsid will occur in the nucleus (AAV, adenovirus) or in the cytoplasm, and sometimes beyond, in the supernatant (MLV, HIV). Culture conditions are also critical for these cells, in order to obtain optimal performance as well as reproducible production. The possibility of using bioreactors is clearly an advantage, and control of expansion quality and of cell performance represent a unique know-how indispensable to the emergence of these technological systems. Other aspects, just as critical, concern vector purification and quality assurance of clinical lots according to exact specifications. Finally, the concept of bioproduction has to be integrated in an overall quality procedure. The same is true for working in a controlled and confined environment. Bringing together these different types of cellular engineering expertise is, naturally, at the heart of transfusion medicine. Therefore, it seems judicious for the domain of blood transfusion to foresee future changes, particularly in the area of biotherapies. Although common sense, or pragmatism, tells us that cell and gene therapy cannot constitute our only basis for development, not taking this therapy into account would be a fundamental strategic error. We must not, of course, see biotherapies as the answer to all our hopes for regenerative medicine in the near future, particularly in respect to diseases for which we have no effective solutions at present. But we would be wise to develop the needed technology, as the specialty advances step by step. The most desirable way to achieve this is for transfusion medicine to work in partnership with hospital/university Centers, the National Research Institute and patient associations, and to invest collectively in the field of productive or regenerative cells, particularly since other, equally expensive, fields such as nanotechnology will become part of the therapeutic and analytic arsenal at our disposal in this new century.

Of course, mastery of the collected and controlled cell remains the focus of transfusion medicine. But scientific indicators are making it clear that biotherapies will gradually become legitimate complementary treatments – as shown by the fact that hematopoietic stem cell transplantation has already opened the way decades ago. It will take time, and perhaps a very long time, for gene therapy to become one of the common tools of the hospital practitioner. But transfusion medicine must show strategic foresight worthy of the promise of this specialty.

References

1. Kren B T, et al. Correction of the UDP-glucuronosyltransferase gene defect in the gunn rat model of crigler-najjar syndrome type I with a chimeric oligonucleotide. *Proc Natl Acad Sci USA* 1999 ; 96: 10349-54.
2. Liu C M, Liu D P, Liang C C. Oligonucleotide-mediated gene repair at DNA level: the potential applications for gene therapy. *J Mol Med* 2002 ; 80: 620-8.
3. Kahn A, *Thérapie Génique: l'ADN médicament*. Paris: John Libbey Eurotext, 1996.
4. Kahn A. *Et l'homme dans tout cela. Plaidoyer pour un homme moderne*. Paris: Nil Editions, 2000.
5. Dawkins R. *The Selfish Gene, 2nd Ed.* Oxford University Press, 1989.
6. Boussif O, et al. A versatile vector for gene and oligonucleotide transfer into cells in culture and in vivo: polyethylenimine. *Proc Natl Acad Sci USA* 1995 ; 92: 7297-301.
7. Seisenberger G, et al. Real-time single-molecule imaging of the infection pathway of an adeno-associated virus. *Science* 2001 ; 294: 1929-32.
8. Zufferey R, Donello J, Trono D, Hope T. Woodchuck hepatitis virus posttranscriptional regulatory element enhances expression of transgenes delivered by retroviral vectors. *J Virol* 1999 ; 73: 2886-92.
9. Arruda V R, et al. Safety and efficacy of factor IX gene transfer to skeletal muscle in murine and canine hemophilia B models by adeno-associated viral vector serotype 1. *Blood* 2004 ; 103: 85-92.
10. Magnan M, Moullier P. *La Génétique, Science Humaine*. Paris : Éditions Belin, 2004.
11. Fischer A, et al. Severe combined immunodeficiency. A model disease for molecular immunology and therapy. *Immunol Rev* 2005 ; 203: 98-109.
12. Chuah M K, Collen D, VandenDriessche T. Biosafety of adenoviral vectors. *Curr Gene Ther* 2003 ; 3: 527-43.
13. Gilboa E, Kolbe M, Noonan K, Kucherlapati R. Construction of a mammalian transducing vector from the genome of Moloney murine leukemia virus. *J Virol* 1982 ; 44: 845-51.
14. Danos O, Mulligan R C. Safe and efficient generation of recombinant retroviruses with amphotropic and ecotropic host ranges. *Proc Natl Acad Sci USA* 1988; 85: 6460-4.
15. Moullier P, Bohl D, Heard J M, Danos O. Correction of lysosomal storage in the liver and spleen of genetically-modified skin fibroblasts. *Nature Genet* 1993 ; 4: 154-9.
16. Maréchal V, Naffakh N, Danos O, Heard J M. Disappearance of lysosomal storage in spleen and liver of mucopolysaccharidosis VII mice after transplantation of genetically-modified bone marrow cells. *Blood* 1993 ; 82: 1358-65.
17. Samulski R J, Chang L S, Shenk T. Helper-free stocks of recombinant adeno-associated viruses: normal integration does not require viral gene expression. *J Virol* 1989 ; 63: 3822-8.
18. Xiao X, Li J, Samulski R J. Efficient long-term gene transfer into muscle tissue of immunocompetent mice by adeno-associated virus vector. *J Virol* 1996 ; 70: 8098-108.
19. Naldini L, et al. In vivo gene delivery and stable transduction of non-dividing cells by a lentiviral vector. *Science* 1996 ; 272: 263-7.
20. Nakai H, et al. AAV serotype 2 vectors preferentially integrate into active genes in mice. *Nat Genet* 2003 ; 1: 1-6.
21. Rivera A, Ferreira A, Bertoni D, Romero J R, Brugnara C. Abnormal regulation of Mg2+ transport via Na/Mg exchanger in sickle erythrocytes. *Blood* 2004 ; 105: 382-6.
22. Miyoshi H, Smith K A, Mosier D E, Verma I M, Torbett B E. Transduction of human CD34+ cells that mediate long-term engraftment of NOD/SCID mice by HIV vectors. *Science* 1999 ; 283: 682-6.
23. Duisit G, et al. Five recombinant simian immunodeficiency virus (SIV) pseudotypes lead to exclusive transduction of retinal pigmented epithelium in rat. *Mol Ther* 2002 ; 6: 446-54.

24. Strang BL, Ikeda Y, Cosset FL, Collins MK, Takeuchi Y. Characterization of HIV-1 vectors with gammaretrovirus envelope glycoproteins produced from stable packaging cells. *Gene Ther* 2004 ; 11: 591-8.
25. Watson D J, Kobinger G P, Passini M A, Wilson J M, Wolfe J H. Targeted transduction patterns in the mouse brain by lentivirus vectors pseudotyped with VSV, Ebola, Mokola, LCMV, or MuLV envelope proteins. *Mol Ther* 2002 ; 5: 528-37.
26. Cardoso J E, et al. In situ retrovirus-mediated gene transfer into dog liver. *Hum Gene Ther* 1993 ; 4: 411-8.
27. Wang L, Nichols T C, Read M S, Bellinger D A, Verma I M. Sustained expression of therapeutic level of factor IX in hemophilia B dogs by AAV-mediated gene therapy in liver. *Mol Ther* 2000 ; 1: 154-8.
28. Wang L, et al. Sustained correction of disease in naive and AAV2-pretreated hemophilia B dogs: AAV2/8 mediated, liver-directed gene therapy. *Blood* 2005 ; 6: 6.
29. Acland G M, et al. Gene therapy restores vision in a canine model of childhood blindness. *Nat Genet* 2001 ; 28: 92-5.
30. Narfstrom K, et al. Functional and structural recovery of the retina after gene therapy in the RPE65 null mutation dog. *Invest Ophthalmol Vis Sci* 2003 ; 44: 1663-72.
31. Horn P A, Morris J C, Neff T Kiem H P. Stem cell gene transfer-efficacy and safety in large animal studies. *Mol Ther* 2004 ; 10: 417-31.
32. Neff T, et al. Methylguanine methyltransferase-mediated in vivo selection and chemoprotection of allogeneic stem cells in a large-animal model. *J Clin Invest* 2003 ; 112: 1581-8.
33. Yanay O, et al. Treatment of canine cyclic neutropenia by lentivirus-mediated G-CSF delivery. *Blood* 2003 ; 102: 2046-52.
34. Beaty R M, et al. Delivery of glucose-6-phosphatase in a canine model for glycogen storage disease, type Ia, with adeno-associated virus (AAV) vectors. *Gene Ther* 2002 ; 9: 1015-22.
35. Bennett J, et al. Stable transgene expression in rod photoreceptors after recombinant adeno-associated virus-mediated gene transfer to monkey retina. *Proc Natl Acad Sci USA* 1999 ; 96: 9920-5.
36. Chirmule N, et al. Humoral immunity to adeno-associated virus type 2 vectors following administration to murine and nonhuman primate muscle [In Process Citation]. *J Virol* 2000 ; 74: 2420-5.
37. Favre D, et al. Immediate and long-term safety of recombinant adeno-associated virus injection into the non-human primate muscle. *Mol Ther* 2001 ; 4: 559-66.
38. Weber M, et al. Recombinant adeno-associated virus serotype 4 mediates unique and exclusive long-term transduction of retinal pigmented epithelium in rat, dog, and non-human primate after subretinal delivery. *Mol Ther* 2003 ; 7: 774-81.
39. Provost NLM, Weber G, Mendes-Madeira M, Podevin A, Cherel G, Colle Y, Deschamps MA, Moullier JY, Rolling P. Biodistribution of rAAV vectors following intraocular administration: evidence for the presence and persistence of vector DNA in the optic nerve and in the brain *Mol Ther* 2005 ; 11: 275-83.
40. Song S, et al. Intramuscular administration of recombinant adeno-associated virus 2 alpha-1 antitrypsin (rAAV-SERPINA1) vectors in a nonhuman primate model: safety and immunologic aspects. *Mol Ther* 2002 ; 6: 329.
41. Nathwani A C, et al. Sustained high-level expression of human factor IX (hFIX) after liver-targeted delivery of recombinant adeno-associated virus encoding the hFIX gene in rhesus macaques. *Blood* 2002 ; 100: 1662-9.
42. Palfi S, et al. Lentivirally delivered glial cell line-derived neurotrophic factor increases the number of striatal dopaminergic neurons in primate models of nigrostriatal degeneration. *J Neurosci* 2002 ; 22: 4942-54.
43. Kordower J H, et al. Neurodegeneration prevented by lentiviral vector delivery of GDNF in primate models of Parkinson's disease. *Science* 2000 ; 290: 767-73.

44. An D S, *et al*. Lentivirus vector-mediated hematopoietic stem cell gene transfer of common gamma-chain cytokine receptor in rhesus macaques. *J Virol* 2001 ; 75: 3547-55.
45. Fischer A C, *et al*. Successful transgene expression with serial doses of aerosolized rAAV2 vectors in rhesus macaques. *Mol Ther* 2003 ; 8: 918-26.
46. Cavazzana-Calvo M, Fischer A. Efficacy of gene therapy for SCID is being confirmed. *Lancet* 2004 ; 364: 2155-6.
47. Fischer A, Cavazzana-Calvo M. Integration of retroviruses: a fine balance between efficiency and danger. *PLoS Med* 2005 ; 2: 10.

The Ethics of Donation:
an Established or an Evolving Practice?

Didier Sicard

In our country, the term "ethical donation" stands for a concept we take for granted. This concept, founded on the three-fold requirement of a "voluntary, anonymous and free" donation, regards as diabolical all importing of blood from foreign countries, that could be even minimally commercialized or make the object of a financial transaction. Thanks to its anonymous generosity, blood donation represents the paradigm of medical ethics.

In fact, blood donation was at the origin of the principle that the human body and its products cannot be considered property, a principle that imposed non commercialization of the body, an imperative formalized by the so-called bioethics laws of 1994, reconfirmed in 2004. Blood donation has long been considered – and still is – a major example of the functioning of an ideal society, because of the notions associated with it: generosity, solidarity, brotherhood, in short, participation in a common human adventure. Not surprisingly, these ideals emerged in France immediately after the Second World War, to mark the rebirth of the country through a renewal of values: blood donation as unifying symbol, representing a common vision, and part of the ideas supported by the "progressive" tendencies of the country.

The Concept of the Voluntary

The anonymous character of blood donations has never been problematic, and the only exceptions to it are donations for a family member. The same cannot be said for the voluntary nature of donations, which was more contested and more often brought into question than is generally believed. In the first few years, two systems existed side by side: one rewarded by "restaurant tickets" and small gifts, the other standing firmly for totally free donations. This point of view was defended by the first associations of regular, volunteer blood donors. These two adjectives, "regular" and "volunteer", clearly indicate commitment as opposed to opportunistic or chance donation, with no real understanding of its significance.

It was this second vision of the "voluntary" that won out. Encoded for the first time in the July 21, 1952 Decree, it guaranteed the "medical and non profit character" of blood transfusion and, implicitly, of voluntary donations. This vision was the focus of blood donation campaigns that allowed developments in surgery and transfusion medicine, as well as the first successful exanguinotransfusions. For example, heart surgery, that requires impressive quantities of blood, stopped being an exceptional feat and became routine practice. In other fields, however, this type of routine has become irresponsible through excessive use (transfusion as a "tonic"!). In the face of growing needs, ensuring donor loyalty became essential for transfusion centers. But how to ensure this loyalty? What was the best way to obtain a regular input of blood, so that practitioners prescribing transfusions, not always aware of supply problems, would not find themselves in dangerous situations of inadequate supply? One answer was to grant donors special status, to glorify them, to make them stand out as good citizens. Donor associations took advantage of this image to acquire greater and greater power, particularly in the political arena. How could politicians refuse the requests of virtuous citizens held up as models? More and more blood was needed. Only donor associations could organize efficient campaigns. Transfusion centers were permanently endebted, trapped in the middle between the growing needs of physicians and the autonomy of donors. Gradually, some ambiguities appeared in business firms: half-days and even whole working days off were granted to donors, they were treated as heroes, given medals and commemorative celebrations, little gifts and banquets where each participant, regardless of his social or political affiliation, identified with all the others: all of them altruistic human beings united by their common involvement in a great cause. The blood donor was seen as committed. A thousand, ten thousand blood donors together are impressive and reinforce this image. Ministers and politicians are intimidated. Transfusion centers are dependent.

A Free Donation

The worthiness attached to blood donation goes beyond its usefulness. This donation became a symbol of brotherhood, of civic values, as well as of good health. The disappointment, and even aggression provoked by refusal of a donor at a transfusion center clearly indicate the sense of public humiliation felt by those who were excluded.

In this context, all the elements were in place for catastrophic events to occur in the 1980s. It was at that time that the HIV infection epidemic started to spread. Blood consumption was at its height, demand was considerable. Mobile transfusion units were set up in cities and in villages all over the country. Blood donation had such a positive image that some donors, "new donors", not those who give blood regularly, wanted to benefit from it and to participate at least once. In fact, the most marginalized persons were the most likely to be attracted to this strongly symbolic, image-enhancing action. The homosexual community, still vulnerable at that time, became very generous and protested strongly when it was excluded as soon as the first signs of possible transfusion-related risk appeared, and the national media picked up the community's claim of unjust discrimination. Drug addicts gave blood to prove that they were not addicts. Prisons opened their doors and provided great quantities of blood that was easy to obtain, renewable and encouraged in the name of possible redemption. Moreover, some subjects, worried about possibly having an infection, were asking transfusion centers to test them for their infection because they could not obtain these tests elsewhere. Unfortunately, we did not yet know, during this initial period of spread of the epidemic, that a subject who has just been infected and who is still seronegative for several weeks is more contagious than ever. It is precisely during this period before antibodies appear that the viral charge is highest.

Safety Requirements

Thus, on the one hand there was the donation as a civic value, and on the other there were those, most envious of this image, who wanted it for themselves, disregarding safety and indifferent to the fate of recipients.* Given that safety concerns had long been focusing on syphilis and hepatitis B, donors were screened mainly based on medical and biochemistry data, rather than on risk of transmission of viral infection to recipients. The 1980 International Code of Ethics governing blood donation insists almost exclusively on donor rights and protection, and only speaks of the recipient in relation to immunisation risk.

Despite the 1983 circular issued by the Ministry of Health, recommending greater vigilance in the choice of donors, the questionnaires given to prospective donors were not very rigorous.

Questions on intimate relations were considered shocking for regular, generous donors, who are certainly less at risk than new donors. These questions that could make them embarrassed and ill at ease are therefore avoided in the name of a certain respect for dignity, so as not to discourage donors. Convivial relations replace expertise, demand takes precedence over critical assessment of the offer.

Clearly, generosity by itself has never been a safety factor. We would do well to reflect on the responsibility of a fragile system in which everything depended on a good will that became a factor of leverage. "Ethical" values of volunteer spirit and generosity were turned into unquestioned power and became the source of a very harmful situation for patients.

Recognition for oneself is not an ethical value; responsibility toward others is. Altruism cannot be the final objective of blood donation. This donation must be constantly re-evaluated in terms of its fundamental character.

Thus, although not commercializing blood remains an ethical value, we need to look at the problem in a larger perspective. Generosity cannot be rewarded by excessive social recognition. This is where the difficulty lies. It can be challenging to solicit altruism by organizing "blood donation days" without creating unduly rewarding visibility. Allowing donor associations, whose members are, by definition, generous, to participate in the efficient organization of donation events should not grant them power in municipal or regional affairs.

A Question of Ethics

This question of the "free donation" (a strangely redundant expression) has long hindered the application of the European Directive of June 14, 1989, which placed stable blood products in the category of products considered medicinal for purposes of marketing authorization. For a product of the human body to be treated like any other product on competitive markets poses a problem of conscience. In the context of a public institution, consent for marketing authorization is conceivable, but on a free market, private or involving shareholders, the donors' sense of "ethics" tends to sound the alarm in this situation seen as a derailment.

But the raw material, blood, does not carry much weight compared to the engineering that becomes more and more necessary to product safety, and that is responsible for the high

---

*This is in no way intended to unjustly condemn volunteer blood donor associations, without whom transfusion possibilities would have been compromised, and who deserve the greatest recognition. Our intention is to underline the power of the image that could attract less scrupulous donors, or donors ignorant of the consequences of their acts. Scientists aggravated the problem by being more concerned with immunological questions than with transmission of infectious diseases.

costs of administering the system. This is why the volunteer nature of blood donation does not stop commercialization of the products derived from it. It could, however, contribute to its safety. For example, the French Fractionation Laboratory does not acquire blood products that have been involved in a commercial transaction. The question of ethics is then displaced and becomes a matter of commercial label.

The issue of non commercialization involves much more than blood products. It also concerns cell therapies, stem cells, gametes and even organ donation. It seems unacceptable for a society to pay donors of such products, although in many parts of the world such remuneration is practiced. Perhaps we will one day openly offer compensation for temporary or permanent injury, in order to avoid a criminal market, particularly prejudicial to poor countries. Ethics are not a matter of waving the flag of trampled principles. It is a matter of acknowledging a debt toward donors, a debt that could someday translate into financial compensation that takes into account possible injury, and that is not clandestine.

Ethical problems can occur in the process of questioning donors. The homosexual community (if indeed it is a community!?) justifiably objected to the exclusion of homosexual donors on the basis of their sexual orientation. Homosexuality is not an automatic exclusion criterion, or if it is, it constitutes *a priori* discrimination disrespectful of sexual difference. However, the homosexual candidate does not have an absolute right to be recruited as a donor. It is the responsibility of the professionals collecting the blood to ensure that the donor does not constitute a danger due to his life style or his risk-taking behavior.

A heterosexual can be a thousand times more dangerous than a homosexual. Nevertheless, the HIV infection that affected homosexuals particularly justifies great caution and vigilance in the questioning of blood donors concerning their sexual behavior. Some countries like the United States chose to confront donors with an ethical responsibility – rather than a penal threat – by asking them to sign a declaration stating that they have answered the questions truthfully and in good faith. This has never been accepted in France.

Informing Recipients

It is very strange that transfusion, once the paradigm of medical ethics, should have become the paradigm of medical risk! Although it is clearly legitimate that a patient be informed in advance of the risks involved in a medical procedure or treatment, the administrative and medical pressure created in the wake of the 1985 events encouraged exhaustive information that can be anxiety provoking. The height of anxiety was probably reached with Creutzfeldt-Jakob disease. It is in fact possible that prionic infection can be transmitted through the blood. After many methodological problems, the prion was discovered to carry infection through the blood in animals. Some British observations reported infection by the new Creutzfeldt-Jakob variant in persons having received blood a few years before the donor showed any signs of such infection. In this situation, ethical considerations are divided between the obligation to inform, transparency, the right of persons to manage their future accordingly, the right of medicine to be informed of the possible risk associated with the person awaiting specific symptoms, and respect for this person who has no choice but to anxiously wait for the possible manifestation of a clinical symptom. Information should make sense, that is, it should be useful, effective, it should help to arrive at preventive or therapeutic solutions. In the case of Creutzfeldt-Jakob disease, none of these possibilities exist, and we can justifiably ask ourselves if the obligation to inform, advocated by some, does not serve primarily to protect doctors and institutions rather than patients. Although it is clear that rigorous traceability is essential, it is not at all clear that individuals can deal with hearing that they were transfused with blood from a person with this disease, given that at present we are totally ignorant of the real risk, which is probably marginal.

Safety Measures

Today, no product is safer than blood, and yet no product frightens patients more...Each year, security measures increase: leukodepletion, nanofiltration, viral PCR (HIV, hepatitis C, hepatitis B), exclusion of transfused persons from blood donation, exclusion of persons having lived in England before 1997, etc. Yet, safety is still limited by the donor/recipient immunological conflict, that remains one of the rare human error factors when accidents occur. Increasing safety is an endless process that makes blood products more and more expensive and limits their use to more and more serious situations. When in doubt, the tendency is to abstain from transfusion rather than to transfuse; this can sometimes have negative consequences, as some recent incidents have shown.

Of course, ethics recommends concern with safety, but not unreasonable concern.

Refusal of Transfusion

Certain communities refuse transfusion as a matter of principle, no matter what the need is. This refusal is based on a literal reading of the Bible, which warns against the consumption of blood... When this refusal is expressed by a patient in serious danger, the doctor is often forced to respond either by excessive constraint or by casual assent. A recent law that entered into force in 2002 concerns the patient's rights and grants this refusal great legitimacy, making it difficult for the doctor to offer serious opposition. Of course, when the patient is a minor, the public authority can justifiably intervene, in an emergency, to allow transfusion. But when the patient is an adult, religious beliefs can take priority over the call for help and the need to be saved. This is why any medical intervention should be practiced with great caution. It is inconceivable to consider the patient as dependent on his community, and equally inconceivable to disregard his affiliation with this community. Rather than act based on medico-legal considerations or based on fear of legal repercussions, it is better to try to act with subtlety and gentleness to convince a pregnant woman with delivery hemorrhage, or a person with a hematologic disease, of the temporary need for transfusion. If consent is obtained, the patient's decision must be treated with strict confidentiality, in order to safeguard his relation with his community.

In any case, refusal of a transfusion must always be taken seriously, no matter what the consequences. The essential difficulty is proper evaluation of the true intention and competence of the person who refuses. This is where the fundamental ethical question lies.

Conclusion

Applying the precautionary principle in the field of transfusion in no way dispenses us of any of our responsibilities. This principle should not be used as legal protection, but as the basis for constant exchanges between science, man and a society where collective reflection and lucid discernment are encouraged. It is the role of the humanities to question biological sciences, in order to prevent the latter from being erected into a monument that precludes further reflection.

Bibliography

- Sicard D. Evolutions éthiques de la transfusion sanguine. *Hématologie* 2001 ; 7 : 272-5.
- Sicard D. Principe de précaution et transfusion sanguine. *Transf Clin Biol* 2000 ; 7 : 219.
- Keown J. The gift of blood in Europe : an ethical defence of EC directive 89/381. *J Med Ethics* 1997 ; 23 : 96-100.
- McLachlan HV. The unpaid donation of blood and altruism : a comment on Keown. *J Med Ethics* 1998 ; 24 : 252-4.
- Keown J. A reply to McLachlan. *J Med Ethics* 1998 ; 24 : 255-6.
- Avis n° 85 du CCNE. « L'information à propos du risque de transmission sanguine de la maladie de Creutzfeldt-Jakob ».

New Fields of Expertise: what Priorities for Tomorrow?

Bernard Cuneo, Philippe de Micco

Today, blood transfusion is at a crossroads. Medical and scientific knowledge have become part of its scope long ago, as have available technologies. Transfusion medicine is now an open and diversified practice at the service of patients. The quality of its know-how, its expertise in production processes, and the great number of scientific projects in which it participates reinforce its involvement in decisions and activities that go beyond the actual scope of supplying labile blood products, whether based on its own initiatives or in response to demand. This evolution can be observed all over the world.

In France, this evolution is particularly evident. "French-style" blood transfusion has given rise to transfusion medicine, whose priority is to satisfy self-sufficiency requirements first, as well as to ensure quality and safety of labile blood product collection, manufacturing and distribution, pertaining to its own field of responsibility, as well as to the many activities of related fields and to research activities, based on the knowledge and expertise it has accumulated in the study and processing of blood cells and bone marrow.

The existence of this large perimeter is an indication of the interactions that will shape transfusion medicine in the next few years. These interactions will require new skills, new production equipment and optimization of collective effort, that is, of the ability of different teams to produce knowledge and shared action whose quality and efficiency are greater than individual results could be. This is certainly one of the main challenges facing us today. All these interactions and innovations can only develop successfully if management of human resources in the field of transfusion facilitates it. The French example is useful for identifying needs, as well as for pointing out some areas to work on in terms of training, knowledge acquisition, professional profiles and cooperation both within the transfusion sector and with the external environment.

Human Resources and Transfusion Activities

Inevitable Professional Developments

Now that different transfusion activities have attained a certain level of quality and of technical and organizational maturity, in order to continue to develop they will have to be able to improve their production processes and, sometimes, the organization of work, by transforming or renewing personnel competence.

- In terms of **collection**, the main change will concern the pre-donation interview, traditionally conducted, in France, by a doctor. Although, over the last few years, studies in the field have confirmed that the presence of a doctor at the collection site is still important to donors, it is inevitable that the roles of doctors and nurses will evolve, for two reasons.

First, procedures are now sufficiently subjected to norms that interpretation and diagnosis of a situation can be performed by a state-certified nurse, while the doctor can play the role of "blood transfusion epidemiologist" or manager of the link between collection pools and blood product needs. It is possible that entrusting interviews to paramedical personnel will contribute to standardization (and therefore to quality and reproducible results), because this personnel tends to follow precise procedures more rigorously.

Second, these developments constitute a positive step toward professional evolution for both these professional groups, whose roles are perceived by the most aware among them to be at a relative standstill. We now have to define the methods of selection and training of nurses considered able to carry out this new function, and to establish for both doctors and nurses the corresponding changes in status and qualification.

- In terms of **the biological qualification of donations**, an activity increasingly linked with technological processes and tools, its evolution will lead to considerable need for engineers and/or technicians to handle equipment maintenance and design, as well as the corresponding evaluations. In transfusion medicine, the abnormal result is the exception. Here too, there will be less and less room for interpretation. When an automated production line functions normally, biologists only have to intervene exceptionally. Interpretation software, based on precise algorithms, does the rest in most cases. Because manufacturers send their own engineers to the installation site, what we need in transfusion medicine is an interface, that is, someone who can discuss the equipment with the engineers.

This being the case, the doctor or the pharmacist/biologist will become the resource person able to provide general information regarding the functioning and development of the technological platform.

- In terms of **processing**, we foresee the development of an industrial-type process. At present, our process at this stage of production is still small-scale. Developments will be major, particularly through reduction of processing steps and increase of control steps (see chapter by Georges Andreu). Recourse to new technologies (for instance, follow-up by means of an electronic chip) will not solve all problems at once. Gradually, the personnel will have to become familiar with new tools, as well as with a new role implicit in their participation in the new production system. It will take time to build and to instil the new mentality without which no new work process can be implemented.

- In terms of **immuno-hematology and distribution**, their respective roles and the need for a close link between them will undergo two major changes. First, introduction of artificial intelligence systems will optimize allocation decisions, not by deciding in the place of the prescribing physician or by replacing the transfusion council, but by providing it with organized data appropriate for decision-making. At the same time, management at a distance of distribution centers could be implemented thanks to automated controls that can be connected to video systems. Second, within the scope of an "enlarged" transfusion council, cooperation between the French National Blood Service (Etablissement Français du Sang : EFS) and health institutions should improve and develop, for the benefit of patients. This cooperation will have to take place on a permanent and regular basis, inevitably leading to better results.

In order to achieve this objective, transfusion medicine must plan and organize the time dedicated by its personnel (doctors, biologists, nurses…) to this interchange, and must enrich their training by providing them with complementary types of knowledge, in order for the level of expertise to constitute a solid basis for closer cooperation between the EFS and health institutions. Unless this is done, the pressing need for such cooperation will remain unrealistic and therefore unrealized (as is often the case for cooperation between different hospital departments). One solution could be for the EFS to institute, under the supervision of its educational council, a sort of "upper level immuno-hematology program" within its continued medical and professional university training program currently under development.

Key Points

Beyond the specific elements related to different activities, we can distinguish several key points characterizing the overall human resources perspective in transfusion medicine activities.

For a long time, transfusion medicine could have been considered a labour-type activity, that is, a field in which often under-qualified persons were hired to carry out activities for which they became trained on the job, as they were entrusted with increasingly more complex tasks, often surpassing the original job description. But despite its concrete reality, this over-qualification did not receive any recognition outside the immediate work environment in which it functioned. In fact, the professional advancement of some of these self-taught employees is now at a standstill, and they will find it difficult to revise the content and meaning of their work, given that often they do not wish to do so because, rightly or wrongly, they have convinced themselves that they are unable to. For these employees, like for those who feel that they are wasting quality initial training by performing repetitive tasks (like certain physicians assigned to collection), and that it is too late, it could be best to stress career advancement benefits to justify a change of position not necessarily connected to higher qualification.

For employees ready to move ahead, the main challenge will be to find their appropriate place, despite the growing role of machines, computer technologies and automation. Traditionally, they initially experience this upheaval in the work environment as "being replaced", but the transition can be successfully managed provided the reasons and the need for the ongoing changes are continually explained, provided leadership responsibilities are not assigned before the persons involved feel ready to handle the technical process (the "machines"), provided these employees are eventually entrusted with control of this process or with continued improvement, provided it is possible to compensate for the "virtual" effect associated with automation and with computer systems that create distance between the worker and the product of his own actions (abstraction), and provided it is possible to concretely and physically repossess the ongoing work [1].

In addition, interface and mediation activities, as well as activities aimed at establishing relations between the different actors in the transfusion system, and between this system and its environment, will become more numerous. But because transfusion medicine has been operating alone until now, having been relatively marginalized within the health system, the personnel, including some managerial staff, will find it difficult to hold these positions or to work smoothly with those who occupy them. Therefore, it will be necessary to train all the personnel to perform these tasks and professional functions in the field of transfusion, although these functions will not always constitute distinct positions, but will enlarge the scope of the employees' work. As for those who will hold actual expert positions, needed within the field or in order to ensure contact with external experts (such as biomedical engineers in hospitals), the structure of the EFS will have to include high-level positions (with corresponding qualification and remuneration) that will not necessarily correspond to managerial or hierarchical functions (the double ladder Anglo-Saxon business system).

Human Resources and New Developments

In addition to traditional transfusion activities, transfusion medicine will also develop its skills by applying them in a wider field, by creating activities for independent applications, and by benefiting from the consequences of these new developments. These developments, already undertaken, function on a larger scale and are part of projects specifically oriented toward future goals. Their consequences and requirements in terms of human resources will be of four types.

Cell Engineering: a Partnership Model

This activity involves, on the one hand, *in vitro* erythrocyte production by hematopoietic stem cell culture, and on the other hand, tissue reproduction – processes that require skills and techniques possessed by transfusion specialists, and particularly by the EFS, ever since they have acquired experience related to blood and bone marrow cells. After knowing how to separate blood components, then how to separate red blood cells, and finally how to use cryopreservation, in the 1980s and 1990s transfusion medicine became able to cultivate stem cells. These skills acquired over time allow transfusion medicine today to participate in reconstructive medicine along with other medical fields, and to gain knowledge it does not yet have. But although these skills exist, the persons who possess them, in transfusion institutions, are not always aware that it would be possible and useful to apply them to new developments, and might not feel they have the legitimacy to undertake such applications. One of the challenges we face is to assign to these persons positions of expertise, but on a new basis, often with new partners and in view of achieving new objectives.

To act with others means to bring together doctors, biologists, biotechnology engineers and pharmacists, as we orient more and more toward developing cellular therapeutic products. One crucial factor will certainly be the relation between the doctor and the engineer, two professionals in search of a new and stable identity. Of course, cooperation with hospitals will be essential, particularly for the clinical phase of product development. Because the necessary investments are very high, and because it is still too early to estimate time requirements and possible return on investment, the projects will also have to include economists, financial experts and marketing specialists who can develop business plans together in an uncertain field where failure is almost as likely an outcome as success, which would consist in being able to treat large numbers of patients. As the history of management of relations between research, development and production in high-tech business firms has shown, success will also depend in great measure on effective project managers (feasibility, opportunity, management, budget...) able to create structures where each actor plays an appropriate role. It might be advisable to have recourse to external expertise, for example to highlight innovations or processes discovered by the EFS (patents...), but transfusion institutions should possess within their own network a level of expertise, related to these new developments, high enough to allow them to understand and be understood by their partners. In this evolution, the required collaboration with pharmaceutical and biotechnological companies should not be perceived as a problem. Currently criticized by some volunteer blood donor associations, by a portion of the EFS personnel and by a segment of the public (not necessarily the most politically aware), this cooperation will have to be elucidated and quality partnerships will have to be created, to form a relationship respectful of the ethical principles of transfusion, and recognized by all to be a win-win situation.

Unless this is done, the transfusion system is condemned to marginalization on a fundamental level (through lack of funds for expensive research), as well as on a practical level (through lack of suitable means of production) [2].

Ethics and Quality Control Management: a Dialogue Model

Transfusion medicine has been very concerned with ethical issues in the past few years, particularly after the tragic events related to contaminated blood. In general, public health is always sensitive to these issues, which go beyond legal and deontological requirements, and which guide decision making when rigorous application of the rules is insufficient to determine appropriate action. Transfusion medicine is evidently among the authorities who discuss and structure ethical questions. This is even more important now, since new developments in the field involve cellular engineering and therapy. The point of view contributed by the transfusion field is essential, given that this field has acquired a rich perspective on these sensitive questions due to its intermediary position between the public (donors), practitioners (those who prescribe blood products, users, researchers), and patients.

Participation in the discussion process is also important because the personnel, some of whom were greatly affected by public blame at the time of the contaminated blood, need to understand the sense and impact of their actions, and to feel that they are in step with society as a whole. This dialogue among existing organisations must be coordinated, so that the chosen representatives of transfusion actors, and particularly of the EFS, can be those who are best suited for the areas discussed (more or less technical, more or less political). It would not make sense to try to create, within the field itself, "experts on ethics", because an institutional code of ethics becomes a compromise as soon as it is brought into the public arena.

On the other hand, technical and regulatory norms, related to ethics, quality control or technical standards, or the rules of competition – all of them influencing each-other – have increased in number, augmenting control and coherence requirements. This means that transfusion centers will increasingly need a new professional, with both legal and quality control qualifications, able to manage relations with all control agencies, whose number is growing, and particularly to be effective during inspections, when it is important to point out the field's own technical and economic requirements to prevent the inspector from imposing excessive standards based on his own procedural reasoning. We must remember that confrontation between different organizations does not guarantee safety; on the contrary, it is by listening and understanding each-other that we will find the right answers. Therefore, the legal/quality expert will have to be a master of dialogue.

Participation in Medical Monitoring: a Professional Model

To the present day, in France, transfusion medicine has been essentially excluded from the authorities and systems ensuring medical surveillance, mainly for corporatist reasons. In countries where the status of transfusion has been restricted to blood-bank dimensions, the situation is often similar. In France, since the 1998 law on health security gave rise to an institution responsible for sanitary surveillance (Institut de veille sanitaire), this tendency has paradoxically deepened. As a result, the French transfusion system will have to prove, through clear accomplishments in its areas of competence, that it is one of the major players in health monitoring in France. In addition to corporatist factors, exclusion of transfusion medicine could be due to insufficient development, over a lengthy period, of evaluation and statistical tools, and of analysis skills in transfusion institutions. Today, the objectives established in transfusion (safety, quality, self-sufficiency...) force us to include in the scope of our activities a complete epidemiological follow-up that can guide internal decisions and inform reflection and analysis related to the external context. Thus, this "urgent internal imperative" is also a requirement for legitimacy and credibility, making it possible to participate in public health systems which need the data and analyses transfusion medicine can provide.

This coincidence of an internal need, produced by the evolution of a professional sector, with an external need leads us to foresee the introduction in the transfusion sector of epidemiologists and biostatisticians familiar with social sciences, given that today it has become undeniable that no public health problem can be understood without using a combined epidemiology and social sciences approach.

Participation in Training and Research: a Qualification Model

Over the years, immuno-hematology practice has naturally developed in "transfusion centers," and with it, related know-how. Hospital/university centers, with a few notable exceptions, invested little in this field to which their practitioners had limited recourse. The creation of the French National Blood Service (EFS) brought together in a unified structure most experts in the field, as well as a large portion of the personnel possessing this know-how.

Thus, it is natural to entrust these actors in the transfusion field with the development and transmission of knowledge in this area. Without creating an actual teaching staff, the EFS will have to produce expert instructors, each one a specialist in his field and trained in teaching methods. This activity has to be evaluated as the need for instructors familiar with new knowledge transfer techniques, and the need for test measurement specialists, gradually become apparent.

Similarly, it will probably be necessary to produce, identify and promote the development of a body of researchers originating directly from the system or recruited from outside the system, to constitute the permanent core of a network of research units, specialized or mixed, whose status will be conferred by external authorities (Inserm, universities). The career profiles and the positions created will be particular to the field; training and selection criteria, as well as conditions for advancement, will remain very close to those in public scientific and technical institutions.

Human Resources and Cooperation

In order for these developments to be implemented successfully, and for these "special" human resources needs to be met, several conditions have to be present; these conditions are related to the collective structures in which they exist, and to their modes of functioning.

Creating *ad hoc* Structures

As we have pointed out, in the near future, cooperation will be increasingly important between transfusion institutions (and particularly the EFS in France) and the structures and professions associated with transfusion developments. This type of cooperation requires that each partner possess a strong, clearly established and recognized identity [3]. It is not possible to establish cooperation between partners with unclear characteristics which partly overlap and which are ultimately interchangeable. In France, the creation of the EFS in 2000 has founded a structure large enough but still manageable, whose parameters are defined by law and are under administrative supervision, but which intends to undertake developments it considers indispensable for the maintenance of its expertise and for the future of the field as a whole. To achieve this, the structure must have a strong institutional presence and identity, in the widest domain of its activities, as well as within its internal organization.

This national Establishment is intended to develop, and its development should take visible and recognizable forms inside and outside the sphere of its activities. At every stage, activities and the structures that support them should be as well matched as possible. Thus, we can imagine that the EFS will eventually develop into an institution dedicated to the cell and to the new cellular technologies, and that its regional structure will comprise sites with specific specializations.

To create stable partnerships, we will need flexible structures or groupings with their own identities that must also be more than a simple joining together of minimal common elements. An example of this is given by the joint efforts, in cell engineering, of health organizations which cooperate by sharing expertise and creating links between institutional positions in order to connect fundamental research stages (mainly in the Inserm), research-and-development (universities, CHUs, anti-cancer centers, the EFS...), production (mainly EFS at a number of *ad hoc* sites), and clinical practice (hospitals).

For transfusion medicine to be included in joint projects, its participation must be considered legitimate by its partners, as well as by the administrative supervisors that set the conditions for its development. Research is a good example. In transfusion medicine even more than in other fields, research can only exist in connection with a project where it is needed. The structures being created at present guarantee the fulfilment of this requirement. Researchers, whether trained in transfusion medicine or coming from other fields to join particular projects, will work within suitable professional structures. At the same time, these joint projects or *ad hoc* groupings will give them access to scientific evaluation, without which a research career is not possible. The personnel will be part of two levels of functioning: participation in structures adapted to various activities (such as health cooperation organizations) and a national structure (such as the EFS) which brings them all together and confers global meaning to their efforts.

Creating Dynamic Interaction

For human resources developments to keep pace with transfusion activities, aside from introducing the structures we described (some global, others specific, some cooperative, others taking the form of partnerships), and which create the common vision necessary for action, we must also introduce human resources policies allowing employees to be well integrated in this common vision and to participate fully in partnerships and joint action. We have to create dynamic interaction.

To do so, three factors have already proven to be essential, and their importance will increase in the near future.

- **Management and internal communication** should allow an organization initially built around safety requirements to maintain initiative, creativity and innovative spirit. Organizing and granting recognition can be difficult. They relate to decision-making processes, to the manner in which tasks are performed, to the priority given to debate and discussion, to what is expected of employees. Managers have their own expectations; they sometimes would rather continue to function on a small scale in order to be involved in all aspects of performance (which made their job more interesting), while their organization tends toward industrialization, segmentation, standardization of norms and procedures. This is even more so in new technology fields, where the proximity of research-and-development highlights the excitement of exploring new terrain.

- **Career management** must create diversified career structures reflecting the career advancement possible in an organization where linear, foreseeable career paths are not appropriate for the diversity of profiles, positions, advancement paths and forms of participation in the activities and operational strategies of the organization. Several career structures will have to be implemented, with connections between them so as to avoid isolating human resources and human resources managers.

- **Training** must guarantee access to rapidly increasing knowledge serving to construct a common foundation solid enough to constitute the basis of a common culture and shared understanding. This involves transmitting an image of the transfusion sector and its development, of corporate relations within the sector, of an operational style, etc.; as well as providing up-to-date training in specific fields. Both are equally important and have to be accomplished. We are no longer in a context where employees have merely to follow instructions. We now expect them to acquaint themselves with the unfamiliar, with the functions of those who hold other positions.

Conclusion

Some fields of endeavour and some sectors are yet to develop in the future, others will become integrated in the transfusion sector which will, in turn, participate in joint projects with other partners. This is the challenge faced by tomorrow's transfusion medicine: to go beyond its limits and use its expertise outside its hard core, wherever it is needed, while carrying out its basic mission which continues to evolve. New fields will certainly emerge, but what will be truly new is that all actors in transfusion medicine will have to include in their perspective that of those with whom they cooperate, in order to form hybrid partnerships and to become associated professionals of a new type [4], the only ones able to identify new horizons and the new frontiers of the science of blood and cells.

References

1. Fusfeld H I. *The technical enterprise*. Cambridge: Ballinger Publishing Company, 1988-320.
2. Freeman C. *The economics of industrial innovation*. MIT Press, 1997, 470.
3. Bourdieu P. *Les usages sociaux de la science*. Paris : Inra 1997, 79.
4. Cunéo B. Les chercheurs industriels : itinéraires et positions. *Culture technique* 1988 ; 18 : 259-72.

Quality Assurance and Transfusion Medicine: what Are the Tools, what Is at Stake?

Gilles Folléa, Caroline Lefort

Quality assurance is defined in the Good Manufacturing Practices for Therapeutic Products for human use, published by the European Union [1] as "a wide concept covering everything that can, individually or collectively, influence product quality. It represents the totality of measures taken to ensure that the therapeutic products manufactured meet quality requirements for their intended use". This definition naturally applies to labile blood products, from design, through development and all the way to follow-up after their administration. The need for a quality management system has been integrated in most national Good Manufacturing Practices for transfusion products, and its application by blood transfusion centers is a legal obligation in countries that have undertaken the organization and/or control of transfusion activities on a national scale [2-7, list not exhaustive]. Good Practices for Blood Products have even been established by the World Health Organization and are very easy to consult [8]. In Europe, Directive 2002/98/EC [9], in force in the twenty-five Member States of the European Union since February 8, 2005, stipulates that "Member States must take all necessary measures in order for each blood transfusion center to create and maintain a quality system based on Good Practices". These stipulations apply to hospital blood banks. They have been published in a "sub-directive" in 2005. Thus, implementation of a quality management system to ensure quality, safety and efficacy of labile blood products is currently a universal rule.

The Council of Europe Guide for the Processing, Use and Quality Assurance of Blood Components describes the foundations of a quality system for blood transfusion establishments [10]. This Guide, like the Good Transfusion Practices in effect in France [2], is based explicitly on ISO norm (International Organization for Standardization) 9001: 2000, in that the quality management systems described are based on a process approach and on continuous, systematic improvement. This approach has been applied for the past five years to all activities and at all locations of the blood transfusion center to which the authors are connected. The present chapter will review briefly the general principles outlined in norm ISO 9001: 2000, and will describe the major aspects of its application to the activities of a blood transfusion center by presenting the main methods used in a quality management system based on this norm.

Norm ISO 9001: 2000 and Labile Blood Products

International norm ISO 9001: 2000 [11] recommends a process-based approach. Examples of the application of this norm in a transfusion center are still rare in the scientific literature [12]. In a blood transfusion center, a process is a type of activity; these activities are clearly identified in the European Council Guide [10] and in Good Transfusion Practices in force in France [2]. This classification differentiates between professional processes (collection, processing, biological testing of donations, storage and distribution of labile blood products), support services (personnel, buildings and material) and management processes (record-keeping, quality policy, planning, internal communication, management of surveillance and measurement equipment, management of non conform products, data analysis and improvements). For each process, and for the interaction between them, this approach aims at understanding and satisfying "customer" needs, regards the process as added value, measures process performance and efficacy, and constantly improves each process based on objective measurements. The term "client", used in the Norm, has to be understood in context. In the totally "not-for-profit" context of non profit blood transfusion centers (the large majority in Europe), it refers to patients receiving labile blood products, to physicians prescribing these products, to personnel involved with transfusion in health institutions, as well as to the health authorities corresponding to the authority defined by Directive 2002/98/EC [9] as competent to grant accreditation to blood transfusion establishments, to inspect them and receive notification of serious adverse reactions and events.

In this dynamic perspective of the quality management system, the principles of the "Deming wheel" (plan, do, check, act), illustrated at *Figure 1*, apply to all processes. The application of these principles to blood transfusion centers has been clearly described in the Council of Europe Guide [10] and in the Good Transfusion Practices in force in France [2].

Of course, these principles can be applied to hospitals blood banks, and to the clinical portions of the transfusion chain in hospitals and clinics. In terms of structuring operations, experience has shown the importance of five tools derived from the Norm: process analysis, goal setting and use of indicators, anomaly management, internal audits and "client" satisfaction evaluation.

Process Analysis

For each type of activity and for the interactions between them, process analysis consists of the reflection needed to define and organize them. This reflection, which is based on the regulations applicable to each process and/or on recommendations in force, must be presented as a set of procedures. The processes defined in this manner in a health institution are illustrated by the process map at *Figure 2*.

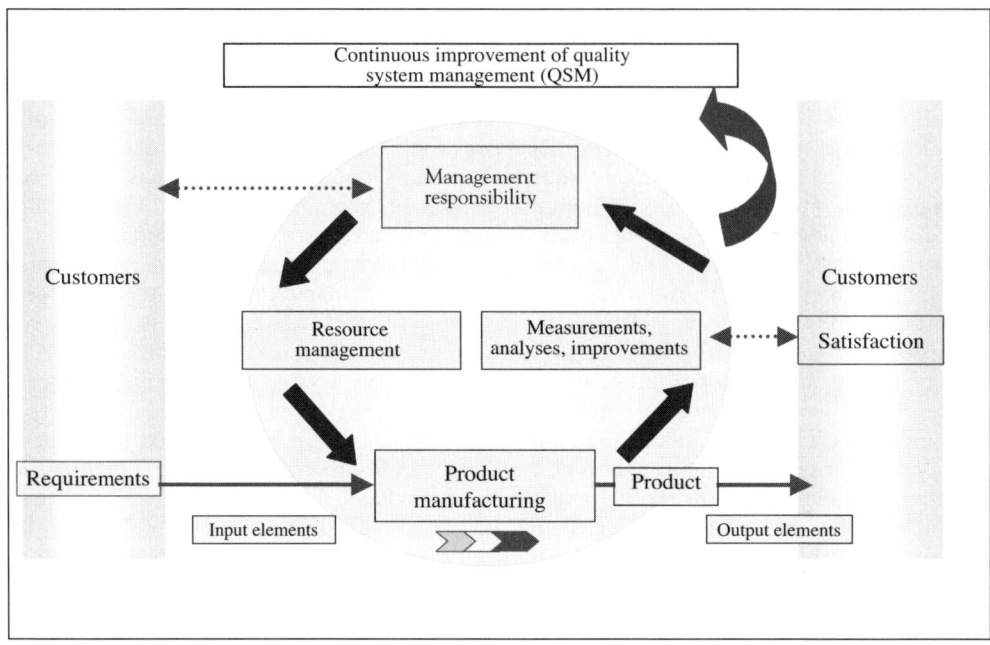

Figure 1. Principles of continuous improvement of QSM defined in norm ISO 9001: 2000 for each process and its interactions.

Documenting the production processes in a health institution must first take into account requirements regarding labile blood products. In addition to national regulations, most of these requirements are described in Directive 2004/33/EC [13], in the Council of Europe Guide [10] and in the summaries of product characteristics recently published by the Council [14]. These requirements serve to define the acceptance and refusal criteria for release of labile blood product, as well as the criteria for the analysis of statistical quality control results for labile blood products. Once these requirements are taken into account, analysis of manufacturing process plans should lead to defining an organizational system that can link collection, processing and biological qualification to labile blood product distribution, and that allows suitable adaptation of collection to patient needs in terms of labile blood products, in order to prevent shortages and to avoid expiration. Analysis of communication with "clients" should lead to structuring, overall, the modes of communication with prescribing physicians and health institutions, with donors and their associations wherever they exist, and with the competent authority or authorities. The Norm implies the definition of another process anterior to "production" of labile blood products: research-and-development, which must satisfy the same quality requirements as those governing design and development of labile blood products.

Analysis of production processes in a blood transfusion center defines the stages of collection, processing, biological qualification, transport of labile blood products, distribution, transfusion and hemovigilance indications (as well as donor repository wherever this exists), organizing them so as to advance the process, and separating homologous products from autologous products, to limit the risk of confusion and error. Control of monitoring and measuring instruments involves having an organized standardization process whose function is to provide the control results for measuring instruments (temperature, volume..) and to

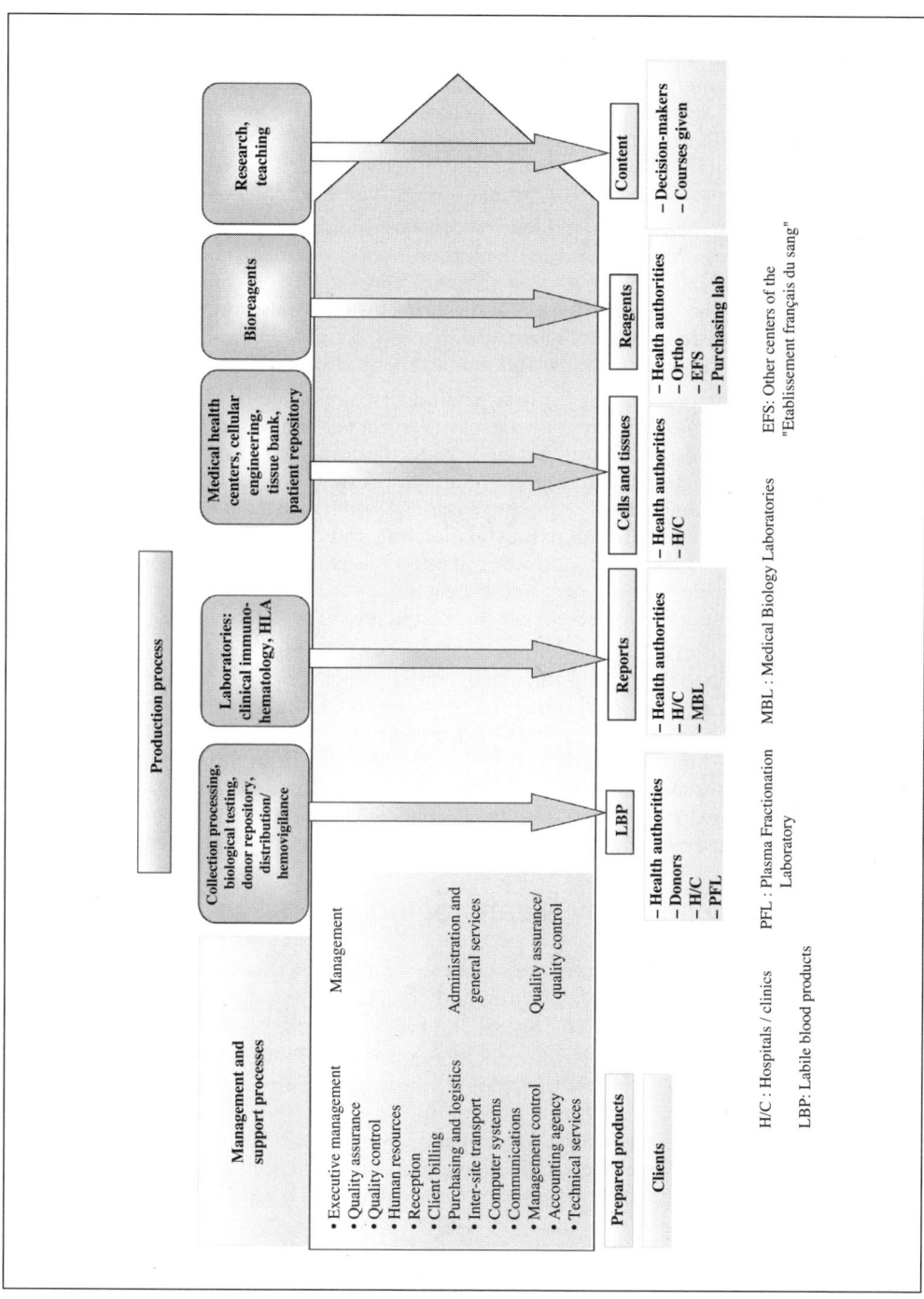

Figure 2. Process flow chart subjected to documented analysis in a blood transfusion center (example drawn from the experience of the transfusion center to which the authors are connected).

conduct the necessary calibration to correct any discrepancies observed, in order to ensure the accuracy and precision of measurements taken within the scope of the activities of the blood transfusion center. Finally, teaching must be considered a production process and must be organized as such in terms of the teaching activities conducted by the blood transfusion center within the French National Blood Service (EFS) (initial training and continued education), in terms of external teaching activities conducted by the transfusion center, and in terms of the respective evaluations of these teaching activities.

For support processes, analysis should lead to determining the organization and methods of initial training, of personnel training for each position, of continued education and of regular competence evaluation. Concerning infrastructures and work environment, analysis should lead to defining the organization and the means of acquisition of consumables and reagents, as well as to defining purchases, qualification, equipment maintenance and management, control of computer systems, and management of biological and toxic waste.

For the management process, the analysis should first define methods of documentation management, as part of the quality management system (Quality Manual, procedures, operations manual, records pertaining to quality, regulations, scientific monitoring...). In addition, objectives, actions, internal communication methods and confidentiality rules have to be defined. Management of products not conforming to standards will also have to be determined, including a procedure for the blocking and recall of labile blood products if necessary, within the scope of the monitoring programs concerned (hemovigilance, material monitoring, reagent surveillance, and biovigilance for human body elements and products used for therapeutic purposes, other than labile blood products and gametes).

This overview makes it possible to define rationally the activities of each blood transfusion center or hospital blood depot, and the management principles of the teams responsible for their application. The process describing the major stages of implementation and control of transfusion medicine procedures in the blood transfusion center to which the authors are connected, presented in the overview, is illustrated at *Figure 3*. In order for the documentation system to be useful and easily accepted, it is important that the documents pertaining to the quality management system be as concise and instructive as possible. Regular review of the documentation system should serve to discard useless documents.

Objectives Monitored by Means of Indicators

In order to implement the processes defined and organized in this manner, the ISO 9001: 2000 norm stipulates follow-up of activities and objectives by means of indicators, and the setting of improvement objectives for each process. Experience has shown that two methods are useful in carrying this out. The first consists of applying quality controls specific to each process; these controls are based on indicators of efficacy and conformity evaluations.

Objectives are set for each indicator. Each operational manager plans and implements the actions necessary to achieve these objectives. Our experience includes quarterly quality control meetings which present and analyze the results of each process, providing a review of relevant indicators, in the presence of executives and process managers, in view of achieving steering objectives. Analysis of the experience acquired after four years of application shows that objectives measured in this manner make it possible to:

– obtain and implement continuous improvement of processes (production, support, management) of the blood transfusion center;

– benefit from shared experiences of various process managers in view of improving each process and their interactions;
– verify the efficacy of corrective measures implemented subsequent to previous meetings;
– inform regularly all personnel of the blood transfusion center of the achievement of objectives associated with the center's missions.

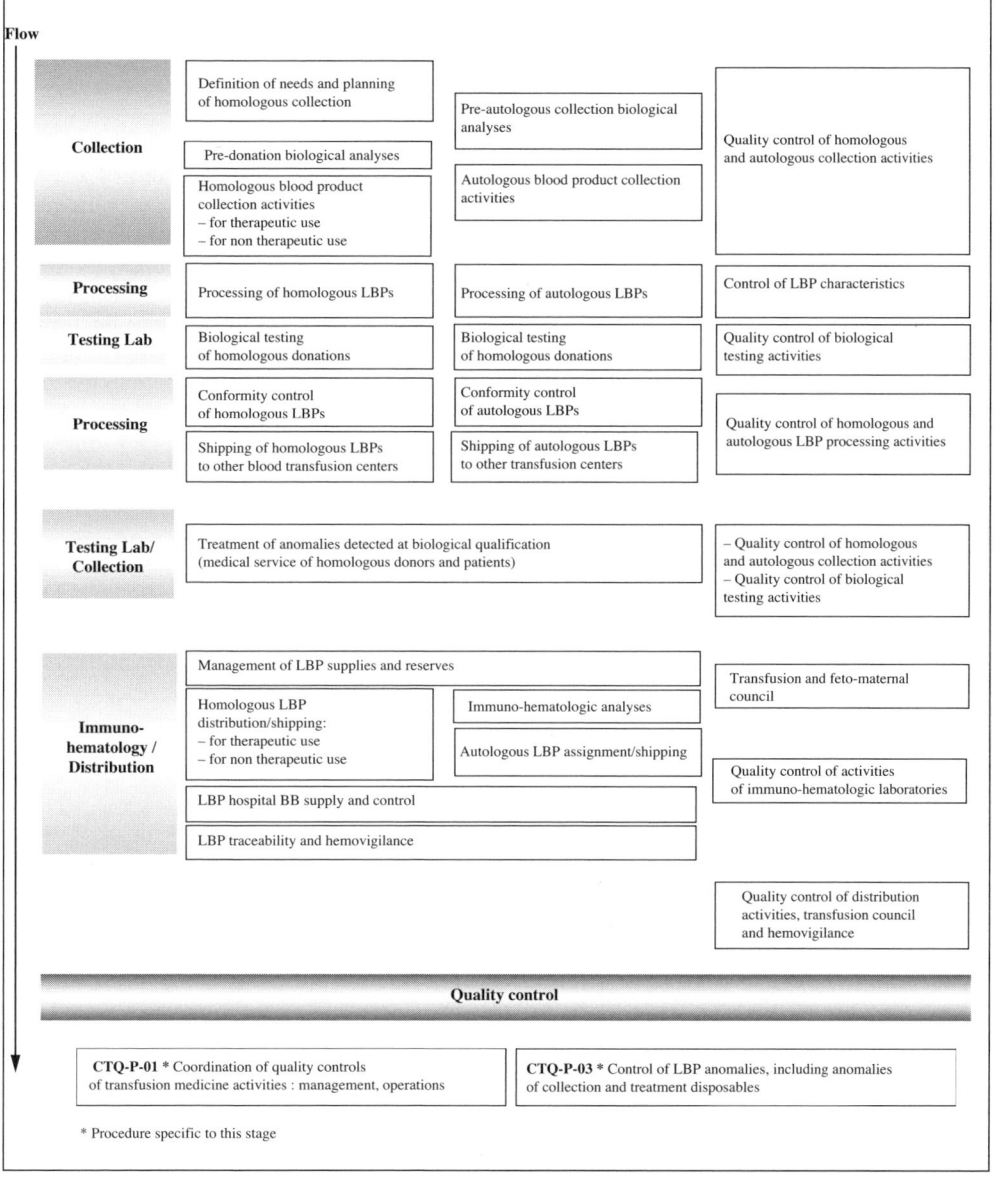

Figure 3. Procedure describing the major stages of manufacturing and control of transfusion medicine processes, taken from the process overview in the transfusion center to which the authors are connected.

The second method is a project management procedure applied to each process. For each project, synthesis of the established objective, of its relation to the center's quality policy (for example, in the center to which the authors are connected: transfusion quality and safety, recognition of competence, efficiency, "client" satisfaction), of the manager(s) responsible for the project, of the schedule established for attaining objectives, and of regular reviews has proven to be very useful to ensure the steering of major projects of the transfusion center. Analysis of the efficacy and quality of each process, and a report on project stages take place at least once a year within the scope of the management review required by the Norm. This executive review also makes it possible to update quality indicators of the processes, and to develop new projects.

To illustrate, the labile blood product supply process consists of matching as closely as possible homologous collections with patient needs in terms of labile blood products, in order to avoid shortages and to prevent outdating as much as possible. *Table I* presents the results obtained in our transfusion center between 2000 and 2004 for self-sufficiency in labile blood products (limitation of external purchases) and outdating rates (surplus not managed). Overall, results are satisfactory, but they point to possible means of improving self-sufficiency in fresh frozen plasma (exclusive processing of quarantined FFP makes rapid adaptation difficult in cases of plasma exchanges requiring large volumes of plasma), and of limiting outdating of red blood cell concentrates, which increased in 2004 following the suppression (regulatory) of transaminase assays in biological testing. Certain measures (refinement of collection adjustments, informing voluntary blood donor associations of supply status by E-mail) were taken in order to improve results in 2005. This type of objective, monitored by indicators, can be applied to all production, support and management processes. The most time-consuming work involves the definition of relevant indicators suited to each process.

Table I. Example of objectives monitored with indicators: application to labile blood product supply process ("Etablissement français du sang" PL 2000-2004).

	Objective	2000	2001	2002	2003	2004
Red blood cell concentrates released	–	105,886	101,714	106,023	108,166	111,003
RBCC purchased externally (shortage)	0	138 (0.1 %)	10 * (0.01 %)	60* (0.06 %)	90 * (0.08)	71 * (0.06 %)
RBCC outdated (surplus not managed)	< 1 %	1,440 (1.4 %)	974 (1.0 %)	935 (0.9 %)	810 (0.7 %)	1,386 (1.25 %)
Apheresis platelet concentrates released	–	10,864	10,623	10,464	9,812	10,393
APC purchased externally (shortage)	0	43 (0.4 %)	2 (0.02 %)	3 (0.03 %)	10 (0.10)	10 (0.10 %)
APC outdated (surplus not managed)	< 1.5 %	327 (3.0 %)	131 (1.2 %)	93 (0.9 %)	117 (1.2 %)	123 (1.2 %)
Fresh frozen plasma released	–	7,997	17,880	20,010	22,981	24,577
FFP purchased externally (shortage)	0	1,645 (20.5 %)	500 (2.8 %)	1,416 (7.1 %)	0	1,275 (5.2 %)

* Objective considered attained given that most red blood cell concentrates purchased externally came from the national blood bank of rare phenotypes for patients belonging to rare blood groups.

Anomaly Management

Reporting and management of anomalies, errors and adverse events are now widely used in human clinical practice [15], and particularly in transfusion medicine [16, 17]. Concretely, we are referring to hemovigilance systems with voluntary [18] or required [19] reporting.

In blood transfusion centers or a hospital blood depot, as in any human activity, anomalies can occur in the course of each process. To manage them efficiently, we use voluntary reporting with classification of anomalies in three categories based on the degree to which they are critical for the product or the service involved. A critical anomaly compromises the safety of a person (patient, donor, employee). A major anomaly compromises the safety of a product or a service (biological analysis results...) A minor anomaly does not compromise the safety of a person, a product or a service.

The following principles have proven to be suitable and useful in anomaly management. Any employee should be able to report an anomaly voluntarily. Only critical and major anomalies are subjected to a management procedure that directly involves the quality assurance Director of the center.

An anomaly report leads to the following procedures: written report, implementation of appropriate corrective measures in a timeframe based on the degree of urgency, analysis of causes of the anomaly, definition and implementation of appropriate corrective measures designed to avoid repetition of the anomaly, follow-up to verify efficacy of these measures, recording into the documentation system of these different steps, and distribution of documents to all concerned. Minor anomalies are treated only at the level of process managers, except when repetitions occur, given that successive repetition of a minor anomaly can constitute a major anomaly.

Complaints from "clients" (prescribing physicians, hospitals and clinics...) are submitted to the same procedure. An additional stage in the quality management system makes it possible to report and treat anomalies that have not yet occurred but are likely to occur, by using preventive measures. Treatment of these "near miss events" has already been described and applied to the clinical aspects of transfusion medicine [17]. Implementation of this prevention stage requires excellent knowledge of the center's quality management system.

In practice, in the blood transfusion center to which the authors are connected, 120 to 140 critical or major anomalies are reported each year; with a proportion of about 15% of critical anomalies and 85% of major anomalies. Of these anomalies, 80% concern the production process, particularly labile blood product processing and distribution. The management review provides the occasion to present a yearly summary of anomalies, corrective measures and their effectiveness, as well as unresolved situations where planned actions were not implemented or did not give results.

Internal and External Audits

An internal audit, or self-inspection, to use the pharmaceutical industry term [1], is an evaluation performed by employees of the center who volunteer for the task and receive special training. Each internal audit must include a questionnaire based on the regulations in effect and on the Norm applying to blood transfusion centers wishing to conform to such quality standards. Each audit must be announced in advance and conducted using the questionnaire, submitted in advance to those who are audited. After the audit, a report is prepared, as well as corrective action forms designed to define ways of improvement in response to the observations made by the audit.

In the transfusion center to which the authors are connected, forty internal audits are conducted each year. On average, each audit produces 3.5 to 4 corrective action forms. Discrepancies observed by internal audits concern support or management processes in over 75% of cases. This being so, these internal audits appear to be a good complement to management of anomalies reported outside internal audits. A summary of anomalies and the measures taken to correct them is presented during the yearly management review.

External audits include accreditation audits and all other audits performed by an institution external to the Center. These audits lead to elaborate corrective measures, implemented and evaluated based on the same principles as those described above. Inspections conducted by regulatory authorities also lead to improvements when actions proposed by each inspection are implemented and followed up by the national authority. Reports prepared as a result of these audits and inspections provide precise information concerning discrepancies and dysfunctions. The reactions recorded and submitted after each audit and inspection describe the corrective measures planned, and communications in response to them indicate whether they are accepted or refused by the institution having performed the audit, or by the national authority that conducted the inspection. The summary of audits and ensuing corrective measures must also be presented and analyzed during the management review. It is desirable that, as is done in the center to which the authors are connected, discrepancies revealed by inspections, and the ensuing corrective measures, be analyzed during the management review from the perspective of their contribution to possible improvement.

Satisfaction Surveys

The ISO 9001: 2000 Accreditation refers to taking into account information regarding "client" perception of the degree to which expectations are fulfilled. To illustrate, in the transfusion center to which the authors are connected, a yearly survey of blood donors is conducted using a questionnaire. In 2003, one of these surveys revealed inadequate visibility of the signage used by voluntary blood donor associations to indicate the location of mobile collection sites. Concerted action taken by each transfusion site in partnership with voluntary blood donor associations resulted in creating a new signage allowing easy identification of each collection site by prospective donors.

Another survey that used a questionnaire was conducted among transfusion actors in a hospital whose labile blood products were provided by the Loire region EFS. This survey has been described in detail elsewhere [20]. The survey revealed the difficulties experienced by hospital actors in situations where labile blood products are requested in an emergency. Establishing a common standard operating procedure for the hospital and the Loire region EFS, involving a precise procedure to follow in case of emergency requests for labile blood products, a procedure which had never been written previously, solved this problem and consequently improved patient safety. Since then, other surveys have been conducted. They always provide new suggestions for improvement, that are interesting and useful.

Quality Assurance in Summary: what Is at Stake?

Each blood transfusion center, each hospital blood bank and each hospital or clinic, in its transfusion medicine practices, must implement a quality management system to ensure the quality of the products and services provided, as well as "client" satisfaction.

From this perspective, quality assurance and, more specifically, the quality management system, are powerful aids in creating the conditions necessary for goal attainment. In this context, the five tools described in this chapter: process review, setting of objectives whose attainment is measured by indicators, anomaly reporting and management, internal and external audits, and satisfaction surveys have proven to be very effective.

Beyond this first quality assurance objective that concerns only products and services intended for patients, competence in using these tools is essential for performing other increasingly important functions. The first concerns management, that is, managing teams in a transfusion center. Regular use of these tools is likely to lead to a progression from quality assurance considered austere and restrictive, to quality assurance that encourages individual responsibility and provides each employee with a better perception of the place of his activities in the transfusion chain, strengthening the coherence of the overall process. In practice, these tools constitute a personnel motivation factor and lead to the acquisition of expertise in using more sophisticated management tools such as process risk analysis, added value analysis, and analysis and preventive treatment of "near miss events". In this sense, a quality management system can evolve into a management-through-quality system, where quality assurance is integrated in the activities of each employee. These tools can also be used to improve efficiency of transfusion chain processes. This is particularly important at a time when control of health costs is increasingly shown to be essential for allowing each country to offer its patients the best medical care possible, by utilizing therapeutic innovations and by controlling emerging risks. In our experience, introduction of a quality management system using the tools described above requires high

initial investment in human resources for a limited time. Beyond that time, the system provides considerable efficiency improvement. In practice, a well integrated quality management system proves to be a cost-saving rather than an added expense factor.

Continued improvement is another desirable objective. A quality management system relies on constant consideration of methods leading to possible improvement.

In practice, such a system is a strong stimulus to innovations that will benefit patients. Experience has shown that the system is quickly and positively integrated by the personnel and the "clients" of the center.

Given these objectives, a well integrated quality management system is likely to create a "win-win" situation for all the actors in the transfusion chain, for patients above all, but also for donors, employees, personnel performing transfusions in health institutions, and for governmental authorities involved in the health of citizens in every country. In this context, a quality management system is applicable on the scale of a blood transfusion center, just as it is on the scale of a National Blood Service. Thus, in 2005, all transfusion centers of the EFS were certified in conformity with norm ISO 9001: 2000, and the process leading to this certification constituted a strong factor for harmonization of practices.

The 2003 report of the Council of Europe concerning collection, qualification and use of blood and blood products in Europe in 2003, based on a questionnaire [21], showed that out of the seventeen European Union countries that answered, sixteen indicated that they possess established and active quality assurance systems.

Among them, two countries in addition to France, Austria and Luxembourg, stated that they have complete coverage through a quality assurance system conforming to norm ISO 9000. In the future, within the scope of the "Daughter European Directive" that recently defined European rules governing quality assurance in blood transfusion centers and hospital blood banks, this type of system could be a harmonization and continuous improvement factor in terms of quality, efficacy and transfusion safety for patients, on a European scale.

References

1. Medicinal Products for Human and Veterinary Use: Good Manufacturing Practice. http://pharmacos.eudra.org/F2/eudralex/vol-4/home.html
2. Arrêté du 10 septembre 2003 portant homologation du règlement de l'Agence française de sécurité sanitaire des produits de santé définissant les principes de bonnes pratiques dont doivent se doter les établissements de transfusion sanguine. *Journal Officiel de la République Française*, 30/09/2003: 16665-78
3. Australian Government. Regulation of blood. http://www.tga.gov.au/bt/blood.htm
4. Santé Canada. Bonnes pratiques de fabrication (BFP) des drogues visées à l'annexe D partie 2, sang et composants du sang humain. http://www.hc-sc.gc.ca/hpfb-dgpsa/inspectorate/sched_d_part2_entire_f.html
5. Sazama K. Current good manufacturing practices for transfusion medicine. *Transfus Med Rev* 1996 ; 10: 286-95.
6. UK Blood Transfusion Services. UK Blood Transfusion & Tissue Transplantation Guidelines. http://www.transfusionguidelines.org.uk/uk_guidelines/ukbts6001.html
7. US Food and Drug Administration (FDA). Current Good Manufacturing Practice for Blood and Blood Components. http://www.gmp1st.com/blreg.htm
8. World Health Organization. Blood products and related biologicals. Good manufacturing practices. http://www.who.int/bloodproducts/gmp/en/
9. Directive 2002/98/EC of the European Parliament and the Council of 27 January 2003 setting standards of quality and safety for the collection, testing, processing, storage and distribution of human blood and blood components and amending Directive 2001/83/EC. *Official Journal of the European Union* of 02/08/2003/2004.
10. Quality system for blood establishments. In: *Guide to the preparation, use and quality asurance of blood components*-11th ed. Strasbourg: Council of Europe Publishing, 2005: 19-32
11. NF EN ISO 9001. Quality management systems – Requirements. AFNOR editions. Paris, December 2000: 1-14. www.boutique.afnor.fr
12. Kalmin ND, Myers LK, Fisk MB. ISO 9000 model ideally suited for quality plan at blood centers. *Transfusion* 1998 ; 38: 79-85.
13. Commission Directive 2004/33/EC of 22 March 2004 implementing Directive 2002/98/EC of the European Parliament and of the Council as regards certain technical requirements for blood and blood components. *Official Journal of the European Union* of 03/30/2004.
14. Optimal Use of Blood. Summaries of component characteristics. http://www.coe.int/T/E/Social_Cohesion/Health/
15. Leape L. Patient safety. Reporting of adverse events. *N Engl J Med* 2002 ; 347: 1633-8.
16. Zimmermann R, Linhardt C, Weisbach V, Büscher M, Zingsem J, Eckstein R. An analysis of errors in blood component transfusion records with regard to quality improvement of data acquisition and to the performance of lookback and traceback procedures. *Transfusion* 1999 ; 39: 351-6.
17. Callum JL, Kaplan HS, Merkley LL, Pinkerton PH, Fastman BR, Romans RA, Coovadia AS, Reis MD. Reporting of near-miss events for transfusion medicine: improving transfusion safety. *Transfusion* 2001 ; 41: 1204-11.
18. Serious Hazards of Transfusion Annual Report 2003. Manchester, UK: Serious Hazards of Transfusion Office, Manchester Blood Centre ; 2004.
19. Andreu G, Morel P, Forestier F, Debeir J, Rebibo D, Janvier G, Hervé P. Hemovigilance network in France: organization and analysis of immediate transfusion incident reports from 1994 to 1998. *Transfusion* 2002 ; 42: 1356-64.
20. Chord-Auger S, Tron de Bouchony E, Moll MC, Boudart D, Folléa G. Enquête de satisfaction des acteurs impliqués dans la transfusion dans un centre hospitalier général: une application de la norme ISO 9001: 2000. *Transfus Clin Biol* 2004 ; 11: 161-7.
21. van der Poel CL, Janssen MP. *Report on the collection, testing and use of blood and blood products in Europe in 2003*. Strasbourg : Editions du Conseil de l'Europe, 2005.

Transfusion Medicine in the Europe of Tomorrow

Gilles Folléa

Today's political context constantly reminds us that we are part of a much larger territory than that of our own country: the European continent. There are thus elections for European representatives, meetings of the European Union (EU) Council... In transfusion medicine, wide distribution of Council of Europe recommendations, and recent publication of four European Directives remind us that European recommendations and mandatory regulations (that is, regulations that must be found to be satisfied at inspection by national health authorities) are in effect in every country of the European Union. Before looking at the future of transfusion in Europe, it is important to review the transfusion institutions currently active on the continent, to present a synthesis of the regulatory framework established by two recent European Directives, and to provide a general description of the *status quo* in terms of the organization of transfusion activities in Europe. These elements can then be used to arrive at future perspectives regarding transfusion in 21st century Europe.

Institutions Regulating Transfusion

These institutions comprise those in the public sector, the European Union and the Council of Europe, and private institutions. Although the Council of Europe has issued numerous recommendations regarding transfusion since 1958, we will look first at the European Union, given that it issues the regulations governing blood products and transfusion in Member States.

The European Union [1, 2]

Countries comprising the European Union, Member States, exert concerted sovereign action in view of bringing to bear, in the international arena, a degree of power and influence that none of them possesses alone.

In practice, shared sovereignty means that Member States delegate some of their decisional power to the common institutions they have created, so that decisions on certain subjects of common interest can be made using a democratic process on a European scale. The European decisional system, particularly as it applies to blood products and tissues, brings together three major institutions: the European Parliament, which represents European citizens and whose members are elected by direct suffrage; the Council of the European Union, which represents Member States; and the European Commission whose mission is to defend the interests of the Union as a whole. This "institutional triangle" sets policies and introduces legislative acts (directives, regulations and decisions) applying to all countries in the EU. In principle, the role of the Commission is to propose new European legislation, and the role of the Parliament and the Council is to pass it.

The European Commission is at the heart of the European institutional system, presented at *Figure 1*; it introduces laws, policies and implementation programs, and is responsible for enacting the decisions of the Parliament and the Council. Like the Parliament and the Council, the European Commission was created in the 1950s by the founding treaties. The term "Commission" designates the members ("Commissioners") appointed by Member States and by Parliament to administer the institution and draw up its decisions, as well as the institution itself and its personnel. A new Commission is appointed every five years, within six months following elections for the European Parliament.

The main role of the European Commission is to submit legislative proposals to the Parliament and the Council. Accordingly, it is the only institution entrusted with drawing

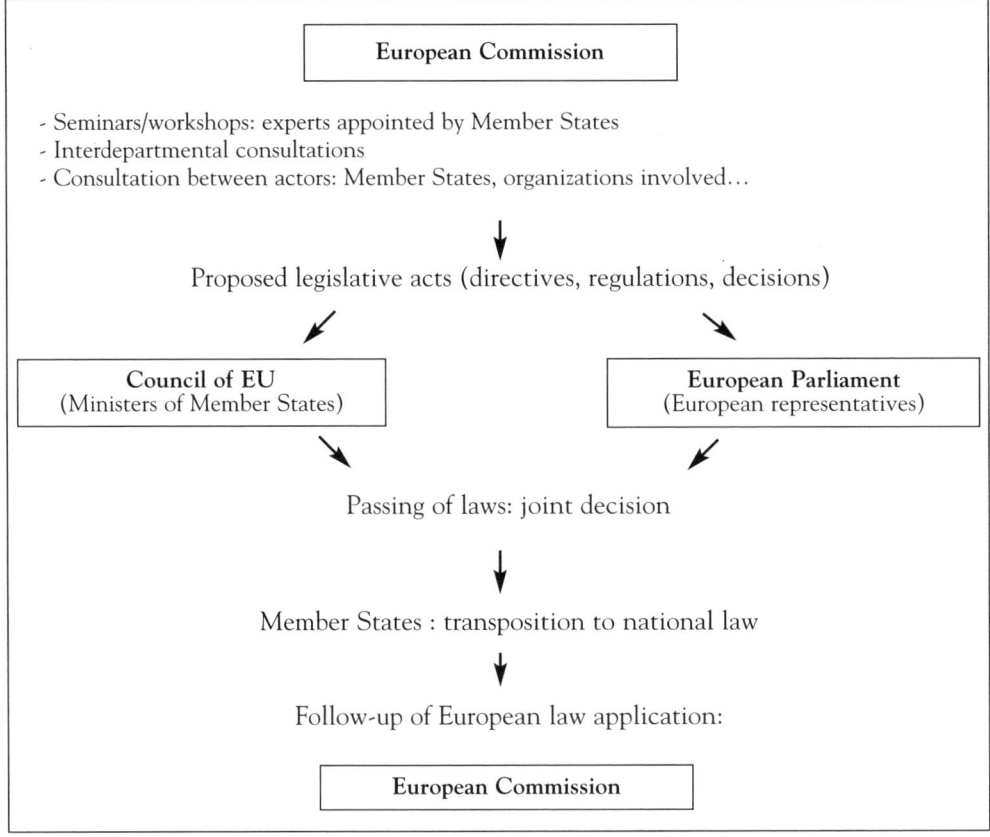

Figure 1. Schematic overview of the functioning of EU institutions for the introduction, application and enforcement of European regulations governing blood products and tissue.

up proposals for new European legislation. These proposals must be designed to defend the interests of the EU and its citizens, not those of particular countries or sectors. Before introducing a bill, the Commission must acquaint itself with the current context and with problems existing in Europe, and must decide whether a European law is the best way to solve them. In accordance with the subsidiarity principle, it must always be presumed that Member States are competent and that the EU is not. The latter must always prove that its intervention is indispensable. The degree of uniformly applied constraint of a European Community measure must be as limited as possible in relation to its efficacy.

In accordance with these principles, the Commission is in permanent contact with many different interest groups, and with two advisory agencies: the European Economic and Social Committee, and the Regional Committee. It also seeks advice from national parliaments and governments. In practice, the introduction of European legislative changes applying to blood and tissues is preceded by workshops and seminars which bring together experts appointed by the health authorities of each Member State, as well as experts called by the Commission. In addition, the Commission solicits advice on planned legislature and legislative texts in progress, from various organizations in the relevant sector. In the field of transfusion, these consultations concern mainly Council of Europe recommendations and the views of the European Blood Alliance (EBA). These consultations lead to the first version of a law (Green Book), submitted to Member States. The proposal that results after interdepartmental Commission consultations constitutes the "White Book". After another consultation among the actors involved, and after more interdepartmental consultations, the Commission submits a bill to the Council and the European Parliament. The procedure for ratifying European laws in this context is a "joint decision", since the Parliament and the Council have equal power to pass these collective laws.

The second function of the European Commission, which could affect the field of blood and tissues, and which falls under its mandate as executive agency of the EU, is the management and application of the EU budget and of policies and programs adopted by the Parliament and the Council. In this role, the Commission has the power to attribute funds for research programs in the field of blood and tissues. It supports activities benefiting the Community, that are coherent with the annual public health program; the Commission can provide grants to cover 60% of eligible costs of the projects considered.

The third function of the Commission is to supervise, with the European Court of justice, the proper application of European legislation in all Member States. When the Commission finds that a country does not enforce a European legislative act, it takes the necessary measures to correct the situation. First, it sets in motion a legal procedure called "infringement procedure". If this procedure does not lead to a solution, the Commission refers the case to the Court of Justice, which has the power to impose sanctions. The decisions of the Court are binding upon Member States and European institutions. Therefore, European legislation, after transposition to national law, is binding upon Member States.

The Council of Europe

The Council of Europe was created in 1945 to connect countries wishing to defend human rights, solidarity and social unity [3, 4]. The Council was created as a European solidarity response to the bursting of dykes in the Netherlands, which caused the death of 1800 people in 1953.

As part of this response, many countries sent blood to the victims; this disaster occasioned the first meeting of the Council of Europe Expert Committee on Public Health, held in July 1954. The result was an agreement signed by seventeen countries on December 15,

1958: European Agreement No.26 on the exchange of therapeutic substances of human origin. The signatories agreed to provide therapeutic substances of human origin to countries in urgent need of them. From the start, the Council stipulated, as a fundamental principle of blood transfusion, unpaid, voluntary blood donation, self-sufficiency and the protection of donors and recipients. Since then, the Council of Europe communicates regularly with health authorities in Member States (46 in 2005) by means of conventions or agreements, recommendations and reports. The best known of these recommendations, regarded by many Council of Europe members as veritable standards, are given in the *Guide for the processing, use and quality assurance of blood components*. The first edition of the Guide was published in 1995. The eleventh edition [5] was published in January 2005.

Table I presents a list (not exhaustive) of documents issued by the Council of Europe relative to blood transfusion, to cell therapy and to organ transplant.

Recently, the Council of Europe has prepared specific monographs called *Summaries of Product Characteristics*; they present, for each labile blood product, definitions, characteristics, rules for collection and processing, rules for labelling, storage and transport conditions, quality assurance rules, follow-up and efficacy rules, therapeutic indications, safe use and potential adverse reactions.

Table I. List (not exhaustive) of recommendations issued by the Council of Europe in the fields of transfusion, cell therapy and organ and tissue transplantation since 2000.
http//www.coe.int/Social Cohesion/Health and Ethics

– Recommendation Rec (2001)4 on the prevention of the possible transmission of variant Creutzfeldt-Jakob Disease (vCJD) by blood transfusion.
– Recommendation Rec (2001)5 of the Committee of Ministers to Member States on the management of organ transplant waiting lists and waiting times.
– Recommendation Rec (2002)11 of the Committee of Ministers to Member States on the hospital's and clinician's role in the optimal use of blood and blood products.
– Recommendation Rec (2003)11 of the Committee of Ministers to Member States on the introduction of pathogenic agent inactivation procedures for blood components.
– Recommendation Rec (2003)12 of the Committee of Ministers to Member States on organ donor registers.
– Recommendation Rec (2004)8 of the Committee of Ministers to Member States on autologous cord blood banks and explanatory memorandum.
– Recommendation Rec (2004)18 of the Committee of Ministers to Member States on teaching transfusion medicine to nurses and explanatory memorandum.
– Recommendation Rec (2004)19 of the Committee of Ministers to Member States on criteria for the authorization of organ transplantation facilities.

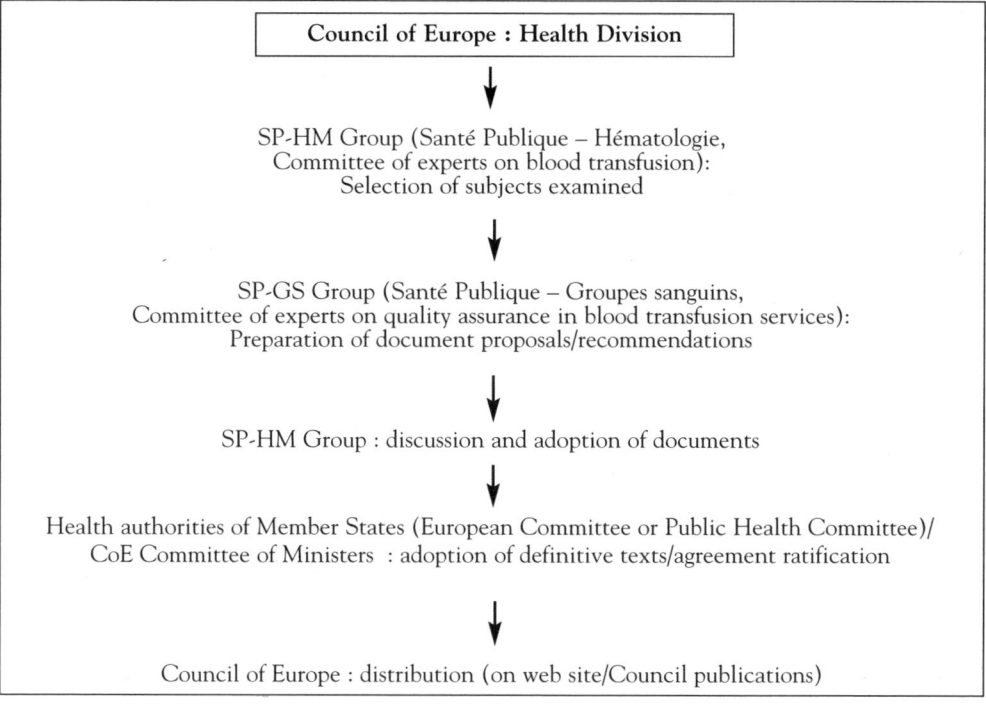

Figure 2. Cycle of preparation and distribution of Council of Europe recommendations and reports in the field of blood transfusion.

Preparation and publication of European documents follow a very precise cycle (*Figure 2*) within the Health Division of the Council of Europe. Subjects to be examined are selected by the Expert Committee on blood transfusion and on immuno-hematology (still designated by the original initials SP-HM: Public Health-Hematology). A specialized expert committee for quality assurance in transfusion services (still designated by the original initials SP-GS: Public Health-Blood Groups) works on these subjects and prepares document proposals. Experts on these committees are appointed by Member States (one per country for each of the two committees). Document and recommendation proposals are submitted to the SP-HM.

After their ratification by this Committee, these documents are submitted to health authorities within the framework of the European Health Committee and, if an agreement must be reached by Member States, to the Committee of Ministers of the Council of Europe.

After their ratification, the definitive texts are widely disseminated by the Council of Europe.

Technical expertise acquired by these Council of Europe authorities enabled the Council to play a major role (see below) in the preparation of Article 29 of Directive 2002/98/EC [6] and in the specification of the technical requirements described in Directive 2004/33/EC [7]. The constant objective pursued by the Council of Europe is to arrive at unified standards for the whole of Europe.

In addition, the Council of Europe organizes and carries out transfusion-related teaching activities, and provides assistance in the structuring of services in Eastern European countries.

Private European Organizations

Among private organizations, the European Blood Alliance (EBA) is undoubtedly the most active. The Alliance was created in 1998 [8] by representatives of the national blood services of nine countries whose common objective was to promote blood product quality and safety, and self-sufficiency based on unpaid, voluntary donations. Today, seventeen countries are members of the Alliance: Germany, Austria, Belgium, Denmark, Finland, France, the Irish Republic, Luxembourg, Norway, the Netherlands, Portugal, Slovenia, Switzerland, England, Scotland, Northern Ireland and Wales (the last four recently constituted a single member: the United Kingdom). Entry into the Alliance of other countries is under consideration: Sweden, Greece, Italy and Spain. In the longer term, the EBA could accept the applications of ten countries which have joined the European Union in 2004.

The Alliance's objective is to contribute to the safety of blood products for European citizens by creating a network of national blood services within the European Union. Achieving this objective involves recourse to four types of action:

– defence of unpaid, voluntary donations, and processing of labile blood products as an indispensable therapeutic tool in the treatment of patients;

– provision of technical and professional support to national and European authorities involved in the setting of norms and issuing of recommendations for labile blood product quality and safety;

– exchange and sharing of information relevant to European Union Member States, on developments in transfusion medicine;

– support of joint projects involving Member States, to promote self-sufficiency and increase the capacities of the EBA and of its members in this field.

Initially, the first objective of the European Blood Alliance was to influence the content of the first Directive of the Council of Europe regarding blood products. In this context, the EBA has defended the following principles most particularly: the principle of unpaid, voluntary donations; limitation of the Directive to fundamental principles; and the description of detailed technical requirements in another document that can be updated whenever appropriate. The work of the EBA in close cooperation with the Council of Europe and the Commission of the European Union has made it possible to achieve these objectives.

The European Blood Alliance has examined other questions in depth. For example, royalties paid to suppliers for implementation of hepatitis C viral genomic screening techniques and pathogen inactivation techniques have been the subject of conferences organized by the EBA. This organization also cooperates with international organizations, particularly the American Association of Blood Banks (AABB) and, since 2004, with the Alliance of Blood Operators (ABO), the Blood Services of the American Red Cross, the Blood Services of the Australian Red Cross, and the Canadian Blood Service. The EBA also has independent relations with the Food and Drug Administration through a Memorandum of Understanding (MOU) in view of harmonizing requirements and decision-making processes, and to promote blood product quality and safety in Europe and North America.

In terms of strategic planning, the priorities established for EBA actions for the 2004-2008 period are:

– influence European legislation governing blood, blood products and blood services, as well as tissues, cells and organs;

– gather and share information regarding the state of the art in the field of transfusion, in order to apply it to transfusion medicine practices;

– follow developments, marketing and price setting for new technologies and new equipment in the field of blood transfusion, to achieve efficacy objectives;

– prepare opinion statements in the form of articles and position papers.

Another private European organization was created in 2002: the European Network of Learned Societies in Transfusion Medicine (EuroNet-TMS).

This Network brings together 6000 professionals from transfusion centers in seventeen countries, sixteen of which are in the European Union.

These are the same countries as those belonging to the EBA, plus Spain, Greece, Italy, Sweden and Switzerland. For Belgium, Finland, the Irish Republic and Luxembourg, national blood societies or Red Cross blood societies have been included in the network, in the absence of learned societies. The main objectives of the European Network of Learned Societies in Transfusion Medicine EuroNet-TMS [9] are:

– provide coherent answers to the issues at stake in the European sphere of transfusion medicine;

– promote medical and scientific developments in transfusion medicine in Europe;

– ensure the highest possible and most up-to-date scientific level in order to set safety and quality standards that will provide uniform transfusion services to European citizens;

– share knowledge and information in Europe;

– develop interfaces with decision-making authorities, taking into account the diversity of European countries.

Work groups within the Network have made it possible to define points of agreement and disagreement on major subjects: organization of transfusion establishments in Europe, price of blood products, role of viral genomic screening for the hepatitis C virus, criteria for clinical use of blood products, donor selection [9], and initial and permanent training in transfusion medicine [10]. All the information provided by Euro Net-TMS has recently been published in a "White Book" [11].

Other private national or international organizations participate in exchanges with the European Commission regarding the preparation of European legislative acts.

These are mainly national and international voluntary blood donor organizations, including the International Blood transfusion Society, the World Health Organization and the International Plasma Fractionation Association (IPFA) which replaced the European EPFA in 2004. The latter was comprised of non profit organizations involved in plasma fractionation, such as the International Federation of Blood Donor Organizations (IFBDO), the European Transfusion Medicine School (ETMS) and the Red Cross.

Finally, a functional network operates alongside these private European organizations. Known as the European Hemovigilance Network (EHN), it was created in 1998 and now has ten full members (Belgium, Denmark, Finland, France, Greece, Luxembourg, the Netherlands, Portugal, the Irish Republic, the United Kingdom) and three associate members (Canada, Norway, Switzerland).

The objectives of the European Hemovigilance Network are :

– facilitate exchange of valid information among members;

– encourage joint activities of members;

– organize training activities for members, in the field of hemovigilance.

In order to achieve these objectives, the following measures have been taken :

– creation and maintenance of a web site (http://www.ehn-org.net);

– introduction of a rapid alert system;
– start of process and official form standardization, through use of a common model;
– compiling and analysis of European data generated by national hemovigilance systems;
– organization of European hemovigilance seminars [12]. This network also provides assistance in the application of Directive 2002/98/EC regarding traceability practices and the reporting of adverse events.

Overview of Regulations

European regulations currently governing blood products are essentially comprised of four directives.

• **Directive 2002/98/EC, January 27, 2003 [6],** commonly called the "mother" directive, was introduced to fill a gap in an incomplete regulatory framework. The 2001/83/EC directive [13] issued on November 6, 2001 had established quality, safety and efficacy requirements for medicinal products industrially manufactured from human blood or plasma, but had not included requirements for human origin plasma and blood cells. The objective of Directive 2002/98/EC is to establish quality and safety standards for human blood and blood components, in order to ensure a high degree of human health protection. Application of the requirements of the directive falls under the responsibility of a competent authority (or several competent authorities) appointed by Member States. An annexe presents the information to be provided by the blood transfusion establishment to the competent authority in order to obtain accreditation; in addition to general information, an organizational chart, quality manual, number and qualification of employees, hygiene measures, premises and equipment, and a list of standardized operational procedures in the fields involved have to be supplied. The blood transfusion establishment cannot make any substantial changes in these activities without prior written consent from the competent authority, which can withdraw this consent if an inspection or control measures show that the transfusion establishment in question does not respect Directive requirements. The competent authority organizes appropriate inspections and control measures in blood transfusion establishments in order to ensure compliance with these requirements. The interval between two inspections or control measures must not exceed two years.

Each blood transfusion establishment appoints a "responsible person" entrusted with:

– ensuring that each blood or blood component unit was collected, controlled, processed, stored and distributed in conformity with the legislation in force in the Member State involved;

– communicating information to competent authorities during the transfusion establishment accreditation procedure;

– application in the blood transfusion establishment of the requirements of the directive governing personnel training and qualification, the quality system, documents, data filing, donor and recipient traceability, and reporting of serious adverse reactions and events.

Concerning data protection and confidentiality, Member States take all necessary measures to ensure that all data, including genetic information, gathered in conformity with the directive, and to which third parties have access, is rendered anonymous, so that the donor cannot be identified.

Concerning blood donation and donors, the directive defines a general framework and refers to Directive 2004/33/EC concerning information to be provided to prospective donors, information to be provided by donors, donor eligibility (acceptance criteria and deferral criteria).

Concerning the voluntary character of donations, the directive states only that all necessary measures should be taken by the Member States to encourage voluntary, unpaid donations. Concerning (biological testing of donations), the directive only specifies, for whole blood and plasma donations, the obligation to determine groups ABO and Rh D, and to screen donors for hepatitis B (HBs antigen), hepatitis C (anti-HCV) and HIV 1/2 (anti-HIV 1/2), adding that supplementary tests could be required for particular blood components, donors or epidemiological situations. Concerning distribution, the directive distinguishes clearly between "distribution" in the sense of supply of blood and blood components to other transfusion establishments, hospital blood banks and manufacturers of blood and plasma-derived products; and "delivery" of blood and blood components destined for transfusion to one patient.

Concerning traceability, the directive indicates that Member States must take all necessary measures to ensure traceability from the donor to the recipient and vice-versa, of the blood and blood components collected, controlled, transformed and/or distributed on their national territories. The annexe specifies requirements for blood component labelling. Data required for traceability is conserved for at least thirty years.

The directive defines hemovigilance as the totality of procedures of organized surveillance regarding serious or unintended adverse reactions and events occurring in donors or recipients, as well as epidemiological donor follow-up. An "adverse event" is defined as an event related to collection, control, transformation, storage and distribution of blood and blood components. An "adverse reaction" can be observed in a donor or a patient; it is related to blood collection or to transfusion of blood or blood components. According to this definition of hemovigilance, Member States ensure that all serious adverse reactions and events are reported to a competent authority, knowing that transfusion establishments have a procedure making it possible to stop the distribution of blood and blood components associated with the report.

The directive refers to subsequent texts that provide a more precise definition of technical requirements and their adaptation to scientific and technical advances (Article 29, to which the Council of Europe made a considerable contribution) concerning in particular :

– traceability;

– information to provide to prospective donors;

– information required from donors;

– requirements for donor eligibility;

– storage, transport and distribution;

– blood and blood component quality and safety;

– autologous transfusion;

– European community norms and specifications relative to a quality system in blood transfusion centers;

– European community procedures for reporting of serious adverse reactions and events.

In conformity with the subsidiarity principle, the directive does not prevent a Member Sate from maintaining or introducing more stringent protection measures on its territory. This directive and the one below have been in force in Member States since February 8, 2005. Existing national norms can be maintained for nine additional months in blood transfusion establishments, in order to allow them to adapt to European requirements.

• **Directive 2004/33/EC, March 22, 2004 [7],** commonly called the first "daughter" directive, provides, particularly in its annexes, precise technical requirements concerning donation and donors, storage and distribution of blood and blood components, and quality control of blood and blood components.

Information to be given to prospective blood and blood component donors is presented in great detail. For homologous donations, this information consists mainly of didactic data on blood characteristics, donation procedure, blood-derived products and benefits to patients, reasons for the medical exam preceding the donation and for qualification of donations, the meaning of "informed consent", exemption, temporary and permanent referral, reasons for deferral, imperative reasons for donors to inform the transfusion establishment of events subsequent to donations that could render previous donations inappropriate for transfusion, the responsibility of the blood transfusion establishment to inform a donor of test results revealing an anomaly that could have consequences for the donor in question. For autologous blood collection, information concerns the possibility of exclusion and the reasons for it, the description of autologous collection procedures, an explanation regarding the fact that autologous blood and blood components might not be sufficient for the needs of the scheduled transfusion, and the reasons for discarding unused autologous blood and blood components, which cannot serve to transfuse other patients.

Information the blood transfusion establishment must obtain from donors at each donation includes donor identification, donor's state of health and his medical history obtained using a questionnaire and a personal interview conducted by a health care staff member, and donor signature. This signature, and the countersignature of the health care staff member on the questionnaire, confirm that the donor has read and understood the information provided, that he had the opportunity to ask questions, that he received satisfactory answers to these questions, that he gave his informed consent to the donation procedure, and that he confirms that, to his knowledge, all the information provided is accurate. For autologous collection, the signature indicates that the patient was informed of the possibility that the blood and blood components could be insufficient for the needs of the scheduled transfusion.

Donor eligibility criteria for whole blood and for blood component collection are given in an annexe. These criteria for whole blood and blood component donations include donor acceptance criteria (age and weight, blood hemoglobin levels, blood protein levels for plasma apheresis donations, platelet levels for platelet apheresis donations), as well as deferral criteria for donors of whole blood and of blood components (permanent and temporary deferral, and deferral in particular epidemiological settings), in view of risk prevention for the donor and for the patient. The annexe also specifies the main exclusion criteria for prospective autlogous donors.

Blood and blood component storage, transport and distribution conditions are presented at Annexe 4. Red blood cell concentrates (and whole blood in case of use for transfusion) must be stored at temperatures between +2 and +6 °C for a maximum duration of 28 to 49 days, depending on collection, processing and storage procedures.

Platelet preparations must be stored at temperatures between +20 to +24 °C for five days, or up to seven days if a bacterial contamination detection or reduction procedure is used. Transport and distribution of blood and blood components at all stages of the transfusion chain must be conducted in conditions guaranteeing product integrity. Autologous blood and blood components must be clearly identified as such, and must be stored, transported and distributed separately from homologous blood and blood components.

The directive defines acceptable results for labile blood product quality control; the required sampling frequency for the entire process is determined on the basis of statistical control of procedures. Thus, red blood cell concentrate hemolysis should not exceed 0.8%

of hemoglobin mass at the end of the storage period. The pH variations of platelet concentrates should not exceed 6.4 to 7.4 at the end of the storage period. The ratio of residual cells in fresh frozen plasma should not exceed 6.0×10^9 red blood cells/L, 0.1×10^9 leukocytes/L and 50×10^9 platelets/L. In addition, collection and manufacturing procedures must be subjected to adequate bacteriological control.

Finally, the directive indicates that Member States must ensure that all controls and procedures specified in the requirements must be validated; that is, objective proof must exist showing that the requirements can be satisfied permanently.

- **Directive 2005/61/EC, September 30, 2005** [14] describes in greater details the EU requirements concerning traceability and notification of serious adverse reactions and events. This directive will be in force in Member States at the latest on August 31, 2006.
- **Directive 2005/62/EC, September 30, 2005** [15] describes in greater details the Community standards and specifications relating to a quality system for blood establishments. This directive has been in force in Member States since October 21, 2005.

Overview of Operations

Since 2001, the Council of Europe publishes an annual report (previously published every two years, between 1989 and 1997) on the control (biological qualification) and use of blood and blood products. The report is based on a questionnaire submitted to Council of Europe Member States (including EU Member States). The 2003 report [16] and other data [11, 12, 17-20] provide a useful picture of the European transfusion context in Europe. Although these data are still incomplete (response rate to the Council questionnaire for 2003 averaged 64%), it is important to present a brief description of current transfusion activities across Europe and their organization.

Analysis [12, 17] points, first of all, to organizational heterogeneity. In the fifteen countries comprising the European Union in 2003, only eight had a unified transfusion system, either a national blood service (France, Netherlands, countries in the United Kingdom and the Irish Republic), or a blood service of the national Red Cross (Austria, Belgium, Finland, Luxembourg). The other countries have blood transfusion centers connected with hospitals, either exclusively (Denmark, Italy) or also connected to some extent with Red Cross transfusion centers (Germany), with regional centers (Spain, Sweden), with a Blood Institute (Portugal) or with a national Center for Hemovigilance Coordination (Greece).

The 2003 report of the Council of Europe [16] provides data on seventeen European Union countries that answered the questionnaire (the other eight did not answer). Out of these seventeen countries, sixteen indicated that their blood transfusion centers possess established and active quality assurance (QA) systems, and fifteen countries reported that 100% of donations are covered by Good Practices. Complete coverage by a quality assurance system conforming to Norm ISO 9000 was reported by three countries (Austria, France, Luxembourg). Complete coverage by another system has been declared to exist in one country (Latvia). A national authority conducts inspections at least once every two years in fifteen countries; in one country, another organization conducts the inspections. (There is only one country where inspections are not conducted every two years.)

Council of Europe data on these seventeen countries show the number of donors to vary between 10.9 to 67.4/1,000 inhabitants, with an average of 33.1 (*Table II*). The Council of Europe considers that a rate below 13/1,000 inhabitants can cause supply problems, and that a rate of 30/1,000 inhabitants is an attainable objective. However, these figures must be interpreted with caution because they do not necessarily distinguish between "active" donors and "inactive" donors in the data bases of blood transfusion establishments. In addition, donors registered in these data bases as having made a first donation vary between 5.6% and 43.1%, and in Denmark first-time donors are only subjected to an exam (with no donation). They can only make a first donation if the results of this exam conform to requirements. The number of whole blood donations, the main source of red blood cell concentrates (RCC) and of plasma for fractionation, except in Denmark (where 99.8% of red blood cell concentrates come from apheresis), varies between 22.9% and 61.8/1000 inhabitants (average : 45.0), with an autologous unit rate between 0% to 4.2% (average : 1.2). In the ten countries where it has been introduced, erythropheresis produces less than 1% of red blood cell concentrates, except in Norway (2.3%) and Denmark as previously mentioned.

The volume of apheresis plasma varies between 0 and 30.3 L/1000 inhabitants (average : 5.1 L), with a ≥ 10L volume in three countries (Germany, Luxembourg, Sweden), witnessing active involvement in plasmapheresis programs in these countries. Supplies of plasma for fractionation vary between 0 and 30.1 L/1000 inhabitants.

Table II. Quantitative data on donors and whole blood donation in seventeen EU countries that responded to the Council of Europe annual survey for 2003 [14].

Country	Inhabitants x 1,000	Donors/1,000 inhabitants	First-time donors %	Whole blood units collected/ 1,000 inhabitants	Autologous whole blood %
Austria	8,174	67.4	8.3	61.8	2.6
Belgium	10,000	26.9	14.5	50.3	0.3
Czech Republic	10,300	35.5	9.1	41.9	4.2
Denmark	5,000	47.4	*	0.2	-
Finland	5,220	32.2	11.3	57	0
France	60,186	25.6	22.4	36.7	2.9
Germany	82,532	28.6	24.1	56.1	3.9
Greece	10,500	34.2	16.2	57.1	0.8
Irish Republic	3,917	-	-	37.2	0
Latvia	2,300	21.2	26.9	24.5	0
Luxembourg	435	31.3	5.6	50.1	1.7
Netherlands	16,193	31.5	6.9	41.5	0.1
Norway	4,577	22.9	13.2	43.6	0
Poland	38,500	10.9	43.1	22.9	0.3
Slovenia	1,964	54.4	10.5	43.2	2.2
Sweden	9,873	30.5	13.3	48.7	0.1
United Kingdom	58,785	29.4	17.2	46.8	0

* No donation at the time of the first coming.

Use of labile blood products is only reflected in labile blood product deliveries to hospitals and clinics, since data on their use in these institutions is difficult to obtain in most countries.

Whole blood transfusion is limited in all countries. Figures shown (*Table III*) for use of red blood cell concentrates vary between 21.6 and 70.8/1,000 inhabitants (average : 43.1). Number of platelet concentrates (PC) transfused varies between 1.04 and 18.9/1,000 inhabitants (average: 6.2); PC/RCC ratio in transfused units varies between 0.05 and 0.40 (average: 0.13) and ratio of apheresis platelet concentrate (APC)/APC+ mixture of platelet concentrates from whole blood (MPC) varies between 0.02 and 0.88 (average : 0.40). Use of fresh frozen plasma (FFP) varies between 3.9 and 20.9 U/1,000 inhabitants (average: 10.3), and FFP/RCC ratio in transfused units varies between 0.10 and 0.96 (average 0.27). 100% leukodepletion is reported by nine of the seventeen countries for red blood cell concentrates and fresh frozen plasma, and by eleven of the seventeen countries for platelet concentrates. Fresh frozen plasma is subjected to safety assurance by quarantine or by inactivation (using solvent and detergent, or methylene blue) in ten of the seventeen countries (100% inactivation in three countries, 100% safety assurance by quarantine in three countries, and by the two procedures combined in one country).

Tableau III. Quantitative data on the use of labile blood products, reflected in deliveries to health institutions in the seventeen European Union countries that responded to the Council of Europe annual survey for 2003 [14].

Country	RCC / 1,000 h	PC (U) / 1,000 inh	PC/RCC (U)	APC/PC (U)	FFP (U) / 1,000 inh	FFP/RCC (U)
Austria	54.7	4.89	0.09	0.57	10.89	0.2
Belgium	47.8	3.80	0.08	0.28	9.23	0.19
Czech Republic	40.2	2.19	0.05	0.75	3.9	0.1
Denmark	70.8	18.95	0.27	0.04	12.15	0.17
Finland	51.9	6.07	0.12	0.02	8.25	0.16
France	32.4	3.32	0.10	0.88	4.41	0.14
Germany	50.2	4.04	0.08	0.66	15.81	0.31
Greece	57.1	12.63	0.22	0.13	14.69	0.26
Irish Republic	33.2	4.22	0.13	0.41	5.66	0.17
Latvia	21.6	1.80	0.08	0.78	20.86	0.96
Luxembourg	45.6	18.42	0.40	0.46	8.55	0.19
Netherlands	37.6	2.92	0.08	0.03	6.89	0.22
Norway	40.1	2.99	0.07	0.31	8.67	0.22
Poland	21.6	1.04	0.05	0.58	9.24	0.43
Slovenia	39.7	11.07	0.28	0.05	16.63	0.41
Sweden	45.1	3.29	0.07	0.41	12.25	0.27
United Kingdom	43.7	4.53	0.10	0.38	6.42	0.15

Biological qualification of donations applies at least the minimum criteria set by Directive 2002/98/EC [6] : detection of anti-HIV-1 and HIV-2 antibody, detection of HBs antigens and detection of anti HCV antibodies, in all seventeen countries. Detection of syphilis is added in sixteen of the seventeen countries (only one of them tests first-time donors). Detection of anti-HTLV-I and II antibody is added in ten countries (only four of them test first-time donors); detection of anti-HBc antibody is added in six countries (only four test first-time donors). Viral genomic screening for the hepatitis C virus is performed on all donations in thirteen of the seventeen countries; viral genomic testing for human immunodeficiency virus is performed in eight out of the seventeen countries, and testing for hepatitis B is performed in two of the seventeen countries. These three viral genomic tests are applied to plasma for fractionation in only two countries.

Prevalences (frequency of positive results for donors tested for the first time) vary from one country to another between 1 and 30 for HIV, and between 1 and 250 for HBV and HCV.

Incidence rates (frequency of seroconversion in repeat donors) vary from country to country between 1 and 50 for HIV, 1 and 400 for HBV, and 1 and 1,000 for HCV. These variations depend in part on methods of detection, on prevalence and incidence of these viral infections in the general population of each Member State, and on the effectiveness of clinical selection of prospective donors. A survey conducted in 2003 in the fifteen countries of the European Union and in Switzerland [18] revealed that prospective donors in different countries are asked very similar questions, but that deferral periods for various contraindications are very different. At present, available data is still too incomplete to allow even approximate evaluation of actual results of prospective donor selection for homologous blood (rates and reasons for deferral).

Hemovigilance is organized within the scope of activities of the national blood service or of another national organization in sixteen countries of the European Union [16, 20]. Reporting of serious adverse reactions and events has become mandatory in all EU countries since October 21, 2005. Until recently reporting was done on a voluntary basis in all the Member States but four. This no doubt explains the great variations observed in frequency of adverse events : between 7 and 350/10,000 [12].

This data highlights the great heterogeneity existing in all transfusion medicine activities, from the donor to the recipient. This situation is difficult to interpret in the absence of more precise data, particularly in terms of satisfaction of labile blood product needs, loss and destruction of labile blood products, as well as frequency of transfusion-related events on the one hand, and absence or delay of transfusion on the other.

European Transfusion Tomorrow

To pave the way for future changes in transfusion medicine, we must first apply the existing European directives. Member States have reported different kinds of problems. Solutions will have to be found so that the minimal norms defined by this European legislation can be applied uniformly in all Member States. Updating of European recent regulations will constitute a second essential step toward the future. Moreover, true harmonization of practices should eventually make it possible for patients in all EU Member States, and beyond the sphere of the Council of Europe, to obtain quality transfusion services of equal effectiveness and safety, in the most efficient manner possible.

This harmonization will benefit from European scale research and training activities.

Application of European legislation

Although current European legislation was drafted with the participation of representatives of all Member States, and although this legislation sets minimum quality standards, application of certain stipulations of Directives 2002/98/EC and 2004/33/EC raises unavoidable difficulties. At the organizational level, designation by Member States of one or more authorities responsible for the application of Directive 2002/98/EC is a problem for States that did not yet possess a national blood service or a national organization in charge of transfusion and/or hemovigilance. Similarly, designation of a "responsible person" constituted a problem –now solved– for Germany, which previously had two such persons (one responsible for production and one responsible for control) [21]. The United Kingdom had to change its regulations to avoid suspension of its transfusion activities due to the stipulation that the pre-donation interview be conducted by a "medical sector professional". Strict transposition of the European Directive would have required that this country entrust doctors and nurses with a function now performed by donor carers under the supervision of a doctor or a nurse [22]. A specific modification of the United Kingdom regulation solved this problem. In terms of donor selection, imposing a pre-donation hemoglobin level of 125 g/L for women and 135g/L for men as a condition for eligibility, a legitimate measure from the public health perspective, particularly for women, poses a problem in the United Kingdom and in France.

In the United Kingdom, the raising of this threshold, which had previously been set at 120 g/L and 130 g/L [23], will unavoidably lead to a loss of donors [22]. This foreseeable loss of donors will occur to a greater extent in France, which had not previously applied this criterion to donor selection. Directive 2004/33/EC has impelled this country to rapidly complete the studies necessary for the rational introduction of this criterion by improving existing methods, that were neither sensitive nor specific [24]. France also will use this opportunity to consider medical treatment of iron deficiency very often associated with anemia in women blood donors [25]. Finally, as a last example in a list that is not exhaustive, in hemovigilance systems based until now on voluntary reporting, introducing reporting to a competent authority of all serious adverse events related to a transfusion chain stage, from collection to distribution, and all serious adverse reactions observed during or following transfusion, will no doubt constitute a difficulty to overcome.

For all these situations, only close cooperation between operators (blood transfusion centers, hospital blood banks) and the health authorities governing them can lead to effective and smooth transposition. Sharing successful experiences among countries should be encouraged, and will no doubt prove useful. Financing of these measures must be assessed and planned in each Member Sate.

Changes in Legislation

Directive 2002/98/EC announced in its Article 29 that certain technical requirements would be addressed specifically in subsequent directives. The first of these was a "daughter" directive (2004/33/EC) that defined a number of requirements (see below).

This was followed by two other "daughter" directives, dealing specifically with requirements regarding traceability, with community norms and specifications relative to a quality system in blood transfusion establishments, and with community procedures for reporting serious adverse events and reactions, including modalities of reporting. In addition to these recent changes in legislation, regulations will have to be updated to correspond to advances in the state of the art.

This work of completion of the first stages of the European regulatory process and of its subsequent development, will be carried out mainly by groups of experts representing Member States before the European Commission. We encourage each State to appoint veritable expert practitioners in the field of transfusion, who are also familiar with the preparation of European regulatory documents, and who work in close cooperation with health authorities responsible for this field in their respective States.

It is highly desirable that the Commission make optimal use of Council of Europe expertise, avoiding wherever possible discrepancies between Council recommendations and

European regulations. In this context, the European Blood Alliance (and other private organizations) should also be encouraged to provide advice, in order to keep Commission requirements from exceeding the specifications provided by the European Union (avoid overly detailed texts), and especially in order to achieve real efficacy/applicability in the interest of patients. Finally, it would be advisable that countries which decide to apply more stringent regulations than those outlined by European legislation avoid excessive measures that do not provide real benefits to patients. Here again, sharing acquired experience among Member States will be a considerable asset.

Harmonization of Practices

Council of Europe recommendations, widely disseminated for many years, and more recently European regulations, which together contributed to the creation and/or development of national blood services, have been and will continue to be powerful harmonizing factors in the activities of transfusion centers and hospital blood banks. However, in order for harmonization to continue, we will have to devise additional tools for collecting the data needed to analyze and better understand organizational and technical differences in the various processes of the transfusion chain, from collection (including soliciting and selection of prospective donors) and all the way to distribution in transfusion centers and hospital blood banks, and to hemovigilance. This data includes results of screening for infectious agents, and epidemiological data concerning general population donors. In our opinion, in blood transfusion establishments, it is donation medicine, still very heterogenous in its practices, from recruitment and informing of donors to selection of prospective donors, that will benefit the most from harmonization of practices. The survey tool for prospective candidate selection, introduced by the European Network of Transfusion Medicine Learned Societies EuroNet TMS [18], and a recent complementary survey [26], should make it possible to measure the impact of Directive 2004/33/EC on harmonization, and should lead to the discovery of shared solutions. In this context, countries that apply ethical principles of unpaid donations and absence of profit for organizations in charge of labile blood product collection, processing, control and distribution should promote the widest possible dissemination of these principles, in order to prevent possible commercial exploitation of these human origin products.

Another portion of the transfusion chain should reap great benefits from European improvements: the portion located in health institutions and, more specifically, at the patient's bedside. In fact, indications for labile blood product transfusion, and important transfusion safety factors for patients in health institutions, have eluded and will probably elude for a long time the influence of European regulations. Indications on transfusion practice are given in Council of Europe Guide [5, p.239-257], and the recent publication of product characteristic summaries by the Council of Europe completes the previous recommendations providing specific indications for each labile blood product. Despite this, it is in this area that we still see many errors that could compromise the safety of recipients [27-30]. The Council of Europe, the European Blood Alliance and the Learned Societies Network are the organizations best equipped to prepare recommendations, distribute them to each Member State and design the tools necessary for observing their impact. In this area, the objective should be very clear : concrete reduction of frequency of human error at each stage of the transfusion chain, and particularly in health institutions, where the health of patients can be affected.

In the same way, these organizations should issue recommendations serving to reiterate and update the indications established for transfusion of each labile blood product. The goal is to reduce the considerable heterogeneity of European indications, demonstrated at least in part by the heterogeneity of labile blood products transfused per 1,000 inhabitants [11, 16]. This reminder of the absolute necessity of respecting recognized indications should contribute, in the future, to renewed efforts toward achieving self-sufficiency.

In fact, the aging of the population and treatment of increasing numbers of patients with leukemia or cancer, at a more and more advanced age and requiring transfusion, could increase the need for labile blood products. Keeping this in mind, we can appreciate that strict respect of recognized indications will contribute to better organize the sharing of these precious resources.

Research

We believe it to be essential that in the future Europe avail itself of more active research in all domains of transfusion medicine. At present, research is most active in the area of epidemiology of infectious diseases transmissible by labile blood products. Every Member State is concerned with prevention of transfusion-related risk, and considerable resources are invested in the pursuit of this research. This research was recently applied to the Creutzfeldt-Jakob disease variant, and resulted in the deferral of prospective donors who had been transfused – a measure that was gradually extended to many European countries. The West Nile virus was also subjected to research, leading to changes in donor selection at the clinical level. But other risks are also the focus of very diversified measures. For example, the risk of *Trypanosomas cruzii* (Chagas disease) and the risk of transmission of viral diseases associated with certain sexual behaviors (sexual relations with partners from, or having lived in, Sub-Sahara Africa). Only examination of the relevant epidemiological data obtained by conducting systematic research will make it possible to assess, to validate and constantly measure the impact of new clinical donor selection procedures, as well as of new tests used to detect viral pathologies (viral genomic screening) or bacterial infection (bacterial screening for labile blood products, and of pathogen inactivation methods. In these areas, the multicenter BOTIA project (Blood and Organ Transmissible Infectious Agents) is a good example of a joint European research project. Countries constituting the BOTIA group are : England, Belgium, Spain, France, Italy and the Netherlands. This project has recently been granted financial support by the European Commission, for a three-year period. The objective of the project is to create a European repository of donor and receiver samples collected before and after transfusion or transplant, to use this repository to determine transmissibility of emergent agent epidemiology, to contribute to the constant improvement of blood donor selection criteria, and to identify the limitations and shortcomings of existing preventive measures [31]. Data produced by this research will be made available to health authorities.

Economic health costs in transfusion medicine constitute, in our opinion, a research topic that has to be developed. Undoubtedly, the objective is to provide Member States with the most efficient solutions, that is, the best solutions in terms of state of the art, offering the highest level of transfusion safety, at the lowest cost. This applies, first of all, to medical activities per se, such as regular reassessment of indications for labile blood product transfusion. Thus, research on thresholds for transfusion of homologous red blood cell concentrates, or on rules defining platelet concentrate doses to be transfused, in view of what has been published [32-34], should allow regular updating of rules for labile blood product use, in order to keep this use to a minimum and increase availability potential. Research on alternatives to labile blood product transfusion and associated therapies, particularly biotherapies (cellular and gene therapies) must, of course, be part of the activities that prepare the future. The same is true of analysis and prevention of labile blood product transfusion complications that are still fatal today, such as immunohematologic incompatibility accidents [30] or transfusion related acute lung injuries (TRALI) [35]. Research must also serve to evaluate the cost/benefit ratio in existing and future organizational systems. For example, this type of research should clarify the nature of interconnections, in each Member State, between blood transfusion establishments and health institutions, to ensure the best transfusion services at all times, without taking the risk of endangering the patient's life due to delay or absence of transfusion [36]. The same scientific principles apply to evaluation of the cost/benefit ratio when a new method or new equipment (including automation and computer systems) is developed and proposed by a supplier, in all areas of transfusion medicine.

Teaching

A report on initial training and continued education in transfusion medicine, drawn up for the purposes of a survey conducted by the European Network of Transfusion Medicine Learned Societies [10, 11], revealed great discrepancies between countries of the European Union. Extremes go from absence of training in transfusion medicine in medical study programs, to absence of a recognized transfusion medicine specialty. Diplomas for practice in a transfusion establishment or a hospital blood bank are very different from one country to another, for doctors as well as for nurses and laboratory technicians. At present, to our knowledge, the Council of Europe and the European School of Transfusion Medicine are the two institutions providing initial training and continued education in different European countries. Nevertheless, in the Europe of tomorrow, transfusion medicine will have to define common modalities of initial training for doctors, pharmacists and scientists working in transfusion establishments, as well as for the nurses and laboratory technicians in these establishments. Common training will also have to be provided to doctors who prescribe labile blood products and transfuse them to patients. Organizing a truly European education in transfusion medicine also involves developing the necessary teaching tools (including access to knowledge and its evaluation through computerized information exchange), in order to ensure qualification of the personnel involved and to check, on a regular basis, the updating of personnel skills in their respective domains. Teaching organized on a European scale will be fundamental to sharing of knowledge and experience, and to the harmonization of practices in all the fields of activity of the transfusion chain.

Conclusion

Professionals in the transfusion field today are inadequately informed regarding the functioning of European institutions responsible for transfusion medicine activities, particularly the European Union and the Council of Europe. It is important that information regarding their role be widely disseminated in every Member State. Awareness of the contribution of European institutions to continued improvement of transfusion activities in the interest of patient safety, and based on respect of fundamental ethical principles applying to blood donation and to transfusion, will lead to reduction of differences between countries, especially regarding indications for use of labile blood products, the reporting of transfusion-related events, and therefore transfusion safety for European citizens.

Acknowledgements

The author wishes to thank Frances Delaney, Karl-Friedrich Bopp, Emmanuelle Jean, Eila Sandborg and Claudio Velati, for providing documents and/or documentary sources that made it possible to prepare this article. The views and opinions expressed are those of the author and do not necessarily reflect those of the organizations in which the author conducts his work.

References

1. Institutions of the European Union. http://europa.eu.int/institutions/index fr.html
2. L'Union Européenne. http://www.senat.fr/europe/diaporama_2004.html
3. Council of Europe. http// www.coe.int
4. Genetet B. *Blood transfusion: half a century of contribution by the Council of Europe.* Strasbourg : Council of Europe Publishing, 1998 : 1-41.
5. *Guide to the preparation, use and quality assurance of blood components* - 11th ed. Strasbourg : Council of Europe Publishing, 2005 : 1-257.
6. Directive 2002/98/EC of the European Parliament and of the Council of 27 January 2003 setting standards of quality and safety for the collection, testing, processing, storage and distribution of human blood and blood components and amending Directive 2001/83/EC. *Official Journal of the European Union* of 02/08/2003.
7. Commission Directive 2004/33/EC of 22 March 2004 implementing Directive 2002/98/EC of the European Parliament and of the Council as regards certain technical requirements for blood and blood components. *Official Journal of the European Union* of 03/30/2004.
8. Leikola J, van Aken WG. European Blood Alliance Founded. *Vox Sang* 1998 ; 75 : 259.
9. Rouger P. Transfusion medicine in Europe. *Transfus Clin Biol* 2004 ; 11 : 11-4.
10. Müller N. Training and education – with a view of the involvement in Germany. *Transfus Clin Biol* 2004 ; 11 : 15-7.
11. Rouger P, Hossenlopp C. Blood transfusion in Europe. *The White Book 2005.* Ronquette MJ, éd. Paris, 2005 : 21-285.
12. Faber JC. Work of the European Haemovigilance Network (EHN). *Transfus Clin Biol* 2004 ; 11 : 2-10.
13. Directive 2001/83/EC of the European Parliament and of the Council of 6 November 2001 on the Community code relating to medicinal products for human use. *Official Journal of the European Union* of 11/28/2001.
14. Commission Directive 2005/61/EC of 30 September 2005 implementing Directive 2002/98/EC of the European Parliament and of the Council as regards traceability requirements and notification of serious adverse reactions and events. *Official Journal of the European Union* of 10/01/2005.
15. Commission Directive 2005/62/EC of 30 September 2005 implementing Directive 2002/98/EC of the European Parliament and of the Council as regards Community standards and specifications relating to a quality system for blood establishments. *Official Journal of the European Union* of 10/01/2005.
16. Folléa G. Donor selection : similarities and discrepancies throughout Europe. Communication. 11th EURO'SAT (Seminars for advances in transfusion). Paris, 21/10/2003.
17. Velati C. Le réseau européen des sociétés savants de Médecine Transfusionnelle (EuroNet-TMS). Communication. Les 10 ans de l'Institut National de Transfusion Sanguine. Paris, 28 juin 2004.
18. Faber JC. The European Blood Directive : a new era of blood regulation has begun. *Transfus Med* 2004 ; 14 : 257-73.
19. Müller N. The EU-Directive from the German point of view. *Transfus Today* 2005 ; 62 : 11.
20. Robinson AE. The European Union : blood safety & quality regulations 2005. *Transfus Today* 2005 ; 62 : 6-7.
21. Boulton F. Threshold concentration of haemoglobin in donor blood. *Vox Sang* 1999 ; 77 : 108-9.

22. James V, Jones KF, Turner EM, Sokol RJ. Statistical analysis of inappropriate results from current Hb screening methods for blood donors. *Transfusion* 2003 ; 43 : 400-4.
23. Boulton F. Managing donors an iron deficiency. *Vox Sang* 2004 ; 87 (Suppl. 2) : S22-S24.
24. Folléa G. Donor selection throughout Europe. Communication XVth ISBT European Regional Conference. Athens 5/07/2005.
25. Baele PL, De Bruyere M, Deneys V, Dupont E, Flament J, Lambermont M, Latinne D, Steensens L, Van Camp B, Waterloos H. Bedside transfusion errors. A prospective survey by the Belgium SAnGUIS Group. *Vox Sang* 1994 ; 66 : 117-21.
26. Andreu G, Morel P, Forestier F, Debeir J, Rebibo D, Janvier G, Herve P. Hemovigilance network in France : organization and analysis of immediate transfusion incident reports from 1994 to 1998. *Transfusion* 2002 ; 42 : 1356-64.
27. Serious Hazards of Transfusion Annual Report 2003. Manchester, UK : Serious Hazards of Transfusion Office, Manchester Blood Centre ; 2004.
28. Rouger P. Evolution des risques transfusionnels en 15 ans (1987-2002). *Ann Fr Anesth Réan* 2004 ; 23 : 1102-6.
29. Lefrère JJ. Le projet BOTIA ("Blood and Organ Infectious Agents"): une biothèque et un observatoire européens des agents transmissibles par le sang ou la greffe d'organes. *Transfus Clin Biol* 2005 ; 12 : 93-4.
30. Hebert PC, Wells G, Blajchman MA, Marshall J, Martin C, Pagliarello G, Tweeddale M, Schweitzer I, Yetisir E. A multicenter, randomized, controlled clinical trial of transfusion requirements in critical care. Transfusion Requirements in Critical Care Investigators, Canadian Critical Care Trials Group. *N Engl J Med* 1999 ; 340 : 409-17.
31. Tinmouth A, Tannnock IF, Crump M, Tomlinson G, Brandwein J, Minden M, Sutton D. Low-dose prophylactic platelet transfusions in recipients of an autologous peripheral blood progenitor cell transplant and patients with acute leukaemia: a randomized controlled trial with a sequential Bayesian design. *Transfusion* 2004 ; 44 : 1711-9.
32. Sensebe L, Giraudeau B, Bardiaux L, Deconinck E, Schmidt A, Bidet ML, Leniger C, Hardy E, Babault C, Senecal D. The efficiency of transfusing high doses of platelets in hematologic patients with thrombocytopenia : results of a prospective, randomized, open, blinded end point (PROBE) study. *Blood* 2005 ; 105 : 862-4.
33. Kleinman S, Caulfield T, Chan P, Davenport R, McFarland J, McPhedran S, Meade M, Morrison D, Pinsent T, Robillard P, Slinger P. Toward an understanding of transfusion-related acute lung injury: statement of a consensus panel. *Transfusion* 2004 ; 44 : 1774-89.
34. Lienhart A, Auroy Y, Péquignot F, Benhamou D, Jougla E. Premières leçons de l'enquête « mortalité » Sfar – Inserm. In : *Conférences d'actualisation 2003. 45ème Congrès national d'anesthésie et de réanimation.* Paris : Elsevier, 2003 : 203-18.

Transfusion Medicine and Hospitals: the Need for Cooperation

The French Experience

Jean-Yves Muller, Philippe Richebe, Véronique Betbèze, Pierre Fialon, Gérard Janvier

Blood transfusion, as a medical procedure, requires, first of all, collaboration between transfusion medicine and hospitals. Implementation of this procedure, and its effectiveness, depend on health institutions functioning in a well-established scientific and economic system. Secondly, there is a relational imperative engendered by the sharing of common structures. In fact, these relations are governed by decisions made in the course of meetings of the Transfusion Safety and Hemovigilance Committee, where questions involving both health institutions and blood transfusion establishments are debated.

The primary objective of collaboration between transfusion medicine and hospitals should be to ensure that the transfusion procedure makes the object of training, and of regular review by the two sectors: health institutions and blood transfusion establishments, particularly in regard to safety, by means of the most complete traceability possible for products that are delivered and transfused. The relation between the two sectors should take into account the financial aspects of blood product prescription, and the two sectors should evaluate professional practices and the effectiveness of prescriptions. These points will be discussed throughout this chapter.

The relation between the transfusion sector and hospitals is based on complementary functions at the medical, as well as the organizational and administrative levels.

At the medical level, the various actions leading to or ensuing from blood transfusion proceed in succession or take place at the same time, in view of attaining two objectives: to treat the patient and to prevent iatrogenic pathologies. Long before arriving at transfusion, prevention of fetal-maternal isoimmunization, which in turn prevents Rh isoimmunization, contributes to preventing potentially dangerous immunization in a future transfusion situation occurring in a life-and-death emergency. Other measures to protect the patient's "transfusion" future are taken during the transfusion itself or during its preparation; they also concern isoimmunization. In every situation, three partners are involved in the transfusion procedure: the health institute which prescribes it, performs it and follows it up, the transfusion establishment responsible for providing blood, and the immuno-hematology laboratory ensuring immunological transfusion safety by defining the immunological parameters of the transfusion product indicated for a particular patient. This three-way partnership is overseen by a hemovigilance system whose mission is to record adverse effects of blood transfusion and to take all necessary measures to improve transfusion practices. The hemovigilance system is inscribed in a supportive legal framework [1-3] and its triangular architecture is represented by clearly mandated actors in blood transfusion establishments, in health institutions and in regional health and social action Agencies: the hemovigilance actors [4].

This network is enhanced by an official structure acting as an interface between blood transfusion establishments and health institutions: the Transfusion Safety and Hemovigilance Committee. The presence of this Committee is mandatory in public health institutions, and is recommended in every private health institution where transfusion is practiced [3]. This structure is mandated to coordinate transfusion policy between the transfusion establishment and the health institution involved. Regional transfusion policy is also within its jurisdiction.

The relation between blood transfusion establishments and health institutions can be analyzed by examining the interface structures that help them to function by making constant adjustments. However, relations between the different partners can also be examined by analyzing the medical situations they face, and the tools created to help them manage each of these situations. In fact, each situation requires that transfusion practice adapt to circumstances, urgency, the possibility of pre-scheduling, location, and distance between actors.

These medical imperatives determine organizational modalities that are set out in detail in a large body of regulatory texts. Finally, institutional constraints and practices make it necessary that links between blood transfusion establishments and health institutions take multiple forms, to suit local circumstances.

But the fact remains that each particular case will have to develop administrative solutions that allow many different situations to conform to the regulatory context, while respecting medical imperatives. This logical sequence that should govern the relation between health institutions and blood transfusion establishments: medical requirements first, then organizational solutions and finally administrative considerations - is not always respected.

When it is not, the weight of administrative structures and the organizational constraints imposed without analysis of medical needs often impede harmonious functioning. At the administrative level, by which we mean the nature and focus of the structures collaborating to administer the transfusion process, we feel it is interesting to see how these structures, different in status, size and management style, can influence the implementation of the transfusion process.

Medical Relations

Medical Basis for Prescription of Labile Blood Products

Medical relations between the French National Blood Service (EFS) and health institutions are designed to set in place tools serving to satisfy the need for labile blood products used essentially in concrete situations, by ensuring availability and solving compatibility problems. The solutions provided must take into account constraints imposed by the biological origin of the product, which limits its availability and is the reason for its inherent risks. Patient safety and efficient use of labile blood products are at the core of medical relations involving blood transfusion. This means that personal interactions within the medical links between structures are sometimes built on uncertain definitions of fields of expertise and responsibilities assigned to each actor.

Principles of good use of labile blood products, in terms of indications, have been outlined in the documents produced by conferences of experts assembled under the aegis of the AFSSAPS. These principles constitute reference documents [5-8] based on evaluation of the medical-scientific evidence considered when drafting recommendations. Based on this evidence, relevance of transfusion indications is perfectly documented, and includes areas of uncertainty.

It is above all the dissemination of these documents serving as medical references, and their adaptation to local situations, that should constitute the basis of collaboration between the EFS and health institutions.

Availability of labile blood products in the right place, at the right time determines the efficacy of blood transfusion and is an essential aspect of medical relations between transfusion establishments and health institutions.

Availability does not constitute a problem when the establishments are close to each other, and when all the expertise of the transfusion establishment is located near the clinical centers of the health institution. But availability becomes a critical issue when the blood transfusion establishment is far from the hospital where urgent need of labile blood products is likely to arise. This problem of distance points out or generates difficulties related to surgery and to emergencies, mainly in four areas:

– advance prescriptions of autologous or homologous labile blood products for potential future use, and particularly for scheduled surgery;

– overprescription, also called precautionary prescription, to anticipate the possibility of more abundant hemorrhage than expected;

– prescriptions for staggered distribution of labile blood products for surgery in a health institution, in view of preventing excessive use by providing supplies at regular intervals only;

– supply of stocks for emergency use, before compatibility tests can be done and the appropriate labile blood products administered to the patient.

These stocks are supplied in accordance with regulations and consist of group O red blood cells. Extending the supply to other blood groups means attributing immuno-hematologic responsibility to the health institution; the extent of this responsibility must, however, be carefully evaluated.

This difficulty of guaranteeing availability of suitable labile blood products regardless of geographic location, clinical context and various types of patient care can be solved by creating coordinated links between blood banks and health institutions, to ensure adequate supply.

Use of safe and efficient transport systems is one possible solution.

When delivery time is not compatible with medical requirements, the most suitable solution is to create blood banks. These are distribution centers overseen jointly by health institutions and by the transfusion organization; they are governed by conventions between these two establishments, as well as by the initial authorization to open. These blood banks are intended to facilitate access to labile blood products. They can take different forms, depending on what is most suitable for health institutions and for blood transfusion establishments:

• **Emergency blood banks:** they provide a limited number of products: group O Rh negative red blood cell concentrates, and group AB fresh frozen plasma concentrates. These products are only provided in emergency transfusion situations that do not allow time for delivery of products from a blood bank.

- **Attribution blood banks:** they have a greater number of labile blood products, to allow attribution of matched products in group ABO, Rh and other groups, depending on phenotype. These banks must possess immuno-hematologic data and software for stock management, traceability and safety control, in conformity with good practice rules governing distribution.
- **Relay blood banks**, where labile blood products already assigned to specific patients by the blood transfusion establishment are stored during the perisurgical period or during a period of transfusion risk.
- **Blood banks serving to transmit blood products to another health institution:** this situation is accepted either on a regular basis or only in a life-and-death emergency. These situations, which are rare, must be governed by conventions between the health institutions involved and the blood bank, which define modes of functioning and the responsibilities of different actors. They are to be used only in geographical areas where no blood bank exists, but where there are health institutions conducting transfusion activities.

These different means of creating blood banks facilitate availability of labile blood products for health institutions located far from distribution sites.

However, they contribute to dispersion and blockage of labile blood product stocks. The health institution and the transfusion establishment must define the procedures between blood transfusion establishments and the blood banks, based on relevant regulations, needs and differences in types of organizations, particularly in terms of personnel training, transport, storage, distribution, emergency management and, if need be, return of labile blood products to the blood bank, so that the health institution can guarantee the transfusion center, at all times, storage conforming and identical to storage provided by the EFS.

Basic principles of transfusion compatibility are also well established.

However, data used to promote knowledge concerning them is not always easily accessible to clinicians. For example, current controversy and debate concerning research on irregular anti-erythrocytic antibodies in relation to dates of transfusion could be clarified by dissemination of the data justifying the recommendations, which would make the latter more understandable. Recommendations now being drafted concerning indications for prescribing pre-transfusion and post-transfusion exams similar to Regulatory Agency recommendations for indications for use of labile blood products, will produce this type of clarifying effect in the future. Decisions will take into account not only the opinion of immuno-hematology experts, but also the experience of different types of prescribers, in order to establish well-founded immunological rules helpful in clinical settings in which their application can be difficult [9]. Application of these rules is one of the goals of transfusion medicine, which dispenses transfusion advice through persons in charge of labile blood product distribution services.

In order for this advice to be safe and appropriate, the health institution must provide the EFS, through prescribing physicians, with data allowing suitable choice of labile blood products: transfusion history, isoimmunization, immunodeficiency, history of transfusion-related reactions, etc.

Transfusion Safety and Hemovigilance Committee

The Committee's role is to ensure, at the local level, medical coordination between the health institution and the EFS. It was created by a circular, issued on July 7, 1994 [3], as an adjunct to the code of Public Health (Art.R.66612-15). Its presence is mandatory in public health institutions that use labile blood products, and is recommended in private health institutions; its creation must be initiated by the Director of the institution. The legally stipulated composition of the Committee includes: the Director of the health institution, the director of the regional transfusion center distributing the blood products, hemovigilance directors of the health institution and the transfusion establishment, medical staff representatives, care givers, and representatives of medical-technical and administrative personnel, particularly those representing the main departments using labile blood products, the regional hemovigilance coordinator, and the head of the regional pharmacovigilance Center for medicinal blood-derived products.

The mission of the Transfusion Safety and Hemovigilance Committee is to monitor the application of transfusion rules and procedures, and to contribute, through its studies and proposals, to the improvement of safety for transfused patients.

The Committee is charged with coordinating hemovigilance actions conducted in the health institution and, in this context, is responsible to the departments involved for including in the patient's medical charts the transfusion file and, if necessary, a copy of a transfusion event report. In view of increasing hemovigilance efficacy, the Committee is also responsible for questions related to collaboration between corresponding systems in the transfusion establishment and the health institution, and more generally, for transfusion information dissemination. The Committee stays informed of the functioning of labile blood product banks; it must be advised of unexpected or undesirable transfusion-related events, and it must design all corrective measures. The Committee offers the medical commission of the health institution a transfusion safety training program for the personnel concerned, and provides the commission with an annual activity report.

Given that one of the functions of the Committee is to adapt national principles to local situations, it would be beneficial to create a National Transfusion Safety and Hemovigilance Committee whose role would be to examine problems encountered by health institutions in the application of general recommendations poorly adapted to certain medical or territorial conditions of transfusion use.

Hemovigilance

The definition of hemovigilance includes concepts of transfusion safety and epidemiological follow-up. In addition to advantages for individuals transfused, this definition allows identification of rare and even as yet unknown consequences of transfusion, that might occur months or years after administration of the labile blood product. Aside from strictly organizational and epidemiological considerations, it is important to ensure that systematic recording of adverse events does not become and end in itself, but continues to aim at systematic improvement of transfusion safety.

Traceability

The hemovigilance mission consists of implementing a double traceability:

– downstream traceability, going from the blood transfusion establishment to the health institution, which traces the use of each donation through the labile blood products and fractionation plasma originating from it;

– upstream traceability, going from the health institution to the regional transfusion center, which can trace the origin and history of each blood product administered, the original donation, the qualification tests, the processing and transformation conditions, and the distribution parameters.

These two types of traceability are completed by a third, which is horizontal; it consists of making an exhaustive list of all blood products received by each patient. For this traceability to be effective, each patient would have to be given a unique identification number, that would make it possible to gather together transfusion data from different health institutions connected with different regional EFS transfusion centers.

However, although in France traceability rates have not reached 100% for all health institutions and all transfusion establishments, labile blood product traceability, at least that of the first two types, accomplished thanks to close collaboration between blood transfusion establishments and health institutions, has nearly reached this objective in only a few years. In this context, hemovigilance plays the role of an active relay system, ensuring transmission of transfusion-related information between the establishments involved.

Today, there is no transfusion event for which we cannot identify, in a matter of hours, based on the labile blood products transfused, all the donations likely to be involved (upstream survey) and all the recipients of other products originating from the same donations (downstream survey). This type of information, when it exists, saves precious time, prevents risk of transcription errors and facilitates surveys. Numerous regional projects of transfusion traceability data exchange are being organized. These transfers are systematized by national guidelines that homogenize methods of file exchange, creating "revolving modes" with systematized data collection fields and reminders of safety rules such as coding, interface contracts and respect of safety and freedom requirements.

The Transfusion Event Reporting Form

This form constitutes a very valuable surveillance tool [10]. Its unique format makes it possible to gather all significant information on the conditions of occurrence of an adverse event during or subsequent to a transfusion, regardless of the degree of imputability of the transfusion. These events are graded according to their severity, and the grade determines their submission to regional or national authorities [10]. Responsibility for use of this document is shared by the hemovigilance systems of health institutions and the EFS, but the obligation to report the event is incumbent on any health professional who witnesses it or has knowledge of it. Relations of data exchange and sharing in real time between the health institution, the regional blood transfusion center, the EFS and the AFSSAPS are facilitated by the existence of a unique Internet information system (e-FIT).

Efficiency of the Hemovigilance Network

This system now makes possible a quantitative approach to the national transfusion event incidence program. It has contributed to attract attention to the scope, in terms of seriousness or frequency, of certain complications: for example, bacterial contamination of labile blood products subjected to preventive procedures starting at the collection stage, while universal pathogen inactivation methods are being applied; complications related to the persistence of attribution errors, or the real risk of vascular overload. These observations have reinforced compliance with recommendations and the application of adequate safety measures both in transfusion centers and in health institutions. Efficiency of this system in identifying new emerging diseases is based on active and targeted training of hemovigilance actors, in order to develop acuity of observation. The importance of this acuity was pointed out by the Center for Disease Control (CDC) in Atlanta in 1981, when AIDS was discovered.

Aptitude for observation of unusual phenomena, and the ensuing reflection regarding them, are inherent to scientific curiosity about all things not yet understood. Without this aptitude, the hemovigilance system would likely be limited to compiling epidemiological data on iatrogenic events that are already known.

Training and Transfusion Medicine Information

In addition to its role in traceability and surveillance, hemovigilance plays a role in training, information and dialogue between transfusion actors. This very practical training is intended to teach all aspects of general transfusion procedures, and to present the local guidelines issued by the Transfusion Safety and Hemovigilance Committee, that must be approved by the Medical Committee of the health institution. This training, in combination with the hemovigilance system of transfusion centers, contributes to transfusion safety, and allows direct involvement of caregivers who perform transfusions and pre-transfusion collection in hospitals, as part of their medical tasks. Each transfusion procedure represents a critical potential point of breakdown in transfusion safety.

Particular attention must be paid to the training of blood bank personnel. In fact, this personnel which often performs transfusion activities, in addition to other caregiving activities, has not received specialized training in transfusion practices as part of their initial training. Close collaboration between the EFS and the health institution must ensure that they receive the necessary training to safely carry out labile blood product distribution, based on regular good practice evaluations.

The Immuno-Hematology Laboratory

This laboratory holds a special place in the analysis of relations between the EFS and the health institution. It is a pivotal actor in transfusion immunological safety: it occupies an intermediary place between the intention to transfuse and the immunological choice of the appropriate product, it acts as a laboratory for pre-transfusion tests given to patients, it orients the immunological choice of blood products based on test results and on available labile blood products, it looks for post-transfusion isoimmunization, and it manages immunological monitoring of successive transfusions in patients receiving repeated transfusions.

This position in the transfusion chain explains its proximity to storage and distribution services, in which it participates closely, including by performing, when appropriate, cross-compatibility tests which compare recipient serum with donor cells that are only available in the transfusion establishment. This intermediary position between the health institution, which entrusts it with the performance of most transfusion-related biological tests, and the EFS which attributes it a key function in the choice of the compatible product, raises certain problems of coordination. These problems are aggravated by the permanent nature of this laboratory activity which, along with labile blood product distribution, must be maintained twenty-four hours a day, because emergency transfusions present the same compatibility requirements as other transfusions.

Difficulties encountered concern test relevance, their relation to transfusion, definition of emergencies and the time required for test result delivery.

The ambivalence of the immuno-hematology laboratory is at the center of these difficulties. As a testing laboratory, it is a traditional hospital lab or a medical biology test lab located outside the health institution and outside the transfusion establishment. But if it acts as a laboratory that ensures compatibility, in real time, between the blood administered and the recipient's serum, it must be close to the distribution center of labile blood products.

It is involved in the emergency biological platform, as well as in distribution services, and must therefore be close to both. Not taking this into account in the development and re-localization of hospital activities requiring blood leads to critical situations and to expensive and often unsatisfactory solutions.

Finally, this activity raises three questions:

– Should immuno-hematology laboratories operate within the sphere of emergency biology, close to users?

– Should immuno-hematology laboratories be located, preferably, close to labile blood product stocks in order to facilitate emergency compatibility tests?

– Should immuno-hematology laboratories be split between their different objectives, even if this means creating second labs in emergency settings?

There is no simple answer to these questions if we consider the overall problem, but it seems that formal collaboration between the transfusion center, via the EFS, and hospitals can lead to the most rational solutions both in terms of safety and in terms of costs. Current developments tend toward a system regulated by national guidelines concerning exchange of immuno-hematologic data between health institutions and immuno-hematology laboratories, regardless of their organizational affiliation (health institution, EFS, medical biology test lab). These exchanges must ensure data availability to allow safe distribution when labile blood products are delivered to a blood transfusion center or to an attribution-type blood bank, and when pre-transfusion controls are carried out in hospital departments.

The main difficulty is to guarantee absolute reliability and coherence in identifying patients, in any structure that generates or uses this type of data. These difficulties can only be solved by harmonization of patient identification elements, or better yet, by the assignment of an identification number unique for each patient in France.

Organizational Relations

Organizations

Organizational analysis is not our primary objective, but we consider it an essential factor for understanding relations between transfusion centers and health institutions.

From a global perspective, these two organizations are very different. The French National Blood Service (EFS) has been, ever since its creation in 2000, a unique, coherent transfusion actor in France. This is the result of a legislative orientation first evidenced by the Law of January 4, 1993, which gave rise to the "Agence française du sang" in 1994. The Law of July 1, 1998 led to the creation of the "Etablissement français du sang" in January 2000. The EFS is a unique national actor performing all operations from collection to distribution of labile blood products. Health institutions take various forms, but we consider them collectively here as being labile blood product consumers. However, their great diversity reflects territorial allocation of means to hospitals, both public and private, and goes hand in hand with great diversity of labile blood product needs, both quantitatively and qualitatively in terms of product diversity, need for assistance and time lapse requirements. The relation between the EFS and the health institution resembles that of a homogenous structure, with the EFS managing transfusion through the intermediary of fourteen regional establishments entrusted with a number of missions. All these centers are subject to uniform rules in terms of production and organization. Regional centers oversee a number of sites that are governed by the territorial rules applying to health institutions. Finally, in a conventional and very strictly regulated manner, blood banks are organized in health institutions located far from blood transfusion establishments. In contrast with this rigorous organization headed by a centralized structure, health institutions, because of the diversity of their missions, are much more heterogenous, and their coordination is understandably more complex and more flexible. This constitutes one of the central problems of the link between the EFS and health institutions: the first speaks with a single voice, while the second has no coordinated expression of its transfusion needs. This organizational difficulty should be examined, in order to arrive at a concerted expression of needs that are initially diverse.

Health Care Organization: Regional Designs

An opportune moment to introduce and regularly adjust this type of coordination could be the planning and adaptation stage of regional health care design, and regional and national transfusion program design.

The objective of regional programs is to organize health care locally in a manner that will maintain and develop proximity activities, progressively introduce technical platforms, and develop health care networks designed to satisfy health care needs in the entire region involved, so as to fulfill public health objectives and implement strategic plans set out in the public health orientation bill and defined for each region [11].

Regional and national programs of transfusion organization [12] are ratified by the Minister of Health on the basis of a bill drafted by the transfusion establishment. Each program defines the collection area for each health institution, the attribution of activities to various transfusion establishments, premises and equipment needed to satisfy blood transfusion needs, and modes of collaboration between transfusion establishments, or between health institutions and transfusion centers.

Coherence between programs is imperative and should be formalized as was done, for example, in the case of regional programs for the organization of third-generation obstetric regional programs, to guarantee the safety of mother and child during delivery; because maternal mortality remains too high, particularly due to third trimester hemorrhage, and particularly at delivery; reducing this mortality rate is now targeted as a public health objective.

Implementation of regional programs of health care organization must guarantee and ensure rapid access to blood cell concentrates, specifically through use of a written protocol describing the sequence of therapeutic measures to implement in these circumstances: in this context, immediate access to a transfusion site nearly is indispensable.

Quality

Given that we have already referred to interface structures, we will now examine the quality structures that should ensure the quality of relations. Electronic relations are representative of existing problems and possible solutions. The "quality" activities implemented in each establishment involved illustrate the overall situation: in general, transfusion establishments conduct quality activities similar to those applied in industry. They aim at the introduction of ISO norms designed to govern "client-supplier" relations. Labile blood product collection, processing and distribution divisions of the EFS, located in transfusion centers or in blood banks are subjected to stringent quality standards defined in good practice processing and distribution rules applying to labile blood products [13].

In the same way, transport and delivery to "clients" within the EFS network are subject to stringent rules.

Immuno-hematology laboratories are governed by the common rules outlined in the "Guide de bonne exécution des actes de biologie médicale" [14].

Hospitals are subject to accreditation procedures based on norms defined by the "Agence nationale d'accréditation et d'évaluation en santé". The initial version outlines general objectives of targeted evaluation in respect to organizations and safety, particularly concerning hemovigilance and transfusion safety (HTS). The second version of this document takes a more systematic approach, focusing on patient care and providing an analysis of services provided, based on assessment of professional practices.

Blood transfusion centers are basically guided toward obtaining the right product, laboratories are encouraged to provide quality results, and hospitals are guided toward horizontal internal actions aimed at better reception and informing of patients.

The hemovigilance system shared by health institutions and the EFS is intended to improve transfusion safety. Initially, its field of investigation was limited strictly to adverse reactions in recipients, given that these reactions were linked with side effects caused or likely to be caused by the administration of labile blood products. Widening the field of study to include surveillance of adverse reactions occurring in donors as well, and the transfusion of products that are inappropriate for recipients, whether or not they produce adverse reactions, produces a system resembling risk management, like the monitoring systems created more recently [15].

Although these procedures have as their ultimate aim better patient care, interface quality must be further improved through joint effort. Transfusion safety and hemovigilance committees only dispose of local power to make proposals and to collaborate in the application of compulsory national regulations. But it must be pointed out that the quality of expert conferences organized by the Regulatory Agency (AFSSAPS has already resulted in the drafting of guidelines on use of labile blood products. Texts produced by the joint efforts of different partners provide indications appropriate for labile blood products. In this field, it is noteworthy that the Quality System was subjected to process quality evaluation.

It would no doubt be beneficial to do the same for all critical aspects of the transfusion establishment/health institution interface. At the organizational level, this would require that hospitals use a coherent method of analysis and expression of their needs, responding to those of the EFS as a single, unified organization. Discussion should be based on type of need, rather than on hospital-by-hospital analysis. Type of need should orient hospital need analysis in specific organizations in fields such as mobile emergency services, hospital emergency departments, hematologic intensive care, etc.

Similarly, creation of a transfusion interface procedure adapted to all settings and designed to be used by three actors: the EFS, the health institution and the immuno-hematology laboratories, should be considered. In order to bring this about, a joint study will have to be conducted on the electronic means needed in hospitals for active transfusion safety. These tools are intended to provide access, in one operation and in real time, to traceability elements.

The question of a unique identification code for patients is a particularly critical and complex issue for solving automated system interface problems. But this problem must be solved if we are to prevent haemolytic accidents due to overlooked or unknown isoimmunization [16].

Information Systems

These systems are organized based on different methods and objectives, to link transfusion establishments and health institutions. Information systems in blood transfusion centers manage the supplies to be distributed and the attribution of labile blood products, create patient files that associate labile blood product distribution data with immuno-hematologic follow-up data, and contribute to product traceability. Health institution information systems manage all aspects of patient medical charts, manage hospital traceability and accompany all transfusion stages: pre-transfusion, during transfusion and post-transfusion.

Because they have different objectives, most current systems only coincide on a few points, of which the traceability imperative is the most obvious, because it requires close cooperation between partners [17].

• The transfusion file

The patient transfusion file, now a legal requirement [1], is an interesting example of difficulties in information system cooperation between health institutions and transfusion establishments. For the latter, this file is part of the computer transfusion file pertaining to all patients transfused based on data concerning laboratory tests and labile blood product attribution. Access to this file is possible using various parameters, but the essential, single element is a unique patient identification number assigned by the blood transfusion establishment based on its own rules. For the hospital, the transfusion file is only one of the elements of the medical chart, which is not always a single document, since a patient treated in different departments of the same hospital can have several charts. In the hospital, a transfusion file is created when transfusion is a possibility, not when transfusion has actually been performed. In fact, as soon as this possibility exists, a number of measures must be taken: examination of patient history relevant to transfusion, clinical data to consider in the selection of labile blood products, pre-transfusion tests, recommended or compulsory, but in any case necessary for the overall transfusion procedure. The patient's medical chart can be accessed using different identity criteria, but its main identifying feature is an identification number assigned by the health institution, having no relation to the identification number given the same patient by the EFS. In addition, until now, hospital identification numbers were not coordinated; each institution used its own identification system. Thus, an important data element entered correctly by the transfusion establishment could be unknown to a health institution when transfusion is prescribed, if personal identity data did not make it possible to associate the patient with his known transfusion number. In the future, electronic dialogue between the EFS and the health institution will have to reach a coherent level of computer system organization and coordination.

• Transfusion protocols

Usually, the immuno-hematology laboratory is part of the EFS. Immuno-hematologic data indispensible for transfusion compatibility is based on these lab results which determine the immuno-hematologic characteristics of the transfusion. Their complexity justifies the fact that the laboratory takes full responsibility for this aspect of blood transfusion, which also requires that the health institution provide the necessary clinical data concerning the patient. In addition to its legal responsibilities, the laboratory is responsible for deciding whether the blood used will be phenotyped or not.

The health institution, which is aware of the clinical situation at the time when the transfusion decision is made, is the only one to possess the information determining the choice of the labile blood product to use, based on indispensable current data. The need for an irradiated or negative for cytomegalovirus product illustrates this point clearly.

Thus, choice of the labile blood product, of its modifications and of its qualifications, depends on specifications known by both the health institution and by the EFS.

This important aspect of the transfusion process is not managed by information systems at present. But it would be possible to do so, given the clear systematization of labile blood product identification, transformation and qualification. An information system functioning like an expert system founded on well-established shared rules is possible to implement.

Transfusion rules applying to each clinical immunologic situation could constitute standard protocols that can be computerized, provided that common norms are defined for the information systems of transfusion establishments and health institutions. This is one of the crucial factors in relations between hospitals and transfusion centers. Blood transfusion centers have coordinated objectives and resources that allow them to advance coherently and at the same pace, particularly in terms of defining norms for electronic systems [18].

The major obstacle to computerizing the therapeutic relation is associated with the great diversity of missions of the hospital actors, the different sizes of hospitals, and their different locations and decisional systems.

Traceability of labile blood products, which also requires sharing of information between blood transfusion establishments and health institutions, is accomplished through considerable effort that could be greatly reduced and made safer by an information system interface.

Problems related to the transfusion file, ensuing from differences in institutional methods, could be eliminated by the use of an efficient EFS/health institution interface.

A solution based on accepting and taking into account different systems of transfusion file management could come from the simple exchange of the data needed for the actions incumbent on all partners involved. Because this exchange requires strict harmonization of the forms in which data is transferred, of prescriptions, of immuno-hematologic results and of specifications for the use of labile blood products - distribution, storage -, it would allow updating in real time of transfusion information from health institutions and from transfusion establishments. This new design would allow each health institution to enter its transfusion files in its own electronic and management system of shared patient medical charts, and to participate at the same time in exchange networks with the EFS and medical biology test laboratories.

A second, more complex solution could consist of the creation of a unique, virtual transfusion file comprising elements of the EFS files and the health institution files, which would receive data from both partners, and which would provide each of them, in real time, the information it needs and which comes from the other partner.

This would constitute a foundation for computer assisted transfusion, that could assist:

– prescription and recording of pre-transfusion tests, which are constitutive elements of a pre-transfusion safety file;

– prescription of labile blood products using prescription rules inherent to clinical and immuno-hematologic data;

– distribution and attribution of labile blood products in a manner allowing product traceability, and traceability of patients receiving them in real time;

– automated transmission of labile blood product distribution and attribution data, allowing control at reception in the department performing the transfusion, carried out in accordance with safety norms, and whose follow-up could be computer assisted;

– follow-up of the transfusion procedure at the patient's bedside, taking into account particularities of each case and leading to computer assistance for the transfusion itself;

– traceability of data acquisition during and after transfusion;

– computerization of post-transfusion actions, patient information, post-transfusion tests;

– electronic recording of events or data that could constitute a permanent, identified transfusion risk, such as the discovery, at any time, of irregular agglutinin.

This design reconstitutes the main stages of already existing computer programs, whose implementation and extension into a network evidently require coordination of exchanges and acquisition of information rights.

Other Organizational Systems

At the level of blood distribution, other designs are possible and are used in other countries. Distribution can be entrusted to the hospital, which acquires a supply of blood from the transfusion center, which then takes on the role of labile blood product manufacturer.

The immuno-hematology laboratory must then be located in the hospital as well.

Although this type of organization can function in countries which have different hospital structures, and in different geographic locations, in France it would have many disadvantages, including dispersion of blood supplies in multiple health care structures, since transfusions are not performed only in hospitals; this would mean losing the critical mass effect of supplies, which allows the major phenotypes to be represented in considerable quantities in the supplies of the different regional transfusion centers.

In terms of actual transfusion, the procedure could be carried out in a transfusion division of the EFS or of the health institution that can perform the transfusion at the patient's bedside. Once again, this type of organization which exists in other countries in some establishments seems rather inappropriate for the diversity of transfusion situations: emergency setting, surgical setting, medical or pediatric setting.

Within the current design, it would, however, be reasonable that in a health care structure only the centers performing a minimum number of transfusions be authorized to carry them out.

This would reduce the need for training and continued transfusion education in health centers performing little transfusion. These centers could temporarily transfer patients needing transfusion to an accredited division, or could have recourse to a mobile transfusion unit that would come to the patient in the health center which does not perform transfusions.

Implementation of transfusion therapies involves, simultaneously or in succession, many health actors practicing in transfusion establishments, in transport services, in health institution blood banks or in clinical units of health institutions. Safety and efficiency, as well as good economic management of transfusion procedures, depend on well-designed organization and perfect coordination of the different actors. This collaboration must take place for each transfusion, in order to provide the patient with the most appropriate and safest product that can answer his substitutive requirements. Collaboration also means planning and maintaining a well-designed organization that can respond to the specific and varied needs of each health institution, functions in an inter-institutional manner, and is formalized through an Agreement established and/or validated by Transfusion Safety and Hemovigilence Committees.

Institutional Administrative Relations

Blood transfusion centers and health institutions belong to the same public jurisdiction, but are governed by different management and administration systems. The EFS is a public organization under direct administrative supervision of the Ministry. Health institutions are public institutions with a Board of Directors in charge of all local institutions. These differences are founded on the existence of different needs. The EFS comprises a number of regional transfusion centers and operates as a national network that ensures great homogeneity of transfusion practices over the whole territory. This organization distributes blood products that originate solely from unpaid, voluntary donations [19].

Hospitals fill needs that correspond to demographic characteristics, taking into account local, regional and inter-regional factors.

Thus, in interactions between transfusion centers and health institutions, the latter are often in direct contact with the regional EFS which, in turn, is governed by the decisions and polices of the national organization. This raises the question of a possible need for more central representation of health institutions from an administrative perspective. This function could be carried out by the hospital directly in contact with the EFS, for all matters concerning horizontal national aspects of local interface problems. Another point of intersection between health institutions and the transfusion establishment could be the regional level, which corresponds geographically to health territories with organizational designs intended to meet health needs. Legal and administrative relations between the two organizations can only be founded on agreements (framework convention); regional structures are often more likely to propose these agreements with health institutions, and agreements are always validated by national authorities.

The complexity of managing relations between the two organizations manifests itself at the level of operational structures, given that in health institutions departments needing transfusion are very numerous and diverse, and their requirements vary greatly. For example, the needs of an emergency operating room, of cardiovascular surgery, of digestive surgery are different from those of a hematopoietic stem cell transplantation department, which are themselves different from the needs of an internal medicine department, of an intensive care department, of an emergency department, of a pediatric or an obstetrics-gynecology department. It is not possible to have a single "transfusion management strategy" in a health institution. However, procedures, rules and organizations can be governed by guidelines. Defining these guidelines is the common task that should be undertaken by the two organizations, in order to find the most rational solutions possible. If all decisions are made by a single administrative structure working in partnership with the EFS, lack of awareness of diversity at the hospital level is inevitable. Transfusion needs in hospitals should be analyzed based on categories: medical, surgical, pediatric, obstetrical - because they have different requirements, including at the immuno-hematologic level. This type of analysis would offer the advantage of bringing unique solutions to problems which obviously cannot be solved in the same way. For example, neonatal transfusion is completely different from transfusion in an adult hematology department. To submit diversified problems to decisions made by a national structure governing hospitals would guide and orient choices and agreements at the local level, to meet overall hospital needs with an EFS local partner subjected to the requirements of the national organization of which it is a part.

A theme-by-theme approach that places category diversity before a common structural origin would be better suited to the consideration of transfusion practice in hospitals. However, agreements should be drafted at the local level between health institutions and transfusion establishments, by Transfusion Safety and Hemovigilance Committees.

Future Collaboration between Hospitals and the EFS

Technological Developments

Some technological developments and the choices made concerning the structures in which they will be integrated will have significant impact on the relations between hospitals and transfusion establishments.

Cell therapy

Cell therapy is no longer an innovative concept, since the earliest experiments were conducted over ten years ago. However, after this first decade, everything remains to be done in terms of design and organization of an innovative cellular biotherapy system. The actors involved are research units that develop therapeutic applications of fundamental discoveries, and health care structures that design innovative protocols allowing clinical evaluation of these therapies. Between the two, there are the actors in research-and-development, in production and in production control. Today, the distribution of these three roles is far from being stabilized. The roles played by different actors are determined by local considerations and particularities which are most often related to the field of expertise involved. This explains the fact that cell therapy units are alternately supervised by research units, university hospital centers, oncology centers, or blood transfusion centers.

But in order for organizations and responsibilities to be understood, it is essential that each actor's role be clearly defined. The EFS transfusion centers are, naturally, experienced in *ex vivo* blood cell collection, production, modification and storage. These activities are regulated by quality criteria based on very stringent specifications.

Involvement of blood transfusion centers in the production of cells intended for therapeutic use seems reasonable given expertise already possessed by the EFS in this type of production. Of course, given the present state of knowledge and material constraints, this activity must be confined to several clearly identified sites. Finally, methods of use, scheduling of protocols and their implementation must be overseen by an expert authority that brings all the actors together; the authority's mission is to select and direct projects based on their technical feasibility and on their financing possibilities. Health institutions and research agencies cannot delegate therapeutic cell processing to EFS establishments unless they participate, as equal partners, in the definition of the programs.

Finally, research-and-development, a crucial and expensive field located between fundamental research and production, must also be examined and structured. Actors involved in this phase of cell therapy include fundamental researchers, cell manufacturers, production controllers, biologists in charge of monitoring, and clinicians. Currently, there is no official position designating the cell therapy function, which does not involve the publication requirements incumbent on researchers, nor to the tasks assigned to clinicians. "Transitional" structures corresponding to the needs of this phase are yet to be created. At this crucial stage in biotherapy development, these structures should offer an administrative, organizational and financial framework based mainly on quality criteria. This intermediary organization between different actors should be based on financing that is the equivalent, for these pre-clinical development activities, to what hospital research projects are for clinical research. But the ultimate destination of the last stages of clinical trials and cell therapy protocols is the hospital setting where the trials are conducted, regardless of the promoter and regardless of the combination of partners connected with the pre-clinical and clinical stages of these trials. In the field of transfusion clinical research, it is reasonable to imagine that the EFS proposes projects to be conducted in conjunction with general hospitals or universities, and conventional university research structures or structures of the "Etablissements publics scientifiques et techniques" (EPST). This does not at all prevent the EFS and its establishments from making contributions to fundamental research within their own structures, or from hosting external research teams.

Developments in Transfusion Therapy

Developments in transfusion therapy will take place based on parameters that are likely to define the field in the future:

– The demand for labile blood products, to which the offer must attempt to adapt, is itself determined by advances in substitutive and blood-saving techniques, and by evolving medical needs.

– Technological advances in ensuring labile blood product safety, which in addition to taking into account health monitoring data on transfusion-related risks, have to foresee increasingly risks related to emergent diseases.

– Technological advances will also no doubt make it possible to reduce immunological risk by providing products that have been made compatible and have low immunogenicity.

These changes will have to be reflected in recommendations regarding indications and modalities for use of labile blood products, as well as economic factors to be considered. It is possible that improvements in ensuring the safety of labile blood products will be achieved at the cost of production cost increases and a decrease in quantities obtained, making the production of cells in *ex vivo* culture economically competitive. The story of the extraction of factor VIII and of genetic engineering factor VIII could perhaps repeat itself in the case of genes.

Concluding Remarks

Transfusion medicine has acquired a homogenous organizational structure oriented to the quality of processed products that guarantee the safety of transfused patients. This has made transfusion medicine a unified structure that coordinates its decisions in a coherent manner based on an internal logic. The body of texts organizing this field is impressive, and leaves no possible room for improvisation, which is, in any case, prevented by a structured control system. Hospitals have reacted to this highly regulated organization by introducing a structure based on a global view of the health care setting vis-à-vis transfusion needs. Given the diversity of hospitals, their participation in a cohesive organizational structure is now the focus of a reorganization program aimed at achieving coherent management. In transfusion practice, these structures must serve to attain at least two major objectives:

– examine and define categories of transfusion needs based on therapeutic objectives in health care departments;
– define possible critical points of breakdown, given this diversity.

Communication, and particularly the introduction of a unique identifying patient code, will considerably modify and facilitate relations between hospital structures and other partners, specifically the EFS. This important stage pf development will encourage electronic links. As a result, communication projects between the EFS and health institutions will further simplify transfusion practices and increase their safety. During this transition period, we have to keep in mind the qualifications of the structures involved, while promoting simplification of all procedures and respect of advanced quality and safety standards.

References

1. Loi n° 93-5 du 4 janvier 1993 relative à la sécurité en matière de transfusion sanguine et de médicament parue au J.O. du 05/01/1993 : 224
2. Décret du 24 janvier 1994 relatif aux règles d'hémovigilance pris pour application de l'article L. 666-12 du Code de la santé publique et modifiant ce code.
3. Circulaire DGS/DH n° 40 du 7 juillet 1994 relative au décret n° 94-68 du 14 janvier 1994 sur l'hémovigilance pris pour application de l'article L. 666-12 du Code de la santé publique et modifiant ce code.
4. Circulaire DGS/DH/AFS n° 24 du 16 mai 1995 relative aux missions des coordonnateurs régionaux de l'hémovigilance et aux orientations de leur action en 1995.
5. Transfusion de plasma frais congelé : produits, recommandations. Agence française de sécurité sanitaire des produits de santé. Août 2002, mise au point février 2003.
6. Transfusion de globules rouge homologues : produits, recommandations, alternatives. Agence française de sécurité sanitaire des produits de santé. Août 2002, mise au point février 2003.
7. Transfusion de granulocytes : produits, recommandations. Agence française de sécurité sanitaire des produits de santé. Juin 2003.

8. Transfusion de plaquettes : produits, recommandations. Agence française de sécurité sanitaire des produits de santé. Juin 2003.
9. Circulaire DGS/DHOS/AFSSAPS n° 2003-582 du 15 décembre 2003 relative à la réalisation de l'acte transfusionnel.
10. Guide d'utilisation et de remplissage de la Fiche d'incident transfusionnel à l'usage des correspondants d'hémovigilance. Version expérimentale 10 mai 2004. Agence française de sécurité sanitaire des produits de santé. Direction de l'évaluation des médicaments et des produits biologiques. Unité d'hémovigilance.
11. Circulaire 101 DHOS du 05 mars 2004 relative à l'élaboration des SROS de troisième génération.
12. Code de santé publique : art L.669.1 CSP.
13. Arrêté du 26 novembre 1999 relatif à la bonne exécution des analyses de biologie médicale. J.O. du 11/12/99 : 18441-52.
14. Arrêté du 26 novembre 1999 relatif à la bonne exécution des analyses de biologie médicale. J.O. du 11/12/99 : 18441-52.
15. Décret n° 2003-1206 du 12 décembre 2003 portant organisation de la biovigilance.
16. Roubinet F, Mannessier L, Chiaroni J, Lauroua P. Aide à la décision en immuno-hématologie : détection des anticorps anti-érythrocytaires. *Transfus Clin Biol* 2000 ; 7 : 513-8.
17. Circulaire DGS/DH n° 94-92 du 30 décembre 1994 relative à la traçabilité.
18. Décision du 6 janvier 2004 du directeur général de l'Agence française de sécurité sanitaire des produits de santé portant modification de la directive technique n° 2 bis de l'Agence française du sang du 24 novembre 1997 relative aux conditions de mise en place de l'informatisation de la traçabilité des produits sanguins labiles, prise en application de l'article R. 666-12-11 du Code de la santé publique.
19. Loi n° 98-535 du 1er juillet 1998 relative au renforcement de la veille sanitaire et du contrôle de la sécurité sanitaire des produits destinés à l'homme. J.O. du 02/07/1998 : 10068.

By Different Roads:

Blood Banks *versus* Transfusion Medicine

Interview:

Francine Décary,

President and Director General, Héma-Québec

and **Patrick Hervé**,

President, "Etablissement français du sang"*

Transfusion medicine, a multidisciplinary field, is organized differently in different countries. Organization based on blood banks is founded on the principle that transfusion activities involve only collection of labile blood products, their biological qualification, their processing or transformation and their storage, in view of delivery to health institutions. Nominative assignment and immunohematology are performed by the hospitals. This type of organization is predominant in Europe and in Canada.

Advocates of this structure stress the very high quality of processed products (close to that of medicinal substances). Such a structure requires more pharmacists and engineers than doctors.

Organization based on the concept of transfusion medicine involves the entire chain of transfusion activities that goes from the donor to the recipient, and includes a considerable transfusion institution/transfusion establishment interface. Nominative assignment and immunohematology are often the responsibility of transfusion institutions, but not exclusively. In addition to these traditional activities, we conduct related activities (treatment centers, cell and tissue engineering, reagent production, research laboratories).

This multiplicity of activities is a specifically French approach. This type of structure requires the participation of many doctors and scientists.

Activities are allocated based on decisions related to the history or the politics of a given country. The editors of the present work were of the opinion that it would be interesting to compare the organization of blood transfusion in France and in Canada, since their operational approaches differ greatly. An interview between two directors of transfusion esta-

---

* Interview conducted by Renaud Albenny, journalist.

blishments, one French, the other Canadian, conducted by an independent journalist, brings to light points of similarity and difference in the orientation that transfusion medicine will take in the years to come.

The people of Quebec and the people of France are connected by strong ties of mutual affection and common interests. Thus, they share a language that each enlivens and enriches by bringing to it its own style, turns of phrase and particular expressions...

The same is true, in a manner of speaking, of blood donation.

Héma-Québec and the EFS speak the same language when it comes to transfusion quality and safety, but each of them speaks it with his own particular accent.

The two "cousins" were born after the terrible tragedy of contaminated blood, are still very young and, aside from being almost identical in age, have surprisingly similar characteristics. They differ mainly in their mission: production of labile blood products for Héma-Québec, transfusion medicine for the EFS.

What does this difference imply in concrete terms? More importantly, what will be its implications for transfusion in the future?

What are the future perspectives for each of the cousins? Where will their paths cross, where will they diverge?

Francine Décary, President and Director General of Héma-Québec, and Patrick Hervé, President of the "Etablissement français du sang" exchange their points of view.

What Is the Context of Transfusion Medicine in your Country?

Francine Décary: We are just recovering from a transfusion scandal whose impact was not as great as in France but which is still connected to ongoing legal suits.

We are in a general context that focuses on the costs of health care. The question that will have to be answered is: What does it mean to have a safe product? Is there a limit to the financial resources that can be invested in this, while other urgent health problems have to be solved? The public still sees blood as being dangerous. As a result, the regulatory Agency requires that we introduce safer and safer methods. Blood supply safety is a major societal challenge.

Patrick Hervé: After the contaminated blood tragedy that shook the whole transfusion field and the French government, we tend to set maximalist standards for transfusion safety.

"Health safety is maximalist."

We are now designing an EFS project followed by an Objectives and Means Contract up to 2009. We have listed all the different measures planned to further increase safety of labile blood products. We plan to detect possible presence of bacteria in platelets, while we wait for an effective technique for inactivation of all pathogenic agents. The cost of these measures is high. The ministry's answer was to say: "Pricing of labile blood products will be adjusted based on the new technologies you introduce."

We need another year to study a new molecular technique that is simpler and less expensive. We have to answer to authorities who are highly fearful of transfusion accidents caused by pathogen transmission.

FD: In France, the scandal affected politicians greatly. In Canada, the repercussions were not as great. In 2005, for the first time, the "Secrétariat du système du sang" organized a public forum on the theme "Transfusion Safety: at What Price?"

In Quebec, the health budget is already restricted. If we decide to bring about marginal reductions of risks that are already extremely limited, it is possible that investments in the transfusion system will hold back the development of other health areas.

PH: I dread the day, which is certainly still far off, when we will have a test for identifying abnormal prion carriers among blood donors. No matter what its cost, we will have to implement it.

Announcing to a donor that he has a prion marker, with no hope of a cure and fatal within five or ten years - maybe more but we can't be sure...will be very difficult.

Promoting prion filters and all the measures intended to eliminate prions from the blood seems much more desirable.

Safety procedures create an anxiety-provoking atmosphere. In the years to come, the main challenge will be to see how society will react to emergent risks such as the prion, West Nile Virus or other unknown viruses.

"The main challenge is to see how society will respond to emergent risks."

What Is the Mission of your Organization?

FD: Our mission is very clear: to efficiently provide safe human blood components and tissues of optimal quality and in sufficient quantity to respond to the needs of the Quebec population; to provide and develop expertise, services and specialized innovative products in the fields of transfusion medicine and human tissue transplantation.

PH: In France , we have a wider mission. First, we have to supply health institutions with the quantity of red blood cells, platelets, plasma...that they need to be self-sufficient.

We do not distribute stable blood products because, since the 1989 European Directive, they have become medicinal products overseen by the Central Pharmacy of Hospitals. The French Fractionation Laboratory was created by the 1993 Blood Law. This lab can only separate ethical plasma, obtained from volunteer, unpaid donors.

FD: In Canada, there is no fractionation plant. We have the product made to order by the Bayer Company in the United States. We do not collect enough plasma to be self-sufficient in intravenous immunoglobulin. But we are self-sufficient in albumin. And we buy and distribute recombinant factor VIII since 1995 for all hemophiliacs.

PH: Our mission is to provide plasma to the French Fractionation Laboratory, so that it can produce plasmatic factor VIII. We are self-sufficient in intravenous immunoglobulin.

FD: Because there are few users or because you collect a lot of plasma?

PH: We collect 650,000 litres of plasma per year. Its cost price is very high.

We are responsible for the whole transfusion chain. We collect, qualify, process, store and distribute labile blood products and, in 60% of cases, we conduct all transfusion-related immuno-hematological testing (IH).

We also have related activities:

1. Biomedical analysis laboratories. In addition to IH, we conduct hemostasis tests, cytology, virology, histocompatibility...

We have about a dozen major laboratories.

2. **Treatment centers**: The EFS has 90 treatment centers for patients. We conduct bloodletting, plasma exchange, extracorporeal photo-chemotherapy, ambulatory transfusion...

3. **Cell engineering**. We process cells for hematopoietic stem cell transplantation. Gradually, we want to arrive at the processing of cells for use in regenerative medicine.

4. **Research activities**, both transfusional and more basic research. At the international level, we are one of the few organizations with such a wide scope of activities.

FD: We serve as a reference laboratory in IH testing. When hospitals have a problem in this area, they contact us. We also have stem cell related activities. We ensure their storage because we apply Good Practices. We also do research.

What is the Difference between Transfusion Models in France and in Quebec?

"In France, we control the entire transfusion chain."

PH: In France, we oversee the entire transfusion chain, from the donor to the patient. We distribute and assign the product to the patient.

In addition, we have a whole set of associated activities.

Within the scope of the Objectives and Means Contract, we conducted lengthy discussions with public authorities. Is it legitimate for the EFS to continue these activities in coming years, although they could be seen as more appropriate for hospitals? Because I believe deeply in the competence of the EFS in the area of cell transfusion, our interlocutors were convinced of our legitimacy and our competence in the handling and collection of cells, beyond blood cells only.

FD: The Quebec transfusion chain is built on three imputability structures. The first and most important is the hospital. It has the laboratory and the blood bank, and it performs transfusions.

The second structure, Héma-Québec, is the provider of labile and stable blood products. It is responsible for the quality and quantity of the products distributed.

The third structure is the Hemovigilance Committee. It oversees the other two in order to ensure that they do not endanger public Health.

Moreover, Héma-Québec will soon have an exclusive mandate for all tissues.

In Quebec, at present, bones, heart valves, corneas, skin…are processed in hospitals anywhere, in the absence of principles of Good Manufacturing Practice, so that quality and safety are not ensured equally in the whole province.

I have convinced the government that in the health sector we are really the only ones who have the expertise in product handling, in biological material procurement and in its qualification, so that it respects the norms and does not endanger the lives of patients.

Héma-Québec will therefore become the sole provider of human tissue. Interestingly, the law that created Héma-Québec placed us in charge of tissues, stem cells and cord blood.

"In the Health System, we are the Good Manufacturing Practices experts."

In Quebec, the attitude was: we want to have a real industry that produces blood cells, placental blood, tissues… We want to make these products about as safe as medicinal products. Quality, quality, quality… all the expertise, intellectual and financial resources are invested in product quality.

Héma-Québec delivers a real medicinal product to hospitals, which use it based on the decisions of prescribers.

Since 1989, blood is legally considered a medicinal product. We operate under federal licence. Tissues are also governed by this legislation. This is why we have become experts in Good Practices.

In Montreal, there are many laboratories interested in stem cells, within the scope of various research projects. We can provide a framework of Good Practices for their projects.

PH: Is it possible that in France we have diversified practices without paying enough attention to Good Manufacturing Practices?

We are somewhat behind Quebec in this respect. We do not have homogenous Good Manufacturing Practices all across our territory. We do our best, but the diversity of existing activities might have the disadvantage of not providing the financial and human resources necessary to attain this safety level close to that of medications.

"Quality! All intellectual and financial means are used to achieve it."

FD: Don't you think you will have to work toward this? For instance, to produce myocardial cells…

PH: We will have to, it's unavoidable. All labs that will produce myocardial cells will follow Good Manufacturing Practices. A European Directive will oblige us to produce regenerative or other types of cells in accordance with Good manufacturing Practices. These are very stringent requirements.

Today, the EFS is examining a business plan to try to understand how to best organize cell therapy. This plan will lead to introducing this activity in a few selected establishments.

Current quality norms make it necessary to group production centers together. We have to go beyond the small-scale scope of academic research, to enter the sphere of applied research and cell production.

FD: Is there not also the risk that if the EFS does not consolidate its activities, they will be conducted by other laboratories of the European Union?

PH: In the future, we will have free circulation of products of human origin in Europe. This is not yet the case today, but we are already exchanging bone marrow grafts and placental blood grafts. And this is only a start. One day, because they will want to ensure the safety and quality of products they transplant to their patients, hospitals will be able to contact any laboratory in Europe that will guarantee the best cell therapy product.

FD: A change of culture is one of the main challenges you will face.

Changing from a classical medical culture to a manufacturing culture is very difficult because the latter has aspects that, at first sight, do not seem scientific or logical. Because the starting material cannot be absolutely controlled, regulation of human products is incredibly stringent.

"What is at stake, is to standardize the process."

To make aspirin, you take a ton of acetylsalicylic acid and you know that the ton is uniform. Sampling is done and the quality of the lot can be guaranteed. But when you collect the blood of four donors, you get four different series of lots. The stakes are in standardizing the process.

PH: Today, we are asked to describe the product injected to the patient. Take a product that has gone through all the stages of processing. At the end of the production chain, what is in the blood bag? What am I injecting to my patient?

Donor A giving blood to recipient B does not give him the same product as the product donor C gives recipient D.

"What am I injecting to my patient at the end of the production chain?"

However, there are norms that ensure that the final product will contain a certain number of active ingredients. In France, this norm could be, for example, the number of cells injected. Below a certain threshold, the risk of the graft not taking and of the patient dying is high. Therefore, it is compulsory to describe product quality.

What is the Structure of your Organization?

FD: We have a hierarchical structure that reflects the direct influence of doctors and scientists. This influence is important in terms of institutional responsibility, but in daily practice responsibility has been delegated to other types of personnel such as nurses and laboratory technicians. This delegation was made possible by the introduction of a normalized manufacturing process (NMP).

"A procedure validated medically and scientifically is carried out by trained personnel."

When a procedure is introduced, we ensure medically and scientifically that it meets the norm. Afterwards, it is applied by personnel trained to perform it. This mode of functioning is illustrated very clearly by the pre-donation interview, which is conducted by nurses.

The Canadian system was designed in this manner in 1947. Doctors were never involved in blood collection in Canada. I think this is an English model. It is not revolutionary for us.

PH: We are coming closer to this model. It's true that we have a highly medicalized culture, with many doctors, some pharmacists and only a few engineers. Over the past few years, because of a cultural change and because of Good Manufacturing Practices, we have seen a continuous increase in the number of engineers and pharmacists. It is important for us to have this type of culture.

As for donation medicine, one of our EFS projects has to do with the gradual replacement of doctors by nurses.

Donor associations insist on the presence of a doctor. There will be a doctor at each mobile collection site in order to reassure and to medicalize. One doctor, instead of three or four. Nurses with State diplomas will replace the others. We will train them, and I think that the pre-donation interview will be of the same quality.

FD: It will be of better quality because nurses receive training that instils absolute respect of the rules.

But I would go even further: why use nurses for the interview? With use of computer systems, you might need them less. Costs would be reduced and the processing of answers would be totally objective.

"In France, we are used to highly medicalized donation."

PH: Donors are not ready for this. In France, we are used to highly medicalized donation. Doctors are even present when donors receive diplomas... It will take time for donors to accept a different structure. To try to convince donor associations is harder than to reorganize teams.

Everyone agrees that we can't continue to function based on the same model.

We will have to change in the years to come. But reflection on these issues started in 2000 and it will take a few years to come to fruition.

Does Quebec Have Automated Pre-Donation Selection?

FD: No, but it would be useful, because we have arrived at that stage.

I consider it too expansive to employ a nurse to perform donor qualification, which is not at all a medical interview any more…I could probably use assistants. But I am not ready to computerize the process, especially at mobile collection sites.

PH: In France, we foresee that in 2007 we will have a single automated program called SAFRAN. All 1600,000 donors will be registered in the same automated system. As Francine Décary has suggested, it would then be possible, through this unified program, to ask everyone, everywhere in France, the same questions in the pre-donation interview.

FD: We could go one step further: the donor seated in front of the screen, with no human intervention. But the difficulty in our field is that validation requires expert systems. The computer would have to be able to make a decision. For our regulatory authorities to approve such a system will be very difficult.

"The next step would be the donor seated in front of the screen."

The possibility is interesting because in pilot projects in the United States, it has been shown that this type of "interview" allows the donor to be more spontaneous and therefore, perhaps more honest.

PH: This clearly shows that much progress is possible. If I would have been asked seven or eight years ago about the role of nurses in pre-donation interviews, I would have said that in France interviews are medical and that it is hard to imagine anything else.

How Important is Research in your System?

FD: At Héma-Québec, research is practically institutionalized. In fact, after the inquiry on contaminated blood in Canada, the Commissioner recommended that the provider acquire a Research-and-Development Division.

When Héma-Québec was created, it was planned that 5% of the operational budget be dedicated to R&D. We have about forty people working in this Division.

"When Héma-Québec was created, 5% of the operational budget was intended for R&D."

PH: For us, the question of research is complicated.

Since its creation, the EFS set up a Scientific Committee to support projects considered essential for the development of transfusion and its associated activities: transfusion research, immunology research, cell therapy research…

Each year, following invitations to tender, the Scientific Committee receives an average of thirty proposals. It selects a third of them and distributes 0.8 million euros among them, a sum granted by the EFS.

The Committee grants the funds but does not organize the research, and does not give it a strategic orientation. As a result, there are a great number of projects but their quality is uneven…

In 2004, a National Research Directorate was created. This Directorate is entrusted with organizing research, with encouraging competence and with identifying promising researchers.

I feel it is important to fight against dispersed efforts in research. A portion of it, whose quality is excellent, is published in prestigious journals. Other research is not published, and it is important to understand why.

FD: Because our research is financed by Héma-Québec, the Board of Directors is in charge of orienting research.

We are smaller than you, but we have also known this lack of orientation during the Red Cross era. Now we say: it is not academic research, it is industrial-type or oriented research that has to be conducted.

"What we need is not academic research, but oriented research."

In the long term, we have two main research orientations:
– *in vitro* platelet production, for which we have a ten-year plan;
– intravenous immunoglobulin production from different monoclonal antibodies.

Within the R&D group, there is a Division totally dedicated to development.

Héma-Québec operates in a manufacturing environment. But we cannot conduct research projects on a production line. Therefore, we recruit donors who do not quality for blood donation, but who wish to participate in research projects: testing of new equipment, of new techniques…

We also have a bio-production Unit because, when Héma-Québec was created, the research group was developing monoclonal antibodies for the blood bank. We have now reached a stage where we have to decide whether we will market some of our products.

We are hesitant to do this.

"Cellular engineering: an important element of our Research."

PH: For us, the important elements of our research include cell therapy, or rather cellular engineering. This is a type of engineering oriented toward regenerative medicine, cellular vaccines for certain types of cancer, lymphocyte clones specific for infections such as CMV, HIV, etc.

Over half of the projects submitted to the Scientific Committee concern cellular engineering.

Our second focus is the examination of types of laboratories that will be responsible for the biological qualification of donations in the ten years to come.

Will nanotechnology and biochips change our present approach to transfusion biology?

What Changes Can the New Technologies Bring About?

"We will encourage development of proteomics."

PH: Proteomics is developing and will continue to develop rapidly. Two or three of our laboratories are working on it. This technique allows much more precise analysis of plasma, platelets and cell biology. We will probably have even more precise quality control techniques in this field. We will encourage development of proteomics in certain laboratories.

Moreover, we are trying to answer another question. Around 2012-2014, will laboratories that qualify blood products have access to nanotechnologies adapted to testing several hundred products a day? I don't know. We have now introduced biochips in several laboratories, but only for limited uses. We will look for an industrial solution. Are nanotechnologies suitable for the needs of establishments like ours? I think that they are. The cost of equipment will be high. Everything will be highly automated. We will have to solve financial, technological and training problems. Expertise has to be acquired. Our personnel will have to be trained. I am starting to discuss this, and I have created a work group which, with the CEA in Grenoble and Genopole in Ivry, is entrusted with examining the feasibility and the specifications needed for laboratories using nanotechnologies. I think this strategy is important.

FD: We have not yet used proteomics. It is not within the sphere of our activities. And we have not yet decided to develop nanotechnologies...

PH: But do think they are useful?

FD: Yes. And I am sure that when they will be fully developed, I will be one of the buyers. But in the meantime, we do not develop them. However, our R&D Division is working with the Génome Québec group to develop a nanotechnology technique that will allow complete genotyping of each blood bag. We have preliminary results...Industrial use might not be far off.

PH: All our efforts focus on quality, on qualification. It is an interesting approach that we have in common.

"To develop a nanotechnology technique allowing complete genotyping of each blood bag."

FD: We have a common objective, but we take different roads to reach it.

Do you Develop New Products?

PH: Francine mentioned *in vitro* platelet production. It's interesting.

As far as the EFS is concerned, we are working with an external researcher to produce *in vitro* red blood cells. Our objective is not to produce the two million red blood cell concentrates that we need every year, but rather to find answers for certain patients with rare blood groups, with immunisations for which we cannot find compatible donors. But it appears possible to take a few bone marrow stem cells from a patient and grow them in culture to produce his own red blood cells.

This researcher has shown that he can produce a quantity of red blood cells just about equal to that of a bag containing whole blood. It will take three or four years for this process to be industrialized. But the approach is interesting.

In Quebec, do you think that in the future you might use a machine that automatically separates red blood cells, plasma and platelets right at the site where they are collected?

"To produce the patient's own red blood cells from a few of his bone marrow stem cells grown in culture."

FD: Yes, our objective for next year is to double red blood cells. We are being delayed by the uniformisation of our projects. As soon as this is done, we will concentrate on the red blood cell objective. At first, we only foresee applying this strategy at fixed blood collection locations. Then we will see if we will include mobile sites. We have never been inclined to take plasma apheresis machines to mobile sites.

What Are your Relations with External Laboratories or Research Institutions?

FD: We collaborate with two groups. First, the Canadian Blood Society research group, our equivalent in the rest of the country.

Previously, we were part of the same entity. The two groups of researchers, who were used to working together, continue to meet regularly.

> "Collaboration extends to social sciences and to research on donor motivation."

In addition, we collaborate closely with Laval University. In fact, we have moved into a new building on the Laval campus. This collaboration also extends to social sciences and research on donor motivation.

We are also working with Laval University on the development of a container that could transport any blood product without modifying the conditions of cold storage or of specific temperature over a period of 24 hours, within a range between +30 °C and -30 °C. Today, the variety of containers is so great that product temperature almost has to be measured every morning in order to choose a container...

PH: In France, INSERM units have been set up in three centers: Besançon, Strasbourg and Brest. They are headed by hospital or university affiliated experts who have created their own structure, whose cost is shared about equally by the INSERM and the EFS.

These units have priority in terms of resource allocation because they ensure good quality research, each one in its own field: one in the area of platelets, another in T-cell immunology, and the third in molecular genetics.

We are also starting to set up Health Cooperation Groups, between hospitals and the EFS. The idea is to unite our efforts in the field of innovative technologies: cell therapy, cellular engineering…The hospital conducts clinical trials, the EFS ensures production. To prepare this, there is basic or applied research, conducted either by a university, an INSERM unit or the EFS.

Is There Cooperation between your Two Organizations?

> "We have a common objective: to supply patients with quality products: blood, marrow, cornea, tissue…"

PH: There are meetings between individuals or teams, but there is no institutionalized exchange. I think we should create it. Although we use different approaches, we have a common objective. We certainly have a lot to learn from each-other.

FD: When I attended the Scientific Workshops in 2003, I realized that collaboration would be very beneficial. Our size is much smaller and we will never have access to so many doctors and experts. It is important for us to take part in these Workshops.

PH: I think that the concentration of medical expertise is partly what motivated the EFS to develop associated activities. Doctors working in our organization eventually want to diversify. They can't be expected to stay in a narrow structure.

It is because of our extensive medical expertise that in the 1980s, when marrow transplantation started, hospitals appealed to transfusion medicine rather than developing the expertise themselves.

In France, like in Quebec, transfusion medicine is located at the crossroads of various specialties: virology, hematology, immunology, engineering…

No other medical discipline brings together such a wide range of diversified expertise.

FD: These varied fields are the inner core. And around this core there is marketing, communication, public affairs...We work in a wonderful field!

> *"We work in a wonderful field!"*

PH: To strengthen our ties, Francine Décary agreed to be part of the EFS Scientific Council.

What Are the Basic Similarities between the EFS and Héma-Québec?

FD: First, our major mission: to provide blood products to the population. This is what makes us get along so well.

No matter where we are, we work in a similar framework. We can talk about nanotechnology, but we will always have to qualify donors...Unless you are already working on a futuristic, painless method of collecting blood...

It's easy for us to talk to understand each-other because we have a common basis. And then there are differences too...

PH: Our perspectives are complementary. We have the same objective: to supply patients with quality products, be it blood, marrow, tissue...

The most important thing is to do everything possible to ensure product quality.

In this respect, neither one of us can tolerate any inadequacies.

We do everything for transfusion safety, but the state of the art in safety is never achieved once and for all. If we had to achieve zero risk with a product of human origin, we could never do it. But in terms of quality, the state of the art is important. This is something on which we both agree.

> *"To ensure self-sufficiency in products needed by patients, and ensure product quality, regardless of its source."*

We have a double objective: first, to ensure self-sufficiency in products needed by patients; second, to ensure product quality, regardless of its source.

Voluntarily, like in Quebec, or a little because we are forced to, like in France, we have to make sure that we work in a Good Manufacturing Practices environment.

Transfusion Medicine in Ten Years: Fiction or Reality?

Patrick Hervé, Jean-Yves Muller

In the past, progress in the field of transfusion medicine occurred in one of two ways:

– Suddenly, as a result of a major scientific or technological discovery or of a dramatic event such as the tragedy of the AIDS virus contaminated blood. Such occurrences bring about rapid implementation of technical and organisational measures compatible with the new state of the art and of knowledge, which are likely to significantly change the structuring of good practices applying to one or more transfusion activities.

– More slowly, by applying lessons drawn from discoveries and crises to the improvement of transfusion practices, quality and safety; and by using them to reflect on the field in general and to bring into question or radically modify its concepts.

Given the succession of events - painful or wonderful, foreseeable or unexpected - that marked the evolution of transfusion medicine, it may seem presumptuous to imagine its future. The field evolves rapidly thanks to progress in biotechnologies, but it remains fragile because it is ever tributary to health crises that can affect it. The contaminated blood tragedy has made the precautionary concept an essential transfusion principle; in the future, we will have to add the notion of reasonable precaution, that we all understand, but that is quite difficult, if not to define, at least to delimit. This was not the case for technical advances, which were applied as soon as their advantages were apparent; the quality concepts adopted successively as our perception of transfusion medicine evolved now constitute a solid foundation for the future. We have no crystal ball, but we have many indicators that allow us to make predictions, with allowances for the usual margin of error. Here again, advances in knowledge have to be taken into account in order to define future perspectives. The concept of hematopoietic stem cells illustrates this evolution in perspectives. Twenty years ago, imagining that we could produce red blood cells *in vitro* was pure utopia. Today, it is scientific reality, and will no doubt be medical reality tomorrow. Today, imagining that in the future bone marrow stem cells from peripheral or cord blood will make it possible to repair any organ is utopia, but what will be the reality tomorrow? We can already state that *in vitro* production of red blood cells is not the end of the fabulous saga that started with arm-to-arm transfusion. The rest of the story will be written by the transfusion medicine of the future.

For the moment, we will review certain elements of progress relevant enough to help us imagine transfusion medicine tomorrow.

Transfusion Safety

Today, it seems that safety has definitely been achieved, although in fact it is the result of technical precision superimposed on biological uncertainty. Safety has grown by taking different paths one after the other. First, there was immunological safety, which was replaced by infectious safety. Today, safety is biological, borrowing elements from both its previous versions, and accepting the notion that biotherapies necessarily include biological and technological risks. Generous donation cannot guarantee everything and, although it is an essential starting point, it does not dispense us from recourse to science and to conscience. We often ask ourselves if more progress has to be made in the area of safety, which is a sensitive public issue. Public health financing requires that we make choices based mainly on what is at stake. The notion of risk has to be considered in the context of how many people are directly concerned, of potential risk for the social milieu and beyond that, of risk for the species. In this regard, development in the near future of viral, bacterial and parasitic depletion or even inactivation for platelet concentrates and therapeutic plasma seems inevitable, provided the effectiveness of these processes is confirmed. However, application of these techniques to erythrocytes is a more removed future prospect.

Reinforced health monitoring is imperative due to the emergence of non conventional transmissible agents. At the start of the 1980s, the very idea that a transmissible blood-borne infectious agent did not necessarily contain a nucleic message was pure heresy. Moreover, it was only when meat pellets were introduced in the feed of herbivores that the prion became a real concern for European transfusion establishments. By revealing the fragility of our certainties, this new catastrophy motivated the creation of projects aimed at developing filters that, in conjunction with specific ligands, could "trap" the prion. But before product filtration, the need to detect these new infectious agents in donor blood led researchers to develop a test serving to detect abnormal prion protein in the blood. Advances in proteomics (molecular level identification of normal and abnormal proteins) should contribute to attaining this objective. But the day we will have such a test, we will face the problem of result interpretation, as well as the problem of informing donors in whom the agent of a terrible, as yet untreatable, disease was detected.

Potential risk related to human origin biological products is persistent. Risk of passage of certain animal species viruses to man through pathogenic mutation requires that we maintain vigilance, particularly given growing intercontinental travel and traffic of exotic animals, which change the epidemiologic context and facilitate dissemination of new pathogenic agents.

The Prospect of Made-to-Measure Transfusion

At first, transfusion was a "uniform, mass" therapy, taking into account only blood group compatibility and supplying only one product: whole blood with all its components, to patients who only needed one of them. Use of blood components was the first step toward personalized transfusion therapy. Will this increasing sophistication continue in the future? The need to prevent immunization risk and infectious hazards, as well as quality and efficiency requirements that are best served by injection of the only blood component needed, lead us to answer yes.

We can already see two tendencies taking shape, that are not mutually exclusive because they answer different needs. First, there are standard corpuscular labile blood products likely to satisfy all emergency transfusion needs; specifications for these products tell us that they should not be associated with any immediate hemolytic risk because they are not ABO compatibility-dependent, nor with any subsequent immunization risk because the antigenic systems involved have undergone chemical camouflage. Second, production of *ex vivo* "personalized, made-to-measure" erythrocytes by expansion of autologous stem cells, or of precursor cells in rare donors susceptible of developing specific anti-public antibodies, has made it possible to solve transfusion dilemmas in complex immunological situations.

These techniques are still complex and expensive, and do not lend themselves to use in daily transfusion practice. Within a few years, technological progress related to biotechnologies should simplify access to "polycompatible" red blood cells in the form of O erythrocytes obtained by enzyme treatment of A and B erythrocytes.

As for rare erythrocyte concentrates obtained by expansion *in vitro* of red blood cell precursors, their place in tomorrow's transfusion arsenal has not yet been defined.

Production of these erythrocytes for large-scale therapeutic use will give rise to problems that will have to be solved. Solving them will lead to considerable progress in finding solutions to acute transfusion problems occurring far from the health institutions and laboratories indispensable until now, and in reducing shortages. But it is still too early to predict all the potential developments, both in terms of medical indications and in terms of impact on the territorial organization of transfusion medicine, in the absence of appropriate therapeutic trials.

Will There Be a More Restrictive Donor Profile?

Sophistication, personalization and increased safety criteria for labile blood products will no doubt have an impact on donor selection.

Risk of infection has already led to deferral of 7 to 20% of prospective donors, depending on the blood collection site. New requirements will lead to donor deferral based on potential risk for them or for recipients. We can already measure the impact of some of these requirements on eligibility for donation. Required minimum pre-donation hemoglobin levels will eliminate a category of "anemic" donors, most of them young women with hemoglobin levels slightly inferior to the limit (European Directive). The proposed introduction of blood count in the donor qualification process would base eligibility to donate on leukocyte count. This could be a useful criterion for deferral of donors with low-grade, non specific infections, including non pathologic hyperleukocytoses in some smokers.

Prevention of risk of post-transfusion respiratory distress syndrome called TRALI (transfusion-related acute lung injury), whose identification is constantly improving, will probably disqualify a number of women immunized by pregnancies, through the use targeted screening to detect antibodies that could be responsible for this rare but dangerous transfusion complication. Designated laboratories will have to specialize in this type of screening, and devise suitable methods to implement and evaluate it.

Travel outside of France will be another deferral criterion, more and more stringent given the propensity for travel to far-off destinations, their diversity and the increase in modes of travel. Specific selection inscribed within a timeframe has already been instituted: cumulated duration of stay in Great Britain, given the risk of bovine spongiform encephalopathy; date of return from Asia for the prevention of SARS; date of return from the United States after travel in areas affected by West Nile virus; return from Guyana, where conditions for the development of *Trypanosoma cruzii*, agent of Chagas disease, exist. Vaccines now being tested could solve some of these problems, making donation possible again for travellers who are now excluded.

These controversial issues clearly show that we are heading toward considerable restriction of donor eligibility, which will result in a different definition of donation, and in particular appreciation of valuable donor categories for whom commercial temptation could arise if we are not careful. Moreover, some European countries are debating possible return to donor remuneration. The European Directive, which recommends unpaid donation, does not make possible payment illegal. We have to remain vigilant. The constraints outlined above are not likely to produce labile blood product shortages in France. Very close links between blood collection sites, inter-regional assistance, daily monitoring of red blood cell concentrates across the national territory, and the remarkable commitment of donor associations "protect" us from this possibility.

Donation Medicine and its Recognition

In the past, blood donation medicine has been unjustly misunderstood at best, and at worst, even looked down upon. Today, donation medicine has become an essential link in transfusion safety, preceding and assisting blood donation: a crucial specialty for reinforcing safety prior to donation qualification. Thanks to broader awareness of infectious risk and of the isoimmune aspects of immunological risk, the doctor in charge of collection teams, working with nurses trained in epidemiology and experienced in the evaluation of donor eligibility, will be considered a scientific expert in the future. His biological risk expertise will enable him to apply his specialized knowledge of the stakes involved in donation eligibility, and in the epidemiology of transmissible diseases. He will contribute a scientific and epidemiologic approach to emergent diseases. He will be asked to provide scenarios of probable future risks. This type of process is already at work in the case of certain exclusions determined on the basis of the precautionary principle. Of course, reasonable limits will have to be defined; the relevance of the principle will have to be evaluated based on eligibility of a biological product, and a reasonable threshold will have to be set for exclusion based on this principle. Today's all or nothing rule - eligible/ineligible - could evolve tomorrow toward a probabilistic statement of risk based on quantified risk assessment involving a large number of parameters identified as relevant to donation eligibility. Aside from the technical difficulties involved, this perspective will have to overcome ethical difficulties before it can become more than mere utopia.

Integrating the Transfusion Network into a Single, Centralized Computer System

This integration is now in progress. The French transfusion network has chosen a unique automated system to be implemented over three years. This unique system will be a harmonization tool for the practices of a unique establishment. The system could be extended to the whole of Europe. The need for biodiversity could succeed in erasing national borders.

Links with health institutions will have to be created despite certain difficulties. Several critical factors will have to be taken into consideration: connected prescriptions, patient identification, automated management of control at reception, computer-assisted transfusion, remote transfusion adapted to blood banks. The pieces of the puzzle will fall into place to fill the current gap. This vertical organization of the transfusion computer system in relation to health institutions should be completed by a horizontal system allowing the sharing of information concerning patients at risk of being victims of a transfusion accident, most often immunological. This possibility is both far removed and important to realize if we want to avoid another drama caused by undetected isoimmunization. The project undertaken by blood transfusion establishments is perfectly coherent with this objective; it is up to health institutions to complete it by contributing to its efficiency.

A New Typology of Transfusion Biology Laboratories

The first automated laboratory process was applied in France to viral genomic diagnosis in July 2001. In two years, new integrated systems will be able to perform analyses using a single blood sample instead of a pool of samples. This single sample test would make it possible to introduce viral genomic diagnosis of the hepatitis B virus; the test increases the sensitivity of the technique and ensures greater safety. If the decision to acquire a system of this type is made, the investment will be very high.

We could ask if such an investment is justified, given a second factor to keep in mind: the introduction of nanotechnologies in the next ten years, both in biological qualification laboratories and in immuno-hematology laboratories. These technologies will require the acquisition of new skills and will lead to the creation of new professions that we have to foresee. We will need partners possessing the knowledge and ingenuity needed to help us advance in these new fields.

In the future, specialized labs will be able to perform thousands of tests each day thanks to micro-array technology for the genotyping of erythrocyte and platelet antigens.

Toward High Level Biotechnology Platforms

Automation of labile blood product production chains will become reality in the next few years. We are developing the first experimental module in two EFS blood transfusion centers. In addition, "intelligent chips" will be used to carry out follow-up of each labile blood product unit, and store all the data concerning the donor and all product characteristics.

Biotechnologies will impose themselves in transfusion medicine. Some countries will advance faster than others, depending on national policies and level of competence. Cell and tissue engineering is an activity worthy of current and future expertise in transfusion medicine.

Concentration of expertise in specialized areas of activity will be indispensable to survival in the context of European competition. These platforms will develop cell and tissue production techniques for therapeutic applications, based on good manufacturing practices. There will be an interface with hospitals within the framework of clinical Research Centres focusing on biotherapies. These activities, highly personalized at the therapeutic level, will probably be of no interest to large industrial groups whose priority is medicinal product technology.

Transfusion establishments will have to be recognized as essential actors in biotherapy implementation, in view of creating a "futuristic" medical discipline called regenerative medicine. Stem cells with different characteristics and origins represent now, and will certainly represent in the future, an important cornerstone for medical progress.

Several European countries, including France, have placed great hope in the promise of hematopoietic stem cells from placental blood. These biotechnology platforms will lead to the emergence of new functions and professional requirements in transfusion, that will call upon pharmacists with production expertise, and on bio-medical engineers and high level researchers able to direct research projects and to oversee the transition between research and production. Although all applications are not yet well defined, we will have to be careful that all these wonderful advances do not degenerate into a strictly commercial operation through the intermediary of profit-making placental blood banks. The danger is great because common pathologies that can generate lucrative business could be introduced in the field of application of these technologies. But the latter will also constitute a therapeutic means of treating rare, even "orphan" diseases, which cannot generate profit and which could be the first to be abandoned if these techniques are commercialized.

Using Transfusion Sparingly: an Objective to Consider in Context

Defining activity indicators is essential for arriving at a clear prospective. The first safety rule in transfusion is to abstain from transfusing if it is not necessary to perform it, not to transfuse what is not necessary, but to provide transfusion when necessary. It is not acceptable to die because transfusion was not provided. Therefore, it is reasonable to imagine that transfusion needs will only increase moderately in the years to come. In fact, over the past ten years, great efforts have been made in all medical fields, and especially in surgery, to reduce blood product prescriptions. Good bedside transfusion practices have been defined (in France). They provide numerous precise recommendations adapted to clinical settings and to emergency situations. These recommendations are based on a very careful review of published work and on evaluation of practices founded on experience.

Decrease in need is also unlikely, given a demographic context that increases the number of elderly patients, and given the concern with providing quality of life for anemic patients by maintaining a hemoglobin level compatible with acceptable social, family and personal life, in the absence of red blood cells and platelets. Nevertheless, the advent of hematopoietic cytokines will probably redefine certain situations. Their discovery, their properties, their synthesis and their entry into the therapeutic arsenal have to be examined to determine their place in the cytopenia treatment chain. Erythropoietin was the first hematopoietic cytokine used to replace blood transfusion in patients with renal failure who are usually very anemic due to kidney damage; this cytokine is synthesized mainly in the kidneys. Since then, thanks to genetic engineering, other cytokines have been produced. GM-CSF, G-CSF and thrombopoietin have been used in settings of hematopoietic stem cell transplantation, either to restore hematopoiesis more rapidly (with very contradictory results), or to improve performance of hematopoietic stem cell collection by apheresis.

But the very high cost of these cytokines must be kept in mind; it is what explains their limited prescription in some European countries and elsewhere.

More recently, a pilot study has shown that it was possible to obtain *ex vivo*, in the presence of a cytokine cocktail, proliferation with hematopoietic progenitor maturation in an autologous transplant setting. Transplantation of hematopoietic stem cells cultivated *ex vivo* could significantly reduce transfusion needs, given more rapid graft take. A clinical multicenter, randomized trial will be conducted in France in the near future.

Confirmation of the first results will translate into significant savings of labile blood products after autologous hematopoietic stem cell transplantation in certain cases.

Collection and processing of platelet concentrates could also eventually benefit from use of cytokines to stimulate thrombocytopoiesis in the donor (injection of thrombopoietin to the donor before cytapheresis), but the advantages and disadvantages of the procedure are not yet known. On the other hand, new conservation solutions for ensuring platelet quality appear to prolong survival *in vivo* of transfused platelets. Their development is at a stage that lets us foresee their use in the very near future.

The "Artificial Blood" Misunderstanding

Artificial blood was announced long ago, but its advent is no nearer now than it was then. In fact, the term is an easy formula that leads to a counterproductive misunderstanding in that it risks discouraging donors. Today, nothing makes it possible to suppose that red blood cell or platelet substitutes will be available for therapeutic use sooner than in ten or twenty years. By definition, a substitute can replace a cell derivative if it has the same biological and functional characteristics, since they would enable it to take the place of the cells it is supposed to replace. But oxygen transporters and platelet membrane fragments are not substitutes; they represent only one aspect of a set of very complex functions and, at best, can only be useful in specific emergency situations. It is interesting to note that some of these pseudo-substitutes can have therapeutic indications that the cell as a whole does not have. These are, therefore, interesting therapeutic products, but they are not blood cell substitutes strictly speaking.

Media headlines like "Tabacco leaves cry hemoglobin tears" or "Sea worm (*Renicola marina*) is donor of universal hemoglobin" only serve to disturb blood donors, who wonder about the future of their commitment. Transfusion medicine will still need erythrocyte, platelet and plasma donors for a long time to come.

Transfusion Medicine in the European Context

Free circulation of labile blood products will soon be a reality. European directives will harmonize practices. Although the principles of unpaid, volunteer donation are not universal in Europe, they are applied in most countries of the Community. Organization of a European field of transfusion will make it possible to achieve self-sufficiency in blood products in all the countries of the European Union, provided there is collaboration. But European-scale transfusion medicine provides many other advantages of which we should be aware.

Harmonization of transfusion safety is one of the major areas on which European authorities are focusing their attention. It is important that a European travelling in Europe should know that, if need be, he can benefit from the same transfusion quality anywhere in Europe. We know that this is far from being the case on the international level. Conditions outside Europe are another issue to be dealt within the future.

Given its size, Europe can also offer university or professional training in extremely specialized areas, on a scale that would not be possible if each Member State had to do it alone. These aspects related to European-scale transfusion medicine have not yet been fully examined. In the near future, we will probably witness the creation of transfusion medicine teaching and research programs reflecting European means and ambitions.

The University: a Key to the Future?

There has been much debate concerning transfusion medicine as an autonomous university discipline, but no concrete measures have been taken. The importance of teaching transfusion and its associated risks has been recognized as a public health matter, just like the teaching of the other substitute therapies. Transfusion medicine is composed of a variety of disciplines, rather than being a single scientific field. Its fundamental area of interest is divided between hematology, immunology, microbiology, biochemistry, genetics, cellular biology, to say nothing of the therapeutic biotherapeutic disciplines that contribute to it. In fact, all the fields of fundamental biology come together to constitute the very broad area of knowledge on which transfusion medicine is built. This is no doubt the best reason for transfusion medicine to occupy its legitimate place within the university. In addition to its fundamental function of conservation and expansion of the cell *in vitro*, transfusion medicine implements quality concepts and industrial certification in a field which is not, strictly speaking, an industry. These practices, conceived in the transfusion setting and carried out to make therapeutic products available, deserve to be examined more closely in the training of medical professionals, regardless of their field of practice.

All professional university programs include research. In transfusion establishments, research has been present for a long time. The place that it holds and the areas on which it focuses have been determined by those who were in charge of it.

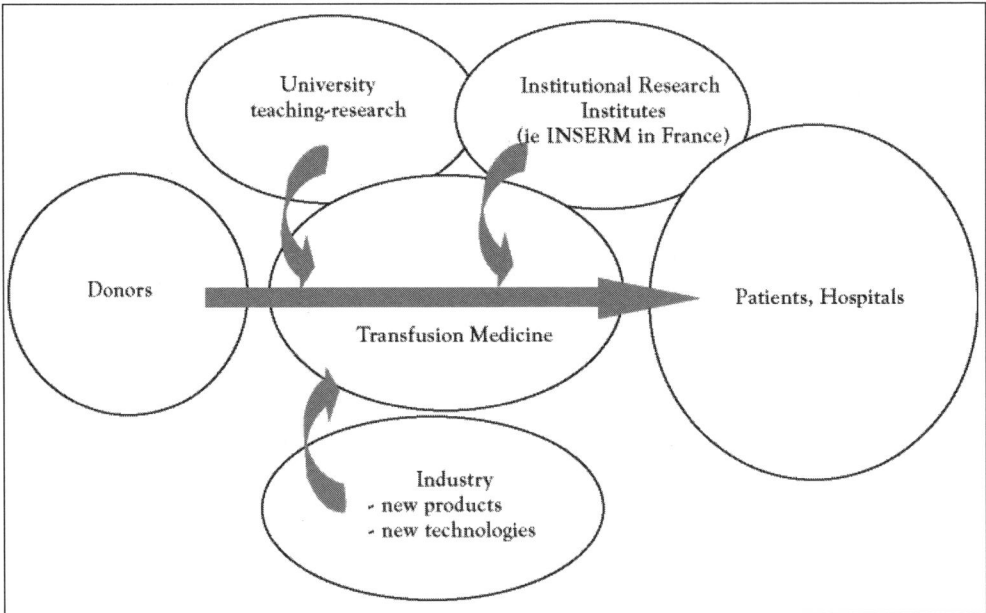

Figure 1. Tomorrow: transfusion medicine as a health and research actor in its environment.

If we ask what makes the specificity of transfusion research, the answers will be many. One of its particularities is that it is located outside institutional research institutes, even when the latter are units integrated in transfusion centers. One of the strong points of transfusion research is that it has access to healthy volunteer donors who are willing to give the blood or cells that are indispensable to many projects. Donation for research is just as valuable as therapeutic donation. One of the problems, no doubt, is the great variety of transfusion themes, which imposes restrictive selection for the purpose of concentrating the resources necessary for an effective research team that needs time and continuity to perform its rigorous and creative work. Institutional transfusion alone does not offer all the potential of transfusion research. Central research orientations will become clear in the future and our work will progress in areas where transfusion medicine is legitimate and irreplaceable, even if we will have to abandon or subcontract some research programs indispensable to the advancement of knowledge.

In addition to these central research orientations, domains of excellence will have to be maintained through collaboration and participation in projects designed with external research teams. Transfusion teams are, of course, involved in major fields such as oncology, transplantation and muscle repair, and are often asked to focus, understandably, on malignant hemopathies or constitutional anomalies of blood cells. These teams possess real know-how in the transition from applied research to clinical practice. This particular expertise makes transfusion centers attractive for setting up the transition platforms essential to the critical development phase which precedes the clinical trial phase. This is probably one of the major roles of transfusion centers; in France, this role serves to fill a detrimental gap between basic research and clinical application, in a field where, as we have already said, the probable absence of commercial profit is likely to discourage potential industrial partners. Objectives and methods of assessment in public health institutions and biotechnology institutions do not encourage this phase of research, and health care institutions are more focused on clinical research, for which they can obtain financing.

Thus, transfusion-center research disposes of many interesting domains to be explored, and of original possibilities of defining its position in relation to institutional research.

This is one of the major challenges of the field in the coming decade.

Achevé d'imprimer par Corlet, Imprimeur, S.A.
14110 Condé-sur-Noireau (France)
N° d'Imprimeur : 92044 - Dépôt légal : juin 2006

Imprimé en C.E.E.